"This book's thoroughness and insightful exploration of child development is groundbreaking and exciting. The clear, engaging writing and comprehensive coverage make it an indispensable resource for students and professionals alike."

Valeska Y. Rivera, *Student, California State University, Los Angeles, USA*

"As a detailed exploration of early childhood development, *Newborn to Infant to Child* offers invaluable insights into the intricate processes that shape human growth from conception through childhood. Its rigorous integration of current research with practical examples makes it an essential resource for students and practitioners alike in developmental psychology and related fields."

Tatiana M. Twiss, *CHAD Senior Student, California State University, Los Angeles, USA*

"This is the book I wish I'd had as a student! Now, as an academic, it is a valuable, concise guide with small nuggets of contemporary insights. Covering all the major conceptual ideas of early child development, this resource provides a neat and engaging outline of the rapid psychological changes humans undergo from the prenatal stage to three years of age. Importantly, the authors have skilfully cut through the research and distilled key highlights in an engaging narrative. This indispensable resource captures the dynamic and sequential nature of early child development, making it a pleasure to recommend to my students and to anyone passionate about understanding the journey of child development."

Ming Wai Wan, *PhD, CPsychol, SFHEA, Division of Psychology and Mental Health, University of Manchester, UK*

"This book is a significant contribution to the field of early childhood development. The authors provide a comprehensive overview of developmental processes across key domains, combining robust empirical evidence with compelling theoretical insights. It is an essential resource for students and researchers in developmental psychology and cognitive science, as well as for practitioners working with infants and their caregivers. I found the chapters on communication and relationships particularly illuminating and plan to incorporate them into my own teaching. I highly recommend this book and anticipate that it will become a foundational text in the field."

Ao Chen, *Associate Professor, Beijing Language and Culture University, China*

Newborn to Infant to Child

This comprehensive and accessible book introduces child development in the first three years of life. Organized chronologically, the book explores three developmental stages – newborn (birth to 3 months), infant (4 to 17 months), and child (18 to 36 months) – covering physical, perceptual, cognitive, language, emotional, and social development at each stage. The book sets this fundamental information in theories of development, contexts of development, research methods in development, and developmental implications for social policies, applications, and interventions.

Key issues, such as the interplay between nature and nurture and interrelations among the several domains of development, are seamlessly integrated throughout. Emphasizing the early years as a unique and critical phase of life, this book features user-friendly elements, like boxes that focus on *How Do We Know This?* and *Application*. Presented in full color, the book also defines key terms in a glossary and offers suggested readings.

Authored by world-renowned experts in child development, this essential edition is ideal for undergraduate courses in psychology, education, child development, nursing, and social work. It also serves as a valuable resource for professionals in early childhood development and education.

Martha E. Arterberry is Clara C. Piper Professor of Psychology at Colby College, Maine. She conducts research in infant perception and cognition and 3- to 5-year-old children's event memory. She is the editor in chief of *Infant Behavior and Development*.

Marc H. Bornstein holds professional appointments with the National Institute of Child Health and Human Development (Bethesda), Institute for Fiscal Studies (London), and UNICEF (NYC). He edits *Parenting: Science and Practice* and *Handbook of Parenting*. Bornstein has published in experimental, developmental, and cultural science as well as neuroscience, pediatrics, and aesthetics.

Newborn to Infant to Child

Understanding the First 1000 Days of Early Childhood

Martha E. Arterberry and
Marc H. Bornstein

Routledge
Taylor & Francis Group
NEW YORK AND LONDON

Designed cover image: Courtney Hale via Getty Images

First published 2026
by Routledge
605 Third Avenue, New York, NY 10158

and by Routledge
4 Park Square, Milton Park, Abingdon, Oxon, OX14 4RN

Routledge is an imprint of the Taylor & Francis Group, an informa business

ISBN: 978-1-032-46439-8 (hbk)
ISBN: 978-1-032-46441-1 (pbk)
ISBN: 978-1-003-38170-9 (ebk)

DOI: 10.4324/9781003381709

Typeset in Berling
by Apex CoVantage, LLC

Access the Support Material: routledge.com/9781032464411

Contents

About the Authors

Martha E. Arterberry is Clara C. Piper Professor of Psychology at Colby College, Maine. She received her B.A. from Pomona College and her Ph.D. from the University of Minnesota. She previously was Professor of Psychology at Gettysburg College, Pennsylvania, and she was a collaborative investigator at the Child and Family Research Section of the *Eunice Kennedy Shriver* National Institute of Child Health and Human Development. Her research interests in perceptual and cognitive development include the study of depth perception, three-dimensional object perception, categorization, and memory. Arterberry is the co-author of *Development of Perception in Infancy: The Cradle of Knowledge Revisited* (2016), *Infancy: The Basics* (2023), and *Development in Infancy* (2024). She also serves as the editor in chief of *Infant Behavior and Development*. For more information about Dr. Arterberry, visit https://www.colby.edu/psych/cognitive-development-lab/.

Marc H. Bornstein holds positions at the *Eunice Kennedy Shriver* National Institute of Child Health and Human Development (Bethesda), Institute for Fiscal Studies (London), and UNICEF (New York City). He earned a B.A. from Columbia College, M.S. and Ph.D. degrees from Yale University, honorary doctorates from the University of Padua and University of Trento, and an honorary professorship at the University of Heidelberg. Bornstein is President Emeritus of the Society for Research in Child Development, and he has held faculty positions at Princeton University and New York University as well as visiting academic appointments in Bamenda (Cameroon), Bristol, Chieti-Pescara, London, Munich, New York, Oxford, Paris, Santiago (Chile), Seoul, Tokyo, and Trento. Bornstein is Editor Emeritus of *Child Development* and Founding Editor of *Parenting: Science and Practice*. He has administered federal and foundation grants, sits on the editorial boards of several professional journals, is a member of scholarly societies in a variety of disciplines, and consults for governments, foundations, universities, publishers, and the media. Bornstein has published widely in developmental science and experimental, methodological, comparative, and cultural science, as well as neuroscience, pediatrics, and aesthetics. For more information about Dr. Bornstein, visit https://en.wikipedia.org/wiki/Marc_H._Bornstein.

Foreword

Philosophers beginning before Plato in the 4th–5th century BCE speculated about the significance of early life for itself and for the course of the lifespan, but formal scientific observations and investigations of newborns, infants, and even children did not begin until the late 19th and early 20th centuries. In different ways, formidable giants of general science, notably Charles Darwin and Sigmund Freud, were largely responsible for these scientific initiatives. In the middle of the 20th century, research into early human life began to blossom, and studies of the newborn, infant, and childhood stages of the life cycle have since become stimulating areas of research across the biological, behavioral, social, and medical sciences. Many investigators, referred to as developmental scientists, now appreciate how much these phases of early life contribute to our knowledge of health and well-being across the balance of the life course. Scientific interest in early development also expanded as a reflection of the emergence of remarkable technological advances for studying newborns, infants, and young children and for helping newborns, infants, and young children born at risk survive and thrive. As a result of this intensified interest and scrutiny, our understanding of early human development increased dramatically. This book focuses on what scientific investigation has revealed about that earliest period of life: phases of the newborn, the infant, and the child. It is also the case from a practical parent point of view that interest and investment in these stages of life are great for their sheer joy, amusement, and fascination. That phenomenologically the infant is quickly emerging from the newborn and the child is quickly emerging from the infant is also compelling . . . and strikes the keynote of our title.

The two of us have taught college-level courses in developmental science. When confronted with the goal of organizing the increasingly vast amount of information about the beginning of human development, the professor must make a fundamental decision. *Do I organize the information by age or by topic?* We opted to organize this book by age, taking what is known as the chronological approach, such that the main sections of the book unfold following three principal chronological stages of the lifespan: the newborn (birth through 3 months) to the infant (4 months through 17 months) to the child (18 months through 36 months). Specific to each stage, we cover the main domains of development: growth and action, perception and thought, emotions and temperament, and communication and relationships. We conclude each stage with a description of the newborn, infant, or child in context. This approach shows how the several domains of development at each stage interconnect and are influenced by larger circumstances in which they are embedded. Altogether, this approach paints a rich and nuanced picture of newborns, infants, and children at each developmental stage of the early life period. In other words, we develop a picture of the *whole child* at each stage. To begin, however, we prepare the reader with an introduction that describes the main theories and methods, structures and functions of development, and we prepare the newborn-infant-child for future development by describing prenatal life.

In this book, we report the findings of many studies, and we highlight the research used in those studies in boxes titled *How Do We Know This?* At the same time, we do not lose sight of the fact that many basic research findings improve the health and well-being of newborns, infants, and children. To this end, we also include boxes titled *Application*. To facilitate readers' understanding and retention of content, we have bolded key terms in the text, listed them at the end of each chapter, and defined them in an accompanying glossary of key terms. For interested readers, each chapter also includes a list of suggested readings.

Acknowledgments

We thank anonymous reviewers of draft chapters of this book for their valuable and constructive input. We are grateful to the editorial and production teams at Taylor & Francis/Routledge, especially to Lucy Kennedy, Molly Selby, and Leah Burton. Many researchers and theorists have shaped our understanding of, and enhanced our fascination with, newborns, infants, and children. Many parents have volunteered their families to help those many researchers and theorists. This book could not have been written without them all.

Martha E. Arterberry
Marc H. Bornstein

CHAPTER 1

Introduction

In 16th and 17th century Britain, picturesque terms like *womb-infant, tenderling, lambkin, lap child, tadpole, cub,* and *hobbledehoy* (and almost a hundred others) entered the English lexicon to describe children, reflecting what seemed to be a new understanding of childhood as a distinct stage of the life cycle worthy of attention (Caller, 2020). There was even recognition of distinct life stages within the age range today we call childhood. For example, *womb-infant* was used to describe the child *in utero*, *tenderling* to describe the very young child, *lap child* or *tadpole* to describe a young child, *hobbledehoy* to describe a lad, and *cub* to describe an older child. In other parts of the world, and in different time periods, terms for *children* and age ranges, or life stages, used to define them have also been applied. For example, the Japanese practice a custom called *meimeisho*, a ceremony which acknowledges the survival of a baby on the seventh day after birth, when the child is finally safely named.

Newborn to Infant to Child focuses on the first three years of life. For convenience, we divide this three-year early life period into three stages: **newborn** (birth through 3 months), **infant** (4 months through 17 months), and **child** (18 months through 36 months). In human development, a **stage** is a set of shared quantitative and qualitative characteristics which differ from those of another stage. Of course, people may disagree about the exact timing of these different stages, but we and many other developmental scientists (like Freud and Piaget) believe that stages provide a helpful organizing framework for thinking and writing about the life course. Stages reflect somewhat steady states in those shared quantitative and qualitative characteristics, and transitions between stages reflect significant changes in human development. Human newborns are relatively undeveloped at birth, especially compared to other species, and the newborn stage is a period of continuing rapid development and regulation of basic biological systems, like feeding, sleeping, and elimination. Starting around 4 months of age, infants become more interactive and make significant gains in motor, perceptual, cognitive, emotional, and social development. In addition, communication (however elementary) emerges, and parents settle into new ways of interacting with their little one. Around 18 months of age, children are able to move, explore, and speak with increasing stability, fluidity, and confidence. Although each of the main sections of this book – on newborns, infants, and children – successively focuses on a specific stage of life, at times we discuss topics that are common to all three stages in the first three years. For facility, when we do, we use the generic phrase **early life period** to describe the first 1,000 days, or the arc of development from birth to 36 months. For variety, we sometimes substitute the terms *period, phase,* or *time* for *stage,*

DOI: 10.4324/9781003381709-1

and we sometimes use the term *individual* generically to describe people in the early life period or in stages after the first three years.

The nine months of prenatal life plus the first the three years of postnatal life encompass only a small fraction of the average individual's life expectancy, and it is fair to ask why we have written a whole book about so brief a period of the lifespan. We think that there are two good reasons for doing so. First, development in the early life period is fast and transformative and represents an ideal circumstance for asking and answering questions about development. The rapidity of development in every sphere of life – from breastfeeding to the introduction of solids, from sleeping at any moment to settling into a regular sleep-wake schedule, from disorganized arm and leg movements to intentional reaching and walking, from vegetative vocalizations to syllables and words – rivets and fascinates watchful parents as well as researchers and clinicians, who ask how and why these developments unfold. Understanding processes underlying development and factors that influence its course not only is compelling in its own right (to *basic science*) but also servers as a means for understanding ways to facilitate optimal development (to *applied science*).

Second, events in this short early life period are acknowledged to have profound influences on the balance of the life course. Philosophers as long ago as Plato (ca. 350 BCE) and scientists from biology and embryology to neuroscience and psychology view the early life period to be uniquely important for several reasons:

1. The immature organism is especially affected by experience.
2. **Neoteny**, the prolongation of the early life period, is especially pronounced in human beings, allowing the developing organism time to adapt to the environment.
3. What is experienced or learned first tends to have lasting influence.
4. The early life period is characterized by an extraordinary facility for learning.

The lineup of developmental scientists who have contended for the importance of the early life period is impressive. Sigmund Freud (1856–1939), the Austrian neurologist and the founder of psychoanalysis, focused attention on this time, asserting that the ways people are treated then establish lifelong traits. Later, Erik Erikson (1902–1994), the German American developmental psychologist and psychoanalyst, contended that the development of trust or mistrust in the early life period profoundly affects the person's future relationships. American behaviorists and learning theorists, like John B. Watson (1878–1958) and B. F. Skinner (1904–1990), stressed the importance of early life period experiences because they occur first, have no competing propensities to replace, and thus facilitate rapid learning. Ethological researchers of animal behavior, like the Austrian Konrad Lorenz (1903–1989) and the Dutchman Niko Tinbergen (1907–1988), and embryological physiologists, like the American Gilbert Gottlieb (1929–2006), all emphasized the special role of experiences in the early life period in terms of **sensitive periods**, times in biological development when organisms are most vulnerable to experience. Additional evidence for the importance of the early life period was advanced by Jean Piaget (1896–1980), the Swiss biologist who theorized that higher-order later intellectual capacities build on simpler early developments. Similarly, early life period biological and behavioral patterns (like temperament) are believed to underlie later, more complex behavior patterns (like personality traits; Chen & Schmidt, 2015; Tang et al., 2020). Modern attachment theorists, like the British ethologist and psychoanalyst John Bowlby (1907–1990) and the

U.S. Canadian developmental scientist Mary Ainsworth (1913–1999), as well as language theorists, like the American linguist Eric Lenneberg (1921–1975), equally assigned great importance to emotional and verbal experiences that occur in the first three years of life as having far-reaching influences over speech and communication. In a nutshell, the first three years are important for themselves and because they set the stage for later life.

PRINCIPAL TOPICS

Acknowledging that the early life period is a time of rapid development that has implications for later life raises important general questions about human development. These questions guide expositions in this book.

1. What is the relation between structure and function in development?
2. Is development best characterized as stable and continuous, or does development follow changeable pathways?
3. What are the relative roles of biology (nature) and experience (nurture) in influencing development?
4. If experiences influence development, are some experiences at some times more auspicious than others?

Structure and Function

At a fundamental level, developmental science is concerned, first, with describing and understanding the status of different **structures** of the developing human (physical components, such as the visual system of the brain) and their **functions** (mental processes and behaviors, such as seeing). Developmental scientists focus on questions of structure and function at different points in the early life period to address questions about the origins of different structures and functions, what they look like at each different stage, and whether and how they change. So for example, with regard to speech, newborns begin life uttering only vegetative sounds, like grunts and cries, to communicate their needs, like hunger. Babbling ("*ba ba ba*") emerges into first words ("bottle"), and later into combinations of words ("more bottle"), to finally, full sentences ("I want more bottle."). Similarly, in motor function, newborns' movements appear jerky and uncoordinated, infants start exploring features of objects by touching them, and children coordinate their hands, fingers, and eyes to gain more advanced multimodal information about their environment.

Individual researchers often focus on one or another structure or function at a given stage in the early life period (e.g., physical growth, perception, or emotions). Some developmentalists study a structure or function in the same individuals across time (in a **longitudinal design**) or in different-aged individuals at the same time (in a **cross-sectional design**; see Box 1.1). Practically speaking, it is difficult enough to study (and to speak about) just one structure or function at one stage, let alone multiple structures or functions at one stage or across stages. However, to paint a complete picture of development, researchers have more and more come to recognize the value of more comprehensive approaches.

Box 1.1 *How Do We Know This?* Two Developmental Research Designs

Two main research designs address questions about development. Each has advantages and disadvantages. **Longitudinal** designs involve repeated measurement of the same individuals over time and constitute a principal method for assessing development. The longitudinal design provides the only means of evaluating stability or continuity in the same individuals. However, longitudinal studies are costly, obviously take a long time to complete, and not all individuals are always available for testing at different ages. **Cross-sectional** designs compare different groups of individuals of different ages. Cross-sectional designs can be completed in shorter amounts of time than longitudinal designs (researchers do not have to wait for individuals to grow up), but cross-sectional designs do not allow developmental assessments of stability or continuity.

When considering the question of how structure supports function, contemporary developmental scientists take a **systems perspective**. Development in the systems perspective is dynamic in the sense that the organization of the system as a whole reflects the activity of different structures and functions. So as any one system emerges (like the changes in physical growth from crawling to standing upright to walking), the emergence and change bring a host of new experiences that influence, and are influenced by, the emergence and changes in related component systems (so the standing child sees the world much differently from the infant who is confined to crawling). Development is dynamic and systemic.

Stability and Continuity

Central to questions of the long-term significance of the early life period is the extent to which structures and functions are consistent over time. **Stability** is concerned with consistency of individual differences over time in the relative individual order or standing of individuals in a group on some structure or function. Activity level in children would be stable, for example, if children who are more active than others when they are young are also more active than others when they are older. Figure 1.1a shows the developmental stability, and Figure 1.1b shows the developmental instability, of a characteristic of individual children in a group over time on a given structure or function.

Continuity is concerned with consistency of the mean level in a group. Figure 1.2a shows continuity, and Figure 1.2b shows discontinuity, either increasing or decreasing, of the mean level of a group over time of a given structure or function. Activity level would show continuity, for example, if a group of children were, on average, as active when they were young as when they were older. **Normative development** is often characterized by discontinuity in a developmental structure or function (Figure 1.2b or c). Thus, the developmental function reflects the changing status of newborns, infants, or children on some structure or function in development across stages.

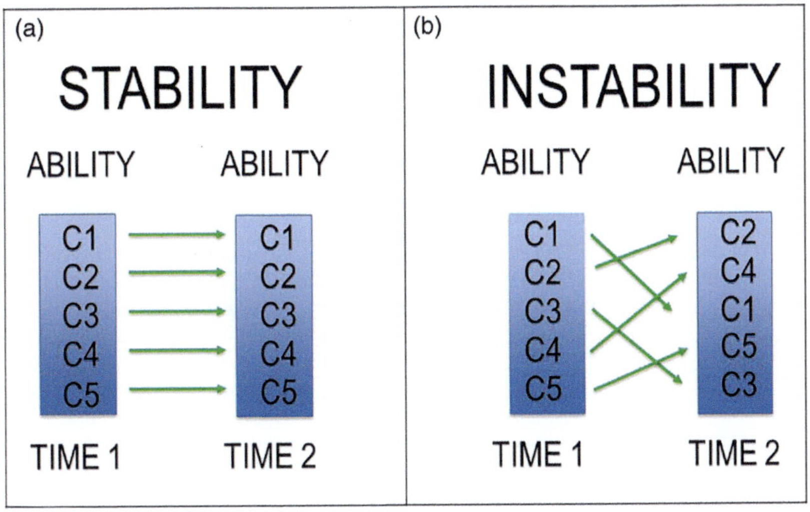

FIGURE 1.1 Stability (a) and instability (b) of individual order in a group of children (labeled C1, C2, etc.) for an ability between two times.

Source: Created by M. H. Bornstein.

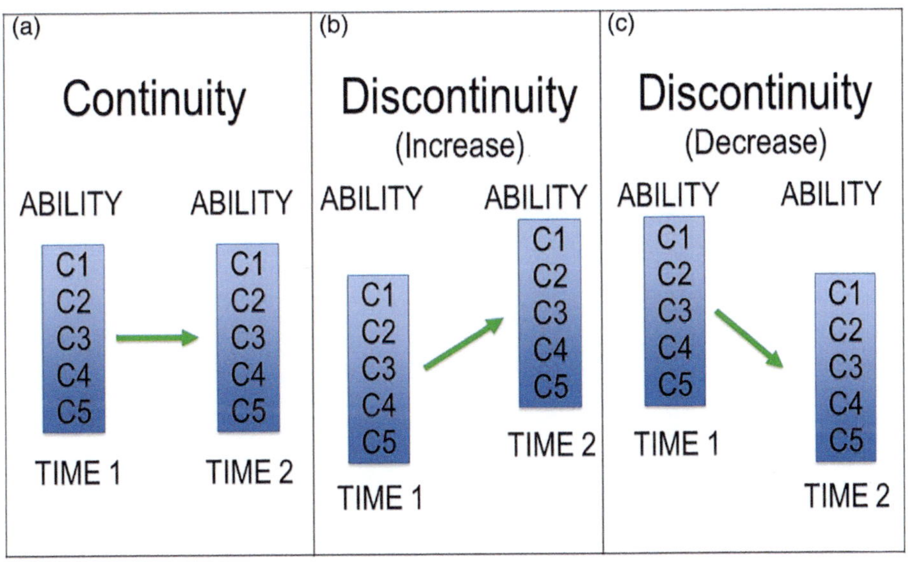

FIGURE 1.2 Continuity (a) and discontinuity (b and c) of group mean level in children (labeled C1, C2, etc.) in an ability between two times.

Source: Created by M. H. Bornstein.

Discontinuity in development can be stepwise or smooth and can unfold differently for different individuals, as shown in Figure 1.3a, but the average of those individual discontinuous developmental functions may give the misimpression of a smooth group discontinuity in development, as shown in Figure 1.3b. The six individuals in Figure 1.3a

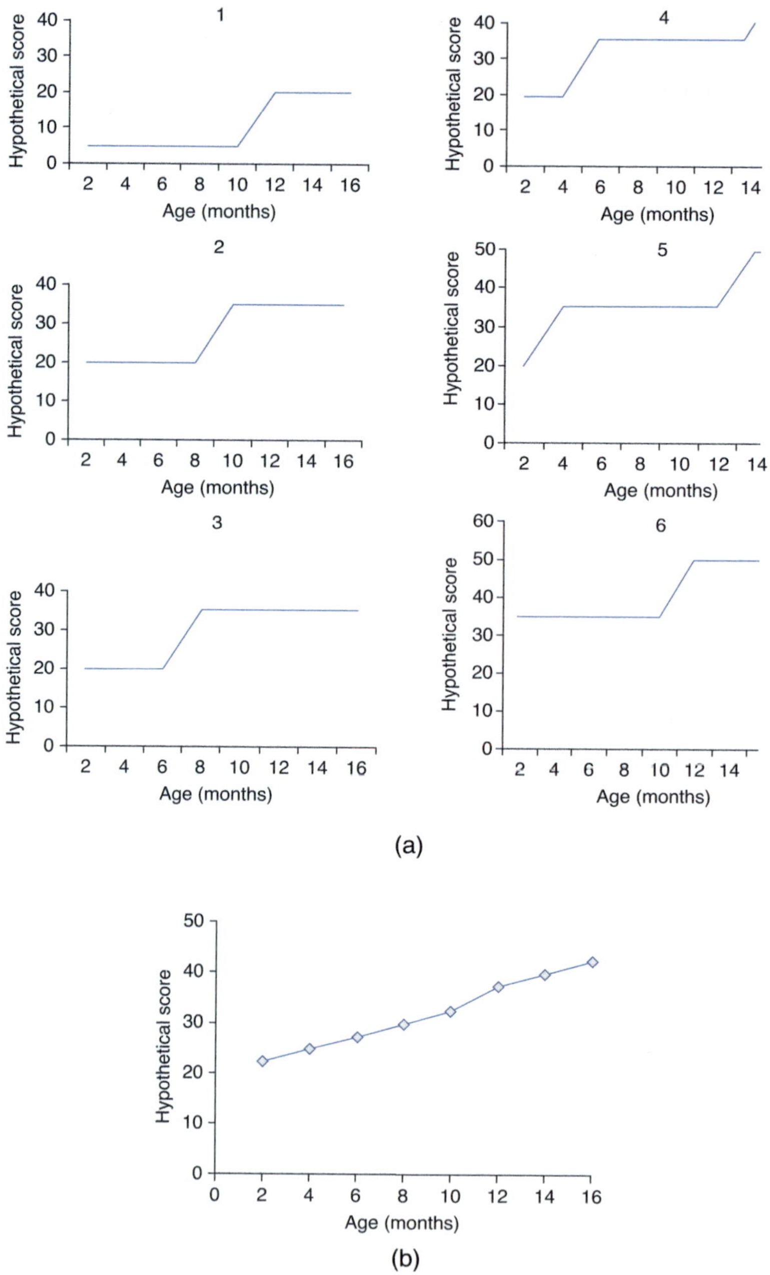

FIGURE 1.3 Individual discontinuity and group discontinuity in the general developmental function. (a) Developmental functions for six individuals; as can be seen, each individual develops in a stepwise fashion. (B) A smooth discontinuous function created by averaging the six individual functions.

Source: Created by M. H. Bornstein.

follow a stepwise developmental path, not showing a change in structure or function up to a certain point in development but showing it afterward. However, averaging the six generates a linear growth function, as shown in Figure 1.3b. Thus, when considering discontinuity in development, which is normative for most structures or functions, the group average might portray a growth pattern quite unlike any individual's growth pattern. Summary portrayals of development at the group level can be misleading about the development of individuals in the group.

A concrete example helps illustrate these points. Emotional availability reflects shared emotional processes and the quality of emotional exchanges between parents and their infants. Emotional availability encompasses both emotional signaling and emotional understanding in relationship partners, as well as the emotional accessibility of one to the other (Emde, 2000). Emotional availability has been referred to as the "connective tissue" in parent–infant relationships (Easterbrooks & Biringen, 2000, p. 123). Emotional availability is evaluated through observations and ratings of parents' interactions with their newborns, infants, or children using the Emotional Availability Scales, which consist of globally rated dimensions (Biringen et al., 2014). Four scales quantitatively assess parent sensitivity, structuring, nonintrusiveness, and nonhostility. Studies employing multiple assessments of the Emotional Availability Scales across time shed light on the stability and continuity of parent emotional availability. For example, one study employed an intra-national and cross-national, prospective and longitudinal design to examine child age and gender, region and country variation in group mean level continuity, and individual differences in the stability of emotional availability in infant–mother dyads (Bornstein, Suwalsky et al., 2012). Altogether, Argentine, Italian, and U.S. American metropolitan and rural residence mothers and their daughters and sons were observed at home when the infants were 5, and children 20, months of age. Between 5 and 20 months, maternal sensitivity, structuring, and nonintrusiveness decreased, but maternal nonhostility and child responsiveness and involvement did not change. The stability of children's and mothers' emotional availability on all dimensions emerged across the 15-month interval for both child genders and across two regions and all three countries.

Questions about individual order and questions about group mean level are both important when trying to understand development. Each newborn, infant, and child is different from every other beginning at conception, and each of us remains an individual throughout development. Most parents are interested in knowing how their own newborn, infant, or child develops an individual personality and intellectual capacity. Researchers, too, find questions concerning individual differences appealing in their own right as well as for what they reveal about general developmental trends. In each chapter in this book, we discuss individual variation as well as normative development.

Studying stability and continuity across stages is challenging. One challenge is how to measure the same structure or function across stages and whether the measures are really measuring the same construct underlying that structure or function (Box 1.2). Development often makes it difficult to tell whether fundamental change has occurred in an underlying construct (such as attachment) or whether an otherwise unchanging construct is expressed in some superficial change in a structure or function (such as crying). Again, the issue is best illustrated by example. Nine-month-old infants may express attachment to their parents by crying, clinging, and seeking to be held. Two years later, however, children's talking may become a more common way to express attachment. (And 15 years later, attachment may be expressed through electronic communication, like texting.) These developmental changes do not necessarily mean that the construct of attachment has changed in strength; instead, they may simply indicate that different structures or functions are used to express them.

Box 1.2 *How Do We Know This?* Reliability and Validity

No matter what the experimental design, studying development in the early life period must adhere to certain general step-by-step scientific requirements. One critical step includes evaluations of the reliability and validity of measures used in the study. Infants are notoriously poor study participants, especially in terms of their consistency. Thus, **reliability** of measurement is a particularly important issue in early life period research. To be valuable and meaningful, a structure or function observed in an infant one day ought to be similar to that observed in the same infant a short time later, or the structure or function would not be a reliable index of the infant. For example, Bornstein and colleagues (2006) evaluated the reliability of infants' and mothers' emotional relationships with one another on the basis of coding of their interactions. Videorecordings of infants and mothers were made at home one week and at the laboratory the next week, and mothers were coded for sensitivity. Individual mothers varied from one another in sensitivity and showed short-term reliability (individual order consistency) across time and context. In other words, those mothers who were more sensitive than other mothers in one week were more sensitive the next week as well.

In addition, measurements need to have **validity** in the sense that they measure what they are supposed to measure. Many assessments contain items, tasks, or tests that themselves bear at least some **face validity** – the measures have an obvious, commonsense association with what they are supposed to assess. For example, measures of maternal sensitivity should assess recognition, concern, and empathy with an infant (and not simple motor ability). Face validity also comes into play regarding decisions about ways to measure structures and functions at different ages. For example, measuring maternal sensitivity to their 1-year-olds might look like placing the infant on the lap to read to together, whereas sensitivity to a 6-year-old might look like arranging the situation so that the mother and child can work independently but close together across the kitchen table. Three other kinds of validity are noteworthy. **Internal validity** is the ability to make causal statements about whether one structure or function caused another to change (discussed later in the context of true experiments). **External validity** is in evidence when structures or functions investigated in one situation generalize in a theoretically meaningful way to other contexts, groups, or stages. **Predictive validity** occurs when a measure of one structure or function (infant attachment) foretells something about a later structure or function (child peer relationships).

Nature (Genetics, Biology) and Nurture (Experience, Environment)

A fundamental and enduring question in developmental science is, *What drives development?* Is development genetically and biologically programmed (nature) or guided by experience and the environment (nurture), or do the two work together in development? The earliest interest in these questions was proposed by philosophers and clergy, who chose clear sides: either nature *or* nurture. **Nativists** argued that mental and moral life are instinctive or inborn, whereas **empiricists** argued that knowledge and ethics are products of experience in the world.

The British philosopher John Locke (1632–1704) exemplifies the empiricist school of thought. Locke asserted that human beings possess no knowledge of the world when they are born. He famously described the mind at birth as a "blank slate" (**tabula rasa**). Instead, Locke contended that mental and moral development reflects what we experience and learn as we grow. Even passing familiarity with a newborn would convince a parent observer that, indeed, this *fetus-ex-utero* "knows" pretty much nothing. The American philosopher William James (1842–1910) advanced a slightly different empiricist view, namely, that the world of the infant is a "blooming, buzzing confusion." There might be something in the newborn mind, but it is definitely a jumble. In James's view, development consists less of acquiring knowledge and more of accruing experiences that organize the mind. In the empiricist view, newborns, infants, and even children, in some ways, are innocent and naive and develop into cognitively and socially thoughtful and ethical mature adults.

By contrast, philosophers in the nativist school decried the empiricist assertion that human beings begin life empty-headed; for them, this view was both morally intolerable and logically indefensible. On biblical interpretation, God would not create mindless creatures "in His image." They also asserted that good or evil must be inborn, because neither could be learned in the short course of the early life period. The French philosopher René Descartes (1596–1650) exemplified this nativist point of view. He proposed that we are born with ideas which start us off in understanding the world, and that the human mind proceeds to impose order on experience. In turn, the British philosopher Thomas Hobbes (1588–1679) and the Swiss social theorist Jean-Jacques Rousseau (1712–1778) were nativists who came down on opposite sides of the question of the original state of good and evil in human beings. For Rousseau, humans in "state of nature" are innocent and good, without envy, distrust, or conflict, and perfectible, whereas Hobbes saw the life of man solitary, poor, nasty, brutish, and short. Thus, from a nativist view, we are born with the foundations of ways to understand the world and morality.

In its extreme form, nativism contends that, if heredity is good, then development and maturity will be good, regardless of whether the experiences or environment in development are good or bad. Similarly, if heredity is bad, then development and maturity will be bad, regardless of whether the experiences or environment are bad or good. By contrast, empiricism argues that, if experiences or environment are good, then development and maturity will be good, regardless of heredity, but if experiences or environment are bad, then development and maturity will be bad, regardless of heredity.

Nativism and empiricism are not relics of distant past eras or confined to philosophical speculation, but both have had advocates across the centuries. For example, Watson famously declared for empiricism:

> Give me a dozen healthy infants, well-formed, and my own specified world to bring them up in, and I'll guarantee to take any one at random and train him to become any type of specialist I might select – doctor, lawyer, artist, merchant-chief and yes, even beggarman and thief, regardless of his talents, penchants, tendencies, abilities, vocations, race of his ancestors.
>
> (Watson, 1924, p. 104)

In stark contrast, the American pediatrician Arnold Gesell (1880–1961), who was "America's Baby Doctor" before the Second World War (and a contemporary of Watson), forcefully supported nativism, writing that "the original impulse to growth . . . is endogenous rather than exogenous" (Gesell, 1954, p. 354), meaning that forces internal to the individual, and not experiences external to the individual, drive development. Some contemporary geneticists likewise focus on biological/genetic causes of mental illness, cancer, and other human afflictions while minimizing the effects of environments, life experiences, or activities of people that may give rise to diseases. For example, Plomin (2018) stated that "DNA differences inherited from our parents at the moment of conception are the consistent, lifelong source of psychological individuality, the blueprint that makes us who we are" (p. ix), while "parents have little systematic effect on their children's outcomes, beyond the blueprint that their genes provide" (p. 85).

Today, these extreme views are being supplanted by the **transactional** framework, which asserts that nature and nurture are inextricably linked and work together over time in the development of the individual, and by **epigenetics,** which argues that experiences modify genetic expression. Developmental scientists no longer subscribe to a rigid dichotomy, believing instead that neither genetic or biological predispositions nor experiences or the environment alone determine the course, direction, or final resting level of development; rather, these life forces continuously influence one another in development. Today, developmental scientists are interested in learning which experiences and environments affect which genetic and biological structures or functions when in development, how they do so, and what their likely outcomes will be.

With advances in mapping the human genome, researchers have been empowered with new tools to unravel more realistically how interactions between genetic makeup and experience shape the course of development. Epigenetics is the modern study of how experience and environment affect when and how genes express themselves (Champagne, 2018). Two people may have the same gene, but their different experiences can alter how and when that gene expresses itself. Similarly, identical twins are never totally and truly identical. They have different experiences even in the same uterus before birth, including access to nutrients on which they might grow or different opportunities to move on which they might develop. Genetics and experiences codetermine development.

Questions about nature and nurture are not solely theoretical and without practical implications. Which theory of development one subscribes to has real-world consequences. If you (or society) believe that intelligence or personality is fixed by genetics, then you (and society) are unlikely to provide experiences that foster greater intelligence or personality adjustment. As neither can be changed, why bother? Genes make all the difference, and experience will have little or no effect. If, however, you believe that experiences are determinative of intelligence or personality, it is incumbent on you (and society) to provide experiences needed to develop optimally, optimally starting in the early life period.

Timing of Experience

The timing of experiences can be determinative in development in addition to the way experiences help shape the trajectory of development. Developmental science has identified three main temporal models of when experiences can affect development. In the "early experience" model, an early experience uniquely affects the individual at that early time, and the effect of that experience continues independent of other, later experiences. For example, infants who grow up in Chicago learn to speak English, and even if they move to Paris later in life, they should be able to continue to speak English. In a second "contemporary experience" model, a later experience replaces or supplants the effects of an earlier experience. Recovery of a structure or function from early experience deprivation is an example. These first two models operate through sensitive periods – that is, experiences at specific times exert effects over development (see Box 1.3). In a third "cumulative experience" model, a given experience influences development because it persists and so amasses in its impact. An example of this model is how the experience of persistent poverty piles up during the early years and can erode adult mental health.

Box 1.3 *Application:* "Fostering" Positive Development

Around the world, some parents find that they are unable to care for their children. This circumstance often results in children being placed for adoption, in foster care, or in institutions, commonly referred to as orphanages. Developmental scientists since the early 1950s have known that institutional care can be detrimental to human development (Spitz, 1965). Following the discovery of dismal conditions in Romanian orphanages, the Bucharest Early Intervention Project charted the effects of extreme deprivation and intervention on development. During the study, half of the infants remained in an institution, and the other half went to live with foster families. Early placement in foster care helped mitigate some negative effects of early deprivation. However, children who were institutionalized and then placed in foster care still lagged behind peers who were never institutionalized (McLaughlin et al., 2015).

Therefore, simply placing children in foster care instead of institutions may not be enough to ensure development and thriving. Foster parents may need help in how to best support their wards, particularly in the area of developing relationships. Empirical research into attachment theory has generated help for foster families in this area. **Attachment** is the early developing emotional relationship between infants and their caregivers. The Attachment and Biobehavioral Catch-Up (ABC; Dozier et al., 2018) Intervention was designed to enhance development in foster children who experienced adversity early in life through increasing parent sensitivity and nurturance and reducing frightening behaviors (Raby et al., 2019). ABC sessions are conducted by trained clinicians, who help parents practice optimizing caregiving, speak with the parents about the supporting empirical evidence, and provide feedback to the parents. The ABC Intervention improved parental sensitivity, resulting in foster children developing attachments quickly to their new caregivers (Bick & Dozier, 2013), and also led to improved vocabulary and cognitive skills in foster children (Lind et al., 2017; Raby et al., 2019).

Thus, the care of children – whether by their biological parents or by others – can set the course for long-term outcomes, for better or worse. Programs that support foster families help reduce negative effects of foster care placement. Additionally, foster-like practices in institutions wherein newborns and infants are reared in small "families" may also yield more positive developmental outcomes (McCall & Groark, 2015).

Gottlieb and his colleagues (2006) distinguished several different actions of experience on development based on the timing of the experience. Figure 1.4 illustrates some different trajectories and outcomes of development depending on the timing of experience. **Induction** is the most dramatic form of experiential influence. It occurs when a particular experience or set of experiences completely determines whether some structure or function emerges in development. Without the experience, the structure or function will not emerge or develop. For example, some newborns have cataracts, which is a clouding of the lens that limits how much light gets into the eyes (and so can transmit information through the rest of the visual system to the brain). Most lenses are replaced within the first year, but even so, newborns with cataracts in both eyes have lifelong impairments in perception (Mondloch et al., 2013). **Attunement** and **facilitation** occur when certain experiences speed up the development of a structure or function, or when the final outcome of development is higher than it would be without that experience. For example, even young infants show remarkable face perception abilities, but around the first year of life, this ability becomes specialized for faces which infants regularly see (Krasotkina et al., 2021). Finally, **maintenance** describes a situation in which experience preserves an already partially or fully developed structure or function and the absence of experience results in loss of the structure or function. For example, all newborns babble. But babbling relies on both hearing speech from others and feedback from one's own speech. In other words, hearing speech maintains babbling and thereby influences later language development.

Section Summary

In this section, we introduced four basic questions about development. They were selected because they are central to understanding development, because of their historical/

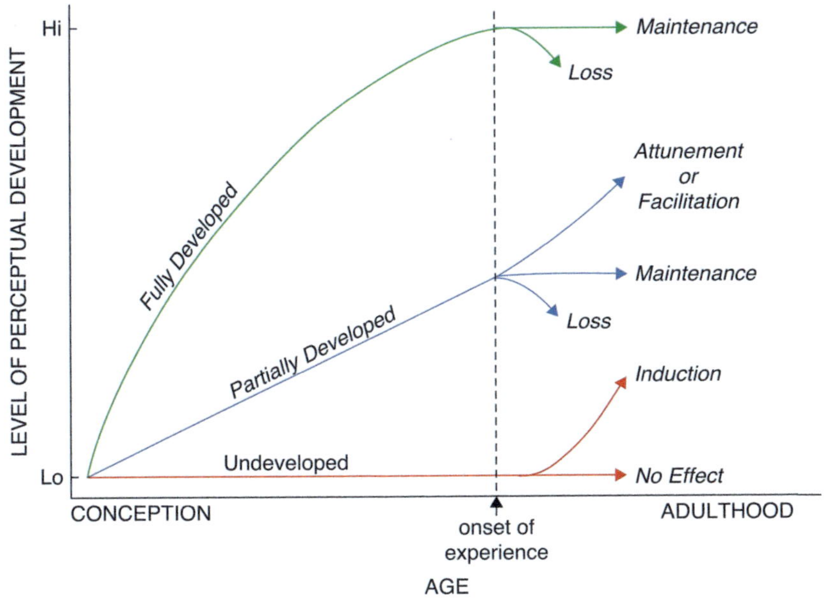

FIGURE 1.4 Possible developmental trajectories and outcomes given different levels of development before the onset of experience and for different experiences afterward.

philosophical precedent, and because they have implications for the health and welfare of newborns, infants, and children. The first question, on the relations between structure and function, explores their association and acknowledges that just because there is structure (legs) does not mean there may always be a function (walking). The second question, on whether development is characterized as stable and continuous, helps us understand how development unfolds and whether there is stability of individual variation and continuity in group mean level across time in a given structure or function. The third question, on the relative roles of genetics and biology (nature) or experience and environment (nurture) in influencing development, unpackages driving forces in influencing the course and outcome of development. The fourth question, on the timing of different experiences, explores the mechanisms of action in shaping development. Responses to these questions infuse each chapter in this book.

FRAMEWORKS OF DEVELOPMENT

There are numerous ways to think about development in more general terms; we have referred to one already – the **transaction framework**. Because of its significance, we elaborate on it and present a second framework, bioecological systems. The transaction framework describes how parents and their newborns, infants, and children mutually influence each other through time. The **bioecological systems framework** lays out the many direct and indirect influences on the development of newborns, infants, and children.

Transaction

The transactional framework of development contends that genes and experience, biology and environment, and offspring and caregivers mutually influence one another through time. That is, nature and nurture work together to shape development in dynamic, interactive, reciprocal, and evolving ways. An important consequence of transaction is that newborns, infants, and children help plot the course of their own development. Figure 1.5 depicts the transaction between child and parent through time. The figure shows three general sources of development: Children contribute directly to their own development (the horizontal arrows), children and parents mutually influence one another at a given time (the vertical arrows), and children and parents influence one another over time (the diagonal arrows). As can be seen in Figure 1.5, the child (C) at an early time influences, at a later time, the parent (P), who influences the child at a still later time. For example, hungry children cue their mothers that it is time to eat, which permits the now-sated children to explore and learn from the environment and to engage more with their mothers. Children also influence the experiences and environments they are exposed to, and they interpret those experiences and environments, and so, ultimately, the ways those experiences and environments affect them and their eventual development. It is also the case that what parents do at one time may not affect their children at the same time but could have an impact at a later time. Similarly, children at one time may have a short- or long-term impact on parents.

To illustrate, consider the emergence of self-produced movement, such as crawling and walking. When infants start moving on their own, they rapidly acquire abilities to explore independently. They also now have control over their proximity to other people, and so they can approach or withdraw at will. As a result, parents may need to adjust their caregiving of crawling and walking infants, because such newly capable infants can now get into trouble on their own – and pretty quickly. Parents must become vigilant about the possibilities that their infants may fall down steps, accidentally knock heavy things on themselves, or eat dangerous houseplants. Much more than before, parents must communicate to infants – primarily through their faces, voices, and gestures – messages that help

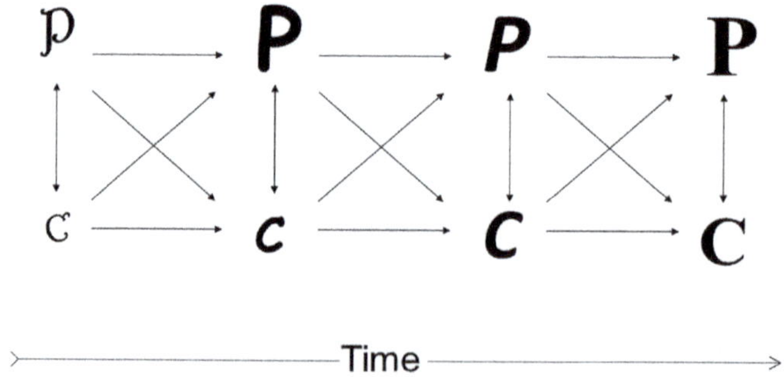

FIGURE 1.5 The transactional framework of development: The child (C) grows and changes and the parent (*P*) changes over time (as indicted by the different fonts) because each also influences the other in a continual reciprocal process of development and change.

Source: Created by M. H. Bornstein and M. E. Arterberry, after Bornstein (2009).

infants regulate their own behavior and learn what to approach and what to avoid. Now, "No!" comes into parents' vocabulary for the first time. Moreover, standing and walking infants seem more grown-up to adults, who, in turn, treat them differently than before those infants were able to move on their own. Thus, newly crawling and walking infants provide opportunities for themselves, such as new ways to explore, and they also change their parents, and these changes, in turn, affect future development.

Systems

Throughout development, effective experiences and environments are not limited to newborns', infants', and children's immediate surroundings. Effective environments for development include peers, schools, social networks, communities, cultures, and even times. The Russian American developmental scientist Urie Bronfenbrenner (1917–2005) proposed a bioecological systems framework that captures the roles of these diverse environments in development (Figure 1.6). In this framework, newborns, infants, and children (with their unique biology) sit at the center of several nested systems. The **microsystem** is most proximal to newborns, infants, and children and encompasses interpersonal relationships and patterns of activities that newborns, infants, and children experience in

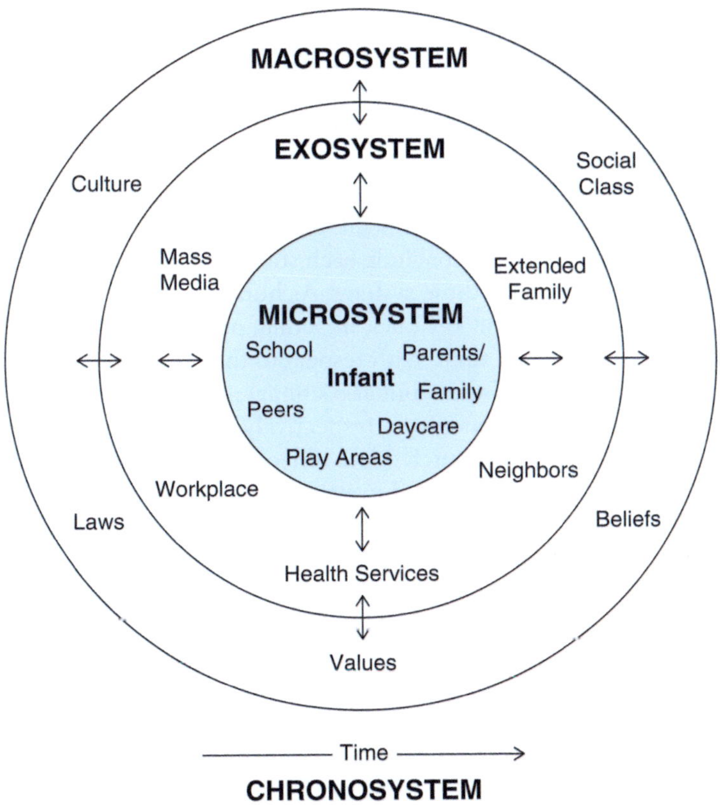

FIGURE 1.6 The bioecological systems framework of development.

Source: Created by M. H. Bornstein.

face-to-face settings. This system includes the immediate environments of family members, peers, day cares, and schools. So for example, infants are influenced by when and how much their mothers speak to them when they are together. A bit conceptually distant from newborns, infants, and children are elements of the **exosystem**, like their parents' workplace, their wider neighborhood, and their family health-care system. Newborns, infants, and children may or may not directly encounter these elements, but elements of the exosystem still indirectly influence their development. So for example, infants are influenced by whether or not their mothers work, the kinds of work their mothers do, the work hours their mothers keep, and the like. The **macrosystem** is the most distant from newborns, infants, and children and encompasses patterns of beliefs, values, and laws of the social class and culture in which newborns, infants, and children are embedded as they grow up. So for example, infants are influenced by the level of wealth their family commands and the customs of the culture they are reared in. Finally, as development literally implies, newborns, infants, and children exist at a given moment as well as at some fixed period in history; the time domain in development is called the **chronosystem**. So for example, infants are influenced by whether they develop in a time of depression or war. As illustrated in Figure 1.6, these spheres of life are embedded in one another. As ordered, these systems stand in increasingly distant relations to newborns, infants, and children, but each system influences development through systems more proximal to the individual. The infant is embedded in a family, which is embedded in a neighborhood, which is embedded in a culture, which is embedded in a historical time. At a given point in development, variables from all these systems contribute to the status and development of structures and functions in and across the early life period. In short, multiple systems do not operate independently of one another; rather, they mutually influence one another (Kerig, 2019).

For each stage of the early life period – newborn, infant, and child – we include chapters on growth and action, perception and thought, emotions and temperament, and communication and relationships. We also conclude each stage with illustrations of the newborn, infant, or child in the contexts of these systems. As human beings grow in many different such contexts, we focus on several key ones, including parents and family, socioeconomic status, ethnicity and culture, and time. With respect to the micro- and exosystems, *parents and family* include mothers and fathers, but also siblings and familial and non-familial caregivers, like grandparents and day caregivers, respectively. With respect to the macrosystem, socioeconomic status (SES) is constructed and reflective of parents' educational achievement, financial income, and occupational prestige. Ethnicity and culture are notoriously challenging to define and to disambiguate as they overlap definitionally and conceptually. For our purposes, we treat *ethnicity* as referring to common linguistic, national, regional, or religious characteristics or identities of a social group, and we think of *culture* as including the beliefs, values, arts, customs, lifestyles, background, and habits that characterize a particular society or nation. With respect to the chronosystem, the lives of newborns, infants, and children are subject to change with multiple scales of time, and developmental science distinguishes micro-time (time changes occurring over the course of a day to over the course of a year), macro-time (time changes across years but within a generation), and historical time (time changes across generations).

Section Summary

The transactional framework of development emphasizes the ways parents and their newborns, infants, and children influence each other and through time. Developmental changes in offspring necessitate changes in parents, just as parents facilitate (or not) changes in offspring. These bidirectional effects can be immediate or emerge over time. The bioecological systems framework highlights both direct and indirect systems effects on newborns, infants, and children, who are embedded in multiple material and social contexts. Larger temporal and cultural forces influence schools, neighborhoods, and the world of work, which in turn influence the adults who closely interact with their newborns, infants, and children.

CONCLUSIONS

The first three years constitute a short period of one's lifespan, but events and developments during this time may have lifelong consequences. Historically, philosophers focused on identifying whether development occurs due to genetic/biological (nativist) versus experiential/environmental (empiricist) forces. Today, developmental scientists acknowledge the complex pervasive interplay between nature and nurture. This transactional perspective highlights how experiences shape the individual and, in turn, how the individual shapes experiences. Studying newborns, infants, and children tells us about general developmental phenomena as well as the significance of the early life period for the balance of the life cycle. Variability among families and the multiple forces of development are captured by the bioecological systems framework. There are near (parenting) and far (cultural) levels of influence on newborn, infant, and child development.

In a given year, approximately 4 million new babies are born in the United States. The wonder is that for the 11,000 newborns who come into the world every day – a number equivalent to the population of a small town – each one is exceptional, special, and unique. The fact that individuals are genetically constituted in unique ways, combined with the fact that each individual encounters unique experiences growing up, means that the paths along which individuals develop are unique and result in all the wonderful differences that make up humanity. Different people naturally understand the world in distinctive ways because of their unique genetic and experiential histories. This developmental perspective has thoroughgoing implications. As the American writer and literary critic Edmund Wilson (1895–1972) noted, for example,

> there is really no way of considering a book independently of one's special sensations in reading it on a particular occasion. . . . In a sense, one can never read the book that the author originally wrote, and one can never read the same book twice.
>
> (Wilson, 1938, p. ix)

In developmental science terms, as individual biology and experience aggregate in life, the result is increasing individual specificity (Bornstein, 2019a).

Through understanding human development, the everyday lives of newborns, infants, and children and their families can be improved. Parents learn how to best care for their progeny, educators provide the best practices for optimal outcomes for their students and medical professionals for their patients, and policymakers evaluate the best programs to support families and society. Not all newborns, infants, and children enter the world in the same way. How development differs among them provides insights into how best to support them to optimize human development.

KEY TERMS

Attachment
Attunement
Bioecological systems framework
Chronosystem
Continuity
Cross-sectional design
Empiricist
Epigenetics
Exosystem
External validity
Face validity
Facilitation
Functions
Induction
Internal validity
Longitudinal design
Macrosystem
Maintenance
Microsystem
Nativist
Natural experiments
Neoteny
Normative development
Predictive validity
Reliability
Sensitive period
Stability
Stage
Structures
Systems perspective
Tabula rasa
Transactional
Transaction framework
True experiments
Validity

SUGGESTED READINGS

Bornstein, M. H. (2019). It's about time! Ecological systems, transaction, and specificity as key developmental principles in children's changing worlds. In R. D. Parke & G. H. Elder (Eds.), *Children in changing worlds: Sociocultural and temporal perspectives* (pp. 277–286). Cambridge University Press.

Bornstein, M. H., Putnick, D. L., & Esposito, G. (2017). Continuity and stability in development. *Child Development Perspectives*, *11*(2), 113–119. https://doi.org/10.1111/cdep.12221

Johnson, S. K., Klimstra, T. A., & Lerner, R. M. (2025). Concepts and theories of human development. In M. H. Bornstein & M. E. Lamb (Eds.), *Developmental science: An advanced textbook* (pp. 3–34). Routledge.

CHAPTER 2

Development Before Birth

Human development begins long before birth, and in this chapter we explore some prominent prenatal influences on the growth of both structures and functions. Long ago, it was believed that the organism-to-be was "preformed" in the mother's egg, waiting to be released, or in the father's sperm, waiting for a medium in which to grow. Modern biology tells quite a different story.

BEGINNING LIFE

Reproduction depends on the process of **meiosis**. This process begins when the reproductive cells (**gametes**) of each parent split, so the successful sperm and fertilized egg will each contain half the number of chromosomes that were present in the original cell. An unfertilized egg (**ovum**) is released by the ovaries and descends the fallopian tube. Membranes of the fallopian tube secrete chemicals that loosen the shell surrounding the ovum, permitting a single sperm to penetrate and fertilize the egg. The resulting 23 pairs of **chromosomes** (the threadlike structures of nucleic acids and protein found in the nucleus of most living cells) carry biological information in the form of genes that compose the genetic makeup of the individual. One member of each pair is contributed by each parent (Figure 2.1). One of the 23 pairs of chromosomes is a pair of sex chromosomes. For females this pair consists of two X chromosomes (XX), and for males the pair consists of one X and one Y chromosome. (XY). Fetuses with two X chromosomes will develop female characteristics, and fetuses with an XY pair will develop male characteristics. Thus begins the uniqueness of each individual. Chromosomes contain genes that themselves are composed of chemical codes of DNA that help guide the development of all future structures and functions.

The endowment of parental chromosomes is the first important event in one's life. However, the **genotype** (the genetic makeup of the individual) does not entirely predict the **phenotype** (the observed characteristics of the individual). Different people with different genetic endowments sometimes can look alike or act similarly, just as identical twins with exactly the same genetic endowment might look or act differently. There are clear genetic contributions to many aspects of development. The phenotypic variability we see in the different people around us, however, springs from several sources because genetic endowment and lifelong experiences *together* shape the characteristics and behaviors of individuals.

DOI: 10.4324/9781003381709-2

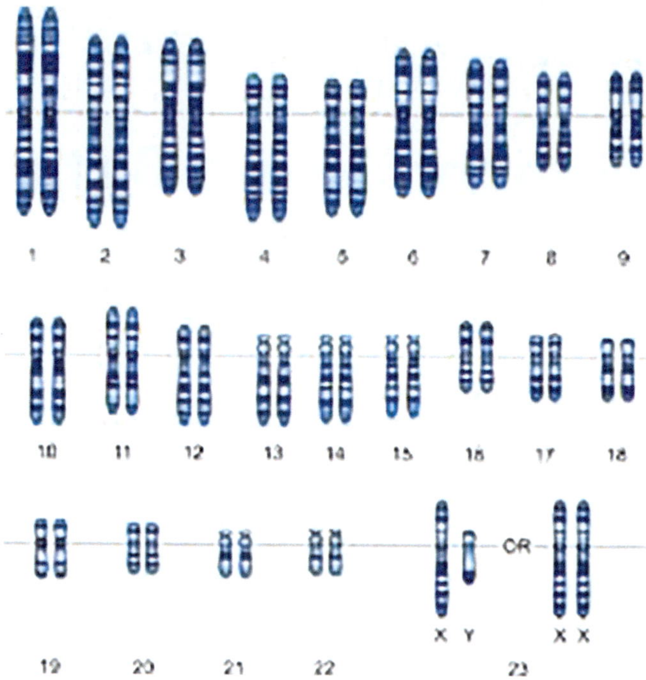

FIGURE 2.1 The human karyotype showing the 23 pairs of chromosomes, including the XY male and XX female.

Birth Disorders

Some birth disorders are genetic and inherited. For example, in the case of hemophilia, a blood clotting disorder, a gene on the X chromosome disrupts the normal process of blood clotting. For most cases of hemophilia, mothers (who are asymptomatic) pass the hemophilia gene on to their sons. Other disorders are caused by malformations in the genes and are therefore congenital. They are typically attributable to spontaneous mutations or to incompatibility of parents' genes. These disorders can be caused by a single gene or by many genes, and they can be transmitted by one parent or by both.

The most common genetic disorders are having an extra chromosome or missing a chromosome. Individuals with **trisomy 21 (Down syndrome)** have 47 chromosomes rather than the normal 46 (23 from each parent). Down syndrome birth rates vary with the age of the parents, with a 1-in-2,000 rate among 20-year-old women but a 1-in-30 rate among 45-year-old women. The prevalence of Down syndrome has decreased by about 60% since the 1970s, the likely result of increased availability and use of prenatal testing (Cheffins et al., 2000). Men with **Klinefelter's syndrome** have two or more X chromosomes and a Y chromosome (XXY instead of the normal XY); this syndrome occurs in about 1 male out of every 500 live births. Males with Klinefelter's syndrome have genitalia that are underdeveloped and average or low-average IQs, but not all males with Klinefelter's syndrome show symptoms. One in every 2,500 female births has **Turner's syndrome**, an X chromosome with no second X (X instead of the normal XX). Turner's syndrome females are short, with thick short necks, broad chests, and nonfunctional ovaries, yet they have typical intelligence and social skills; but as with Klinefelter's syndrome in males, the symptoms in Turner's syndrome for females can vary (Suzigan et al., 2011). The majority of congenital birth defects are not genetic but rather are caused by environmental factors, such as infections or poor nutrition (discussed later).

Prenatal Testing

The chromosomal structure of a fetus can be evaluated using a variety of procedures. Early chromosomal assessment is possible through **chorionic villus sampling** (CVS; Shim, 2014). *Villi*, which also contain fetal tissue, are protrusions of the membrane which surrounds the fetus and later becomes the placenta. CVS can be done as early as 8 to 10 weeks of conception. In **amniocentesis**, amniotic fluid is drawn off through the abdominal wall of the mother. Fetal cells are then cultivated to be observed and assessed individually. The procedure is typically done around the fourth month after conception. Both CVS and amniocentesis are used to diagnose congenital defects, such as muscular dystrophy, spina bifida, and Down syndrome, and to screen fetal DNA for inherited disorders, such as sickle cell anemia and hemophilia (Alfirevic et al., 2017; Peyvandi et al., 2011). Amniocentesis is used in genetic testing when a pregnancy is considered to be at risk, for example, when there is a family history of genetic anomaly or the mother is over the age of 35. CVS and amniocentesis are associated with some risk, with a 1-in-400 chance (or 0.5–1% of all tests) leading to spontaneous abortion (Simpson, 2012). In addition, CVS has been linked to slightly elevated rates of limb deficiencies when sampled before 10 weeks of age (Shim, 2014).

Less invasive techniques for prenatal testing also exist. Expectant mothers can undergo a blood test that measures **maternal serum alpha-fetoprotein** (MSAFP). Assessed during 11 and 13 weeks' gestation, this measure has an 80–90% success rate for identifying chromosomal disorders, such as Down syndrome (Carlson & Vora, 2017). A noninvasive assessment option is **ultrasound imaging** (Figure 2.2).

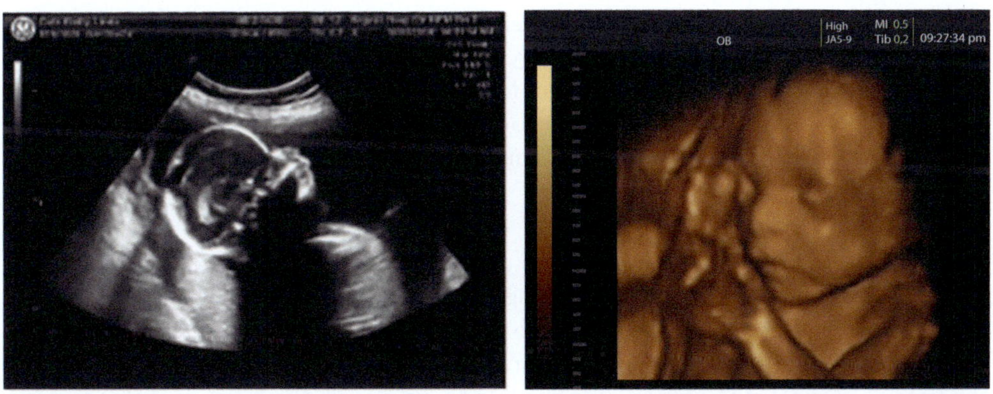

(a) (b)

FIGURE 2.2 Two ultrasound images: (a) A low-resolution ultrasound that can be used to assess the integrity of the fetus, including sex (around 22 weeks' gestation), limb length, and structural integrity of the heart. (b) A high-resolution ultrasound that can be used to identify more specific structural differences, such as facial features if one suspects a fetus might have Down syndrome.

In this common procedure, sounds are sent into the pregnant woman's body from a probe applied to the abdominal skin. A computer analyzes sound pulses that are reflected back and uses them to map structures within the body (Ding et al., 2020). Under current practice, pregnant women typically start with MSAFP testing, followed by ultrasound and possibly CVS or amniocentesis.

Parents undergoing **in vitro fertilization** (when the egg and sperm are united outside of the mother's body and then introduced into the uterus after fertilization) have the option of a single cell being tested for genetic or chromosomal abnormalities before the embryo is transferred (Sravya et al., 2024). Whole genome sequencing of a human fetus also uses noninvasive techniques (Janssen et al., 2024).

Stages of Prenatal Development

Three main stages of prenatal development have been distinguished: the period of the **zygote** (conception to 2 weeks), the period of the **embryo** (2 weeks to 8 weeks), and the period of the **fetus** (8 to 40 weeks). Dating conventionally starts from the mother's last menstrual period rather than the time of conception, which is typically about 2 weeks later. Note that pregnancy from the mother's perspective is more often divided into three equally spaced trimesters (0–12 weeks, 13–25 weeks, and 26–38 weeks) that do not map onto these stages of prenatal development.

The Zygotic Period

The **zygote** is the initial union of the ovum and the sperm, the fertilized egg. This first stage lasts from the moment of conception through the time that the new organism (**blastocyst**) travels toward the uterus, where it implants itself in the **endometrium** (the nutrient-rich lining of the uterus). Multiplication of cells proceeds rapidly during this period. By the end of the very brief zygotic period, human cells have already begun to differentiate, that is to assume specialized roles, depending on their location. For example, some cells will form brain neurons, and others will form the circulatory system. Simultaneously, other parts of the blastocyst develop into support systems for the fetus, most notably the placenta. The **placenta** connects the body of the developing organism to the body of the mother and permits the exchange of nutrients and waste via channels in the thick, tough, tubular **umbilical cord**.

The Embryotic Period

The period of the **embryo**, the second stage of prenatal life, begins when those hairlike structures, the villi, anchor the blastocyst to the uterine wall. The embryonic period is critically important for the differentiation of organs, limbs, and physiological systems. Even by the time of uterine implantation, it is possible to distinguish three layers of the developing individual: The **ectoderm** (from the outer layer of the blastocyst) will form the skin, sense organs, and central nervous system (brain and spinal cord); the **mesoderm** (from the middle layer) will form muscles, the blood, and the circulatory system; and the **endoderm** (from the inner layer) will form the digestive, respiratory, and internal organs. Particularly

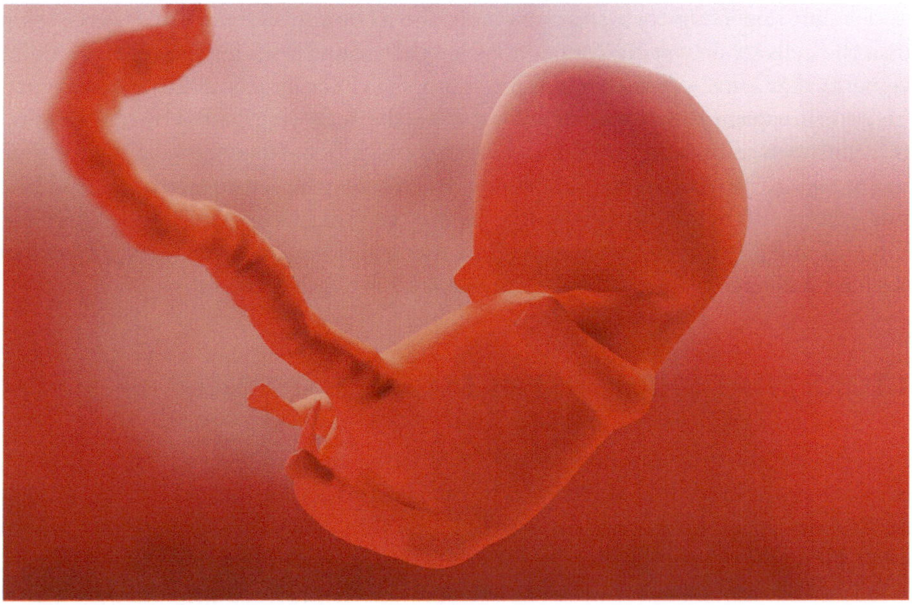

FIGURE 2.3 Side view of a 5-week-old embryo showing the proportionally larger head compared to the rest of the body.

notable by the 14th day is the appearance of the **primitive streak**, which is the first overt stage in the development of the central nervous system.

During the embryonic period, many organs become distinguishable from one another, although they are not fully developed. The embryo is strangely proportioned: The head, for example, constitutes a much larger portion of total body size than it will at any other time in life, between one-third and one-half of the entire length of the embryo (Figure 2.3). Less clearly visible, but no less remarkable, are the tongue and teeth buds. Arms and legs, although tiny, are recognizable as well; there are even fingers and toes. The embryonic stomach produces digestive juices, the kidneys filter blood, and the heart beats. The least developed organs are those which constitute the respiratory system, probably because they are not functional so long as the embryo remains in the fluid environment of the womb.

The Fetal Period

The period of the **fetus** begins when the differentiation of major organs is complete, around two months after conception, and is marked by the first appearance of bone cells. The fetal period is a time of increasing function and great change in bodily proportions. The organs existing at the beginning of the fetal stage only crudely resemble the forms they will later take. In addition, connections among different organs are forged during the fetal period, so a more integrated and coherent functional organism emerges. We can see arm buds in the embryo, for example, but during the fetal period, the arms lengthen, joints develop, fingers separate and grow nails, and a complex network of veins develops to nourish the cells while muscle connections lay the groundwork for the finely coordinated movements that arms will later make.

Functional capacity increases steadily during the fetal stage. After three months, the fetus begins to swallow and urinate, and various reflex behaviors emerge. By four months, fetuses are felt to move *in utero* (**quickening**); by six months, fetuses are capable of breathing and crying; and by seven months, fetuses may survive in the extrauterine environment (**the age of viability**), although with recent medical advances, even younger premature babies have a chance of survival (as discussed later in this chapter).

FACTORS THAT SHAPE PRENATAL DEVELOPMENT

The time before birth is a period of rapid and extensive development, as well as one of enhanced susceptibility and so danger. In other words, a lot can go wrong, given how vulnerable the developing organism is to external influences during this time. An important consideration is how the development of specific systems in the fetus is affected by intra- and extrauterine experiences. An example of self-provided intrauterine experience comes from studies of nonhuman preparations like chickens. When chick embryos are immobilized, the chicks suffer muscle and joint abnormalities after birth, perhaps because their own movements before hatching normally help determine which neuronal connections will grow and which will not in the course of their development. Human fetuses are extremely active. Spontaneous motor activity occurs in cycles of about 1 to 4 minutes, beginning early in the second trimester of pregnancy, remaining stable up to and shortly after birth. How active a fetus is predicts state, cognitive function, and emotional regulation after birth (Bornstein et al., 2002; DiPietro et al., 2015). Fetal motor activity is an individual-level characteristic with implications for postnatal expression of variation in motor development and temperamental qualities of activity level: More active fetuses become newborns, who display more optimal motor and/or reflex performance (DiPietro et al., 2002, 2010) and a range of temperament attributes that access regulatory behavior (DiPietro et al., 1996, 2002). Many prenatal experiences facilitate development, but not all experiences do; and of course, individual differences are pervasive in all these factors.

Other experiences or factors may harm prenatal development. Some include maternal characteristics (e.g., age, diet, and stress) as well as the contraction of diseases, ingestion of drugs, and exposure to environmental toxins. During prenatal development, the embryo and fetus are protected from many insults because the placenta filters harmful agents (**teratogens**) and prevents some, but not all, from causing injury. However, others pass the placental barrier: Diseases, drugs, and environmental toxins pose particular threats.

Maternal Characteristics

Maternal age is one important characteristic that affects fetal development: Younger and older women are at increased risk of birth complications. Mothers 17 years and younger are at risk of higher rates of preterm births (at less than 32 weeks' gestation) and other complications (Khashan et al., 2010). Similarly, women who are 35 years of age or older are at higher risk for such births, prolonged labor, excessive bleeding, diabetes, and pregnancy hypertension than are younger women (Luke & Brown, 2007). In many low-resource countries, older maternal age is a risk factor for child mortality (Bizzego et al., 2021).

Diet is another maternal characteristic that affects the developing fetus. Women whose diets are well balanced experience fewer complications during pregnancy, have shorter labors, and bear healthier babies (see Box 2.1). In particular, malnutrition during pregnancy, especially deficiencies in protein, zinc, and folic acid, have been linked to central nervous system dysfunction, including neural tube defects (spina bifida), prematurity, and other birth defects (De Marco et al., 2011). The timing of malnutrition during pregnancy also appears to affect the type and degree of ill effects fetuses sustain. More severe consequences (e.g., neural tube defects and hydrocephalus – a buildup of fluid in the brain) are associated with severe malnutrition that begins early in pregnancy, whereas malnutrition that begins later in pregnancy is associated with low birth weight.

Still other psychological, familial, and sociological factors influence prenatal development. For example, stress affects maternal hormones, which, in turn, affect the fetus, and mental health disorders in pregnancy are a factor in the early postpartum (Schofield & Schofield, 2025). Chronic stress during pregnancy is associated with premature labor and birthing complications (Paz et al., 2011), and maternal negative affect in pregnancy

Box 2.1 *Application:* Maternal Diet and Exercise

The health of the mother before, during, and after pregnancy has significant impact on her offspring. In this chapter, we discuss a number of ways things can go wrong in a pregnancy and how the developing individual can be harmed during the nine-month journey from conception to birth. A number of potential problems can be avoided if expectant mothers take care of themselves. Mothers who are of a healthy weight before conception, eat a balanced diet, and exercise regularly experience fewer complications with their pregnancies, and they bear healthier babies. Once pregnant, mothers need to be mindful of weight gain – not too much and not too little. The Academy of Nutrition and Dietetics (2019) provides guidance for mothers who are underweight or overweight. Mothers' weight gain is correlated with fetus weight, and increased weight in the mother is related to increased fat cells in offspring – which may put them at risk of weight-related diseases later in life. The nutritional content of food is also important. Folic acid, iron, calcium, B vitamins, and other minerals, such as zinc and copper, are especially important during pregnancy. Most prenatal vitamins have the required nutrient supplements, and women are encouraged to begin vitamin usage when they are planning to become pregnant and to continue while breastfeeding (Dean et al., 2014). One way to control weight is to exercise during pregnancy. Recommended activities include walking, swimming, running, aerobic dancing, and riding a stationary bicycle. In addition to keeping mothers fit, aerobic exercise also helps the baby's cardiovascular functioning (Wowdzia et al., 2023).

In all these ways, planning is an important step toward ensuring a successful pregnancy and a healthy child. A healthy lifestyle before getting pregnant – nutrition, exercise, weight control – sets the stage for optimal prenatal and postnatal experiences for both mother and child.

predicts cytokine levels, which, in turn, predict birth outcomes even in a low-risk population (Takács et al., 2024). Because low socioeconomic status is associated with factors such as poor nutrition, high life stress, and inadequate medical care, the children of impoverished women tend to have poorer outcomes, such as low birth weight or higher incidence of preterm births (Blumenshine, 2010). Pregnancy in itself can be a stress-provoking experience, especially for first-time mothers and even among low-risk women (Lynn et al., 2011), which can also impact newborn birth weight, gestational age, and health status at birth (Doktorchik et al., 2018; Palomo-Gómez et al., 2024).

Disease

Sexually transmitted diseases and diseases such as smallpox and measles can cross the placental barrier and negatively affect prenatal development. For example, women who contract German measles (rubella) during the first trimester of pregnancy (when fetal central nervous system structures such as the eyes and ears are rapidly developing) have a 50% risk of bearing babies who have cataracts or hearing loss. Fortunately, as part of childhood immunizations in high-socioeconomic-status countries, infants receive a vaccination for rubella, so that most adult women and their fetus should have protection. As a result of worldwide vaccination efforts, cases of rubella dropped to 97% from 2000 to 2018, thus significantly reducing the number of babies born with rubella-related impairments (World Health Organization, 2019).

A disease for which there is no vaccine (yet) is HIV/AIDS. The human immunodeficiency virus (HIV), which produces acquired immunodeficiency syndrome (AIDS), passes the placental barrier to infect the developing fetus. In 2018, over 1 million children under the age of 9 worldwide were HIV-positive (UNICEF, 2022), the vast majority of whom acquired the disease from an infected mother during pregnancy or through breastfeeding. Although these numbers are alarmingly high, the situation is radically different in high-socioeconomic-status regions of the world, such as North America and Western Europe, likely the result of widespread public health service efforts for pregnant women to obtain routine, voluntary testing for HIV and the use of antiretroviral drugs in HIV-positive women during pregnancy and delivery and for newborns of infected women. Without such drugs, the mother-to-baby transmission rate of HIV is about 15–45%, which drops to less than 1% when HIV-positive pregnant women are given antiretrovirals (Dao et al., 2007). However, even if infected children do not contract HIV before or after birth, they may have other health problems due to compromises to their immune system (Tobin & Aldrovandi, 2013).

Tobacco, Alcohol, and Illicit Drugs

Many pregnant women still smoke tobacco, drink alcohol, and/or use illicit drugs (Gosdin, 2022; Oga et al., 2018). Nicotine from cigarette smoking is believed to constrict placental blood vessels, temporarily depriving the developing fetal brain of oxygen, stimulating the cardiovascular system, and depressing the respiratory system. Women who smoke have a higher incidence of spontaneous abortions and preterm deliveries, and their offspring experience higher incidence of low birth weight and intrauterine growth retardation

(Hackshaw et al., 2011). Smoke exposure during pregnancy places children at risk of poor cognitive functioning (Mezzacappa et al., 2011; Motlagh et al., 2011). Similar outcomes have been documented for marijuana use during pregnancy (Goldschmidt et al., 2008; Gunn et al., 2016).

A well-studied example of the sensitivity of the fetus to everyday drugs concerns alcohol. **Fetal alcohol spectrum disorder** (FASD) is considered the leading cause of developmental delays with a known etiology. Women who drink excessively during pregnancy experience higher incidences of spontaneous abortions, stillbirths, and preterm deliveries (Patra et al., 2011). Diagnostic criteria for fetal alcohol syndrome (one type of FASD) include pre- or postnatal growth retardation as well as central nervous system abnormalities, such as **microcephaly** (a smaller-than-normal brain; Figure 2.4), that results in neurological impairment, including severe motor impairment, seizure disorders, hearing and vision abnormalities, and sleep difficulties (Satterfield-Nash et al., 2017). Seizures, low muscle tone and motor impairments, cognitive impairments, attention deficit and hyperactivity, and craniofacial abnormalities, such as a narrow forehead, small nose and midface, and a low nasal bridge, are also common (Vaurio et al., 2011). Some children exposed to alcohol prenatally do not display characteristic structural abnormalities, yet they show deficits in a number of areas, including cognition, social interaction, communication, and personal living skills (Caputo et al., 2016; Jacobson et al., 2011). Chronic maternal alcohol intake appears to contribute to overall lower levels of brain volume (Lebel et al., 2011), and opioids destroy nerve cells in the developing fetal brain (Boggess & Risher, 2022; Brubaker et al., 2009). An example of profound brain damage is prenatal exposure to the Zika virus. This virus is transmitted by mosquitos. In 2015 and 2016, an outbreak in Brazil resulted in many babies being born with abnormalities (Wheeler, 2018), the most common of which was microcephaly.

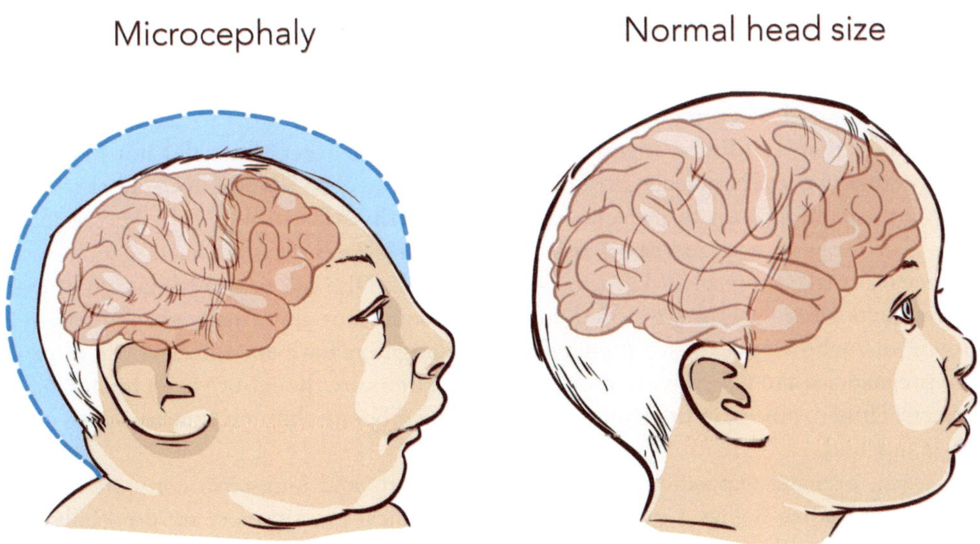

FIGURE 2.4 Profile of two babies showing the difference in head size and the neural configuration that occurs with microcephaly.

Drugs such as cocaine, heroin, and other opioids also affect prenatal development and postnatal functioning. These substances also transfer easily from mother to fetus: Traces of cocaine can be found in the urine of newborns, and newborns can be addicted to heroin or methadone (Eyler et al., 2001). Epidemiological studies reveal linkages between prenatal cocaine abuse and increased rates of spontaneous abortions, stillbirths, and premature separation of the placenta, as well as preterm birth. Prenatal cocaine exposure also leads to low birth weight, reduced head circumference and body length, high levels of irritability, poor state organization, and increased risk for **sudden infant death syndrome** (SIDS; Gouin et al., 2011), an unexpected death in the first year of life. Longer-term effects of cocaine exposure include modest intellectual and language deficits (Bandstra et al., 2010; Lambert & Bauer, 2012). Addicted newborns begin withdrawal from their addiction within one to three days after birth, called **neonatal abstinence syndrome**. Withdrawal symptoms can be severe and include tremors, irritability, vomiting, diarrhea, and sleep disturbances (Reddy et al., 2017). Prenatal heroin exposure is a risk factor for HIV infection because addicts frequently share needles. Long-range effects of opioids appear to include lower IQ and attentional and behavioral problems (Ornoy et al., 2010).

Fortunately, discontinuing drug use may lead to improvements in child development. Scherling (1994) reported that 40% of children whose mothers used cocaine pre- and postnatally had IQ scores of 85 or lower (where a score of 100 is average). By contrast, only 15% of children scored at this low level when their mothers stopped using cocaine postnatally. It is likely that mothers who discontinue drug use postnatally parent better and rear their children in safer environments than mothers who remain on drugs (Liebschutz et al., 2015). Such maternal and material improvements might, in turn, improve child development.

Seemingly harmless drugs can also have simple to catastrophic consequences for developing individuals, even when parents and physicians are acting in the best interests of the mother and the fetus and the drugs have no observable effects on the mothers. In the late 1950s and 1960s, European physicians sometimes prescribed the sedative thalidomide for pregnant women suffering from morning sickness. Those women who took thalidomide during the period when fetal limbs were differentiating gave birth to babies with limb buds rather than full limbs. Ingestion of thalidomide at other times did not have such tragic consequences (Newman, 1985). Another example of an adverse drug effect resulted from a medication used to prevent miscarriage, diethylstilbestrol (DES). The insidious effects of DES, such as increased risk of rare cervical and vaginal cancers, took about 30 years to make themselves known. Less frequently, DES led to the formation of cysts in the ducts where sperm are stored, low sperm counts, or abnormally shaped sperm in grown men who were exposed prenatally. DES daughters have an increased risk of problem pregnancies and infertility, and even their daughters are thought to be at higher risk of cancers. Thus, exposure in the grandmother may reverberate through generations to affect the grandchild.

Clearly, prenatal exposure to drugs has both short- and long-term consequences for developing human beings. Consequently, today, medical practitioners are especially cautious about prescribing (even over-the-counter) medications to pregnant women. Caution also applies to herbals and botanicals. Not much is known about their potential effects on prenatal development yet, but their use in alternative or complementary medical approaches to managing pregnancy is common in some countries, cultures, and communities (Illamola et al., 2020). Finally, not all women who use legal or illegal substances will admit to doing so because of stigma, which limits the extent to which interventions can help reduce potential pre- and postnatal impacts.

Environment

The physical environment also poses toxic hazards for fetuses. For example, PCBs (polychlorinated biphenyls), DDT, mercury, and lead have adverse implications for prenatal development (AL-Gubory, 2014; Parithathvi et al., 2024). PCBs are synthetic hydrocarbons that were used widely in industry before being banned in the United States in the 1970s. Residues of PCBs are still present in the soil, water, and air and can be ingested by eating fish from contaminated lakes. Prenatal PCB exposure is linked to lower birth weight, smaller head circumference, shorter gestation, poorer autonomic and reflex functioning, and long-term deficits in memory and language (Dzwilewski & Schantz, 2015; Jacobson & Jacobson, 1994). DDT and other organochlorines (as these types of chemicals are called) have been commonly used as pesticides in farming and for mosquito control. Although outlawed in a number of high-socioeconomic-status countries, DDT is still used for malaria control in some low-socioeconomic-status countries (Pathak et al., 2011).

Timing and Comorbidity

Teratogens are altogether insidious, but what is a *teratogen* and what is not has been difficult to discover because of the selectivity and time-boundedness of their consequences. In other words, some teratogens do not have easily detectable, systematic, or pervasive effects. Other factors further complicate detection; the **dose–effect relation** is one. The most straightforward mechanism of teratogen action is a linear model, such that greater amounts (in dosages or exposures) are associated with greater effects, making the effects of the would-be toxin clear (Needleman & Bellinger, 1991). However, some substances need to reach a threshold (or a certain level) before the toxic effects emerge or even have positive effects at low levels but toxic effects at high levels (Calabrese & Baldwin, 2003). The threshold model explains the effects of alcohol consumption. Patra and colleagues (2011) found that the dose–response relation for low birth weight and small for gestational age showed no effect up to 10 g of pure alcohol (equivalent to an average of 1 drink/day), and for preterm birth no effect up to 18 g of pure alcohol (about 1.5 drinks/day). Above those thresholds, the risk of birth complications increases as consumption increases.

Studying the effects of diet, drugs, and other environmental influences (such as lead exposure) on the developing organism is further complicated by several other factors. One is that the impact of such toxins varies as a function of when in development they are introduced (e.g., drinking in the first trimester of pregnancy vs. the third trimester). A **sensitive period** is defined as a time during which the organism is especially vulnerable to external influences that alter or modify its structures or functions, often, though not always, in an irreversible fashion (Bornstein, 1989; Hensch & Bilimoria, 2012). Sensitive periods are programmed organism–environment interactions that occur between the time a structure or function emerges and the time it reaches its mature state. Typically, they encompass the epoch during which the structure or function is undergoing its most rapid development. For example, the eyes develop most rapidly in the second month of pregnancy, and so the visual system is especially vulnerable during this period. All the major organ systems differentiate early in gestation, and therefore, as organ development slows toward the end of gestation, the likelihood of gross structural malformation as a result of external factors declines. With respect to many teratogens, older fetuses are at less risk than younger ones (although oxygen deprivation, for example, might be more important to the older fetus). Consequently, the effects of a toxin depend as much, or more, on timing than on the nature of the toxin itself: Two different toxins could have very similar effects at the same phase of prenatal life yet neither affects development at other stages.

Prenatal experiences might have immediate effects, as indicated by prenatal exposure to cocaine and heroin on neonatal functioning, or they might also show long-term **sleeper effects**, as indicated in IQ deficits and behavior problems later in life. If exposure to teratogens continues beyond the prenatal period, risk to the child might not decline. For example, parents who smoke postnatally place their children at risk of bronchitis, pneumonia, and asthma due to the effects of secondhand smoke.

Finally, it is difficult to identify the effects of a single teratogen, because one risk factor, such as alcohol use, may occur simultaneously (**comorbid**) with another, such as smoking, poor diet, and substandard housing with lead exposure (Lambert & Bauer, 2012). Animal studies, in which researchers can exercise a high level of control and fewer ethical concerns, can identify the impact of an isolated toxin, such as the way nicotine induces DNA damage or how caffeine impacts cardiac development in mice. In studies with humans, statistical techniques are used to try to isolate the effects of one teratogen from another (LaMaestra et al., 2011; Mezzacappa et al., 2011). Moreover, it is likely that babies exposed prenatally to a nonoptimal environment will continue to experience a nonoptimal environment after birth. For example, drug abuse by mothers often co-occurs with poverty, poor prenatal care, poor postnatal nutrition, parental psychopathology, and parental neglect. Newborns of drug-addicted mothers experience multiple short-term foster placements, separations, and/or repeated moves (Chassin et al., 2019). As a consequence, it is difficult to determine whether developmental delays in children are a product of one or more prenatal exposures or postnatal contexts of development.

Feeling and Thinking About the Fetus

Not all prenatal development is risk. Parents can set the stage for positive early interactions before their newborn arrives. Mothers (and, to some extent, fathers) often develop expectations for their newborn based on fetal prenatal behavior, such as activity levels, and expectations they have for newborns of different genders. For example, after finding out their child's sex via ultrasound well before giving birth, parents have described female fetuses as "finer" and "quieter" than male fetuses, and described male fetuses as "more coordinated" than female fetuses (Sweeney & Bradbard, 1988). Another way parents prepare for their newborn, infant, or child is by attributing mental states to the fetus, a process called **mind-mindedness** (Meins et al., 2011, 2012), which includes thinking about their fetus's thoughts, feelings, and desires and adjusting or responding to them appropriately (Bigelow et al., 2023; Foley et al., 2022).

CONCLUSIONS

Prenatal development begins with the union of the ovum and the sperm. During the nine months of gestation, the organism undergoes significant changes, first as a zygote (conception to 2 weeks, characterized by cell division and implantation into the uterine wall), then as an embryo (2 to 8 weeks, characterized by the foundation of all organ structures), and finally as a fetus (8 to 40 weeks, characterized by refinement, growth, and weight gain). During the embryonic stage, the organism is maximally vulnerable to harmful agents, or teratogens, such as poor maternal diet, diseases, drugs, and environmental toxins. Isolating the effects of teratogens is difficult because they tend to co-occur, such as poor diet, smoking, drug use, and stress. Also, some effects of teratogens may not be immediately apparent because they appear long after exposure.

To this point, we have mentioned several contexts of prenatal development, including parental influences, SES, and culture. It is important to note that systems of diverse sorts condition the development of the newborn, infant, or child even before birth.

KEY TERMS

Age of viability
Amniocentesis
Blastocyst
Chorionic villus sampling
Chromosomes
Comorbid
Dose–effect relation
Ectoderm
Embryo
Endoderm
Endometrium
Epigenetics
Fetal alcohol spectrum disorder
Fetus
Gametes
Genotype
In vitro fertilization
Klinefelter's syndrome
Maternal serum alpha-fetoprotein
Meiosis
Mesoderm
Microcephaly
Mind-mindedness
Neonatal abstinence syndrome
Ovum
Phenotype
Placenta
Primitive streak
Quickening
Sensitive period
Sleeper effects
Sudden infant death syndrome
Teratogens
Trisomy 21 (Down syndrome)
Turner's syndrome
Ultrasound imaging
Umbilical cord
Zygote

SUGGESTED READINGS

Broderick, A. V., & Neiderhiser, J. M. (2019). Genetics and parenting. In M. H. Bornstein (Ed.), *Handbook of parenting, Vol. 2: Biology and ecology of parenting* (3rd ed., pp. 123–165). Routledge.

Coall, D. A., Callan, A. C., Sartori, J., & Chisholm, J. S. (2019). Prenatal parenting. In M. H. Bornstein (Ed.), *Handbook of parenting, Vol. 2: Biology and ecology of parenting* (3rd ed., pp. 166–219). Routledge.

SECTION I

The Newborn

Birth to 3 Months

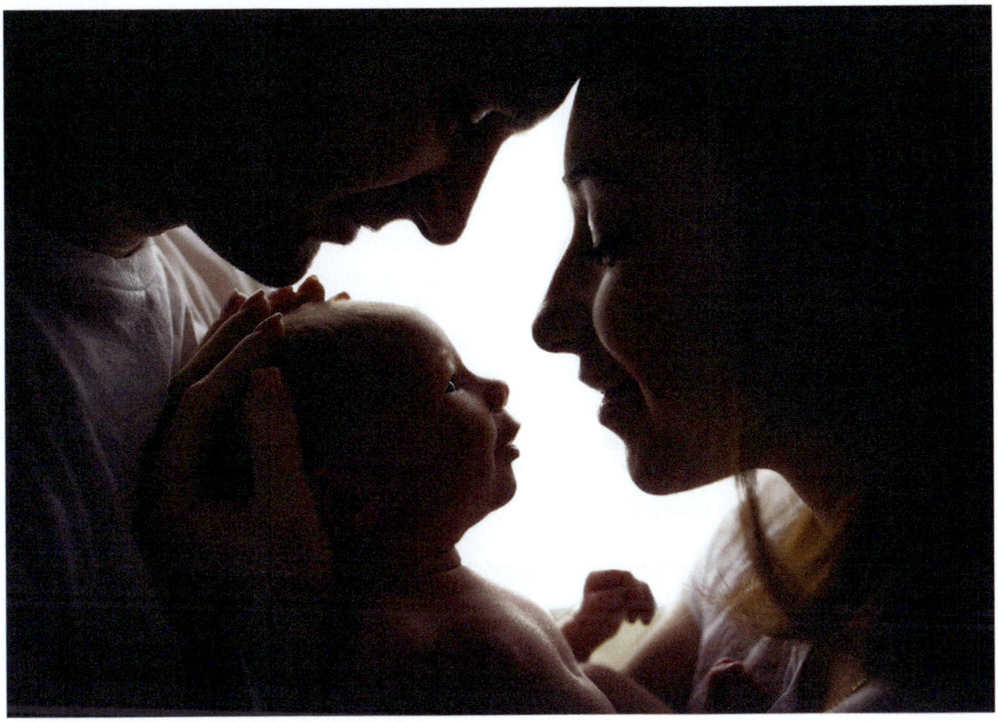

A tremendous amount of development occurs before birth that lays the foundations for immediate development in the newborn, the infant, and the child and the future development of the individual across the balance of the life course. This section of *Newborn to Infant to Child* describes growth and action (Chapter 4), perception and thought (Chapter 5), emotions and temperament (Chapter 6), communication and relationships (Chapter 7), and contexts of development (Chapter 8) in the newborn. To begin, meet mom Mia, dad Noah, and baby Leo.

Mia and Noah had Leo, their first baby, when Mia was 32 and Noah was 34 years old. They were older than the U.S. average age for the birth of a first child (today around age 28) because they spent most of their 20s in college, establishing careers, and of course, dating! When they married and decided to have a child, they adjusted their lifestyle in areas such as diet,

DOI: 10.4324/9781003381709-3

exercise, and managing stress. Leo was born after 38 weeks' gestation, just on time. After a long but uneventful labor, Mia and Noah were thrilled that they could take home a healthy baby boy the very next day. However, the first month with Leo was challenging. Leo seemed to sleep all day and stay up all night – or at least cry a lot at regular intervals throughout the night. Even sharing responsibilities, Mia and Noah found it hard to manage all that their little one demanded – feeding, soothing, diapering – on interrupted sleep.

All things considered, Mia and Noah can count themselves fortunate. Even healthy babies and prepared parents find adjustment to their new responsibilities taxing in many ways. Also, the paths to parenthood are very individual. Some people are ready to be parents but have difficulty conceiving. Others find themselves pregnant unexpectedly but may not have the support or resources to prepare for becoming a family. Still others, despite their best preparations, conceive babies who are born preterm or with an unexpected genetic or congenital condition, like Down syndrome or spina bifida. Still other new parents have followed lifestyles that jeopardize their newborn's health, such as having abused substances and exposed their baby in utero.

In a typical day, Leo spends a lot of time sleeping; however, when awake, he is looking, listening, and even beginning to "think." Mia notices that when she speaks to Leo in the special tones of "motherese" (infant-directed speech), Leo seems to look more intently into her eyes. Noah likes to sing the same song to calm Leo, and over time Noah has noticed that Leo settles more quickly when Noah starts to sing their special song. When these new parents just stand near his crib, they notice that Leo likes to stare at the ceiling fan or, when the wind is blowing, look out the window at the rustling leaves on a tree, and they think that Leo is attracted to movement. Mia breastfeeds Leo, and she has noticed that as she comes near when it is time to feed him, Leo begins to smack his lips, like he anticipates being fed or smells her special scent.

Leo makes a lot of funny faces, even when he is asleep. Mia and Noah wonder what these might mean, if anything. Does Leo feel happiness? They can tell when he is not happy, because he cries – a lot. When he is upset, Mia and Noah troubleshoot to try to figure out what is wrong. Does his diaper need to be changed? Is he hungry? Is it gas? Eventually, Leo calms down, until the next time.

Mia's and Noah's decisions about parenting come from a variety of sources, including baby books, internet parenting blogs, grandparents, and friends. They wonder about the right way to do things and whether what others do will work for Leo. They want to raise a strong, independent boy, but Leo seems happiest when he is in close physical contact with his parents or grandparents.

CHAPTER 3

Newborns

Growth and Action

The early life period is a time of rapid growth, and each day brings dramatic changes. At first, children do not reach, and then they can pick things up with their fingers. At first, they do not turn over, and then they can get out of bed themselves. At first, they do not follow pointed fingers that indicate something, and then they point fingers to do so themselves. At first, they only grunt, gurgle, and cry, and then they say words. All these advances come because of the interplay between physical maturation, particularly of the nervous system, muscles, and anatomical growth, and experiences. Here we describe rapid changes in motor development in the first months of postnatal life.

Developmental scientists tout the importance of understanding nervous system, physical, and motor development for two good reasons. First, the principles of development in these systems provide models for other domains of development. The terms *innate* and *congenital* and the distinction between the two are an example. The term **innate** applies to structures and functions that are inherited, but they may or may not be fully mature at birth. By contrast, **congenital** applies to structures and functions that are present at birth but are not inherited. Some characteristics are innate but not congenital because they emerge in later years of development, as at puberty. Down syndrome is congenital because it arises from too many chromosomes, but it is not inherited. The second reason that nervous system, physical, and motor developments are important is that, on the systems view, development in these domains influences the emergence and growth of other domains. Newborns may at first try to grasp small objects using the palm and the whole hand, but as fine motor skills improve, infants pinch objects using the thumb and the forefinger together. This gross-to-fine motor transition marks an advance that enhances exploration, learning, and cognition.

This chapter looks at birth and at topics related to nervous system, physical, and motor development shortly after birth as important issues in themselves. Later chapters show how these systems of growth and action support perception and thought, emotions and temperament, and communication and relationships.

BIRTH

After approximately 280 days of gestation (at least for first-time middle-income mothers with uncomplicated, spontaneous labor and deliveries), some unknown factor causes the

DOI: 10.4324/9781003381709-4

mother's pituitary gland to release a hormone (**oxytocin**) that, in turn, precipitates muscular contraction and expulsion of the fetus from the uterus. The uterus is actually a muscle that expands during pregnancy. **Labor** involves those involuntary uterine contractions, beginning at the top of the muscle, that literally force the fetus down and out of the birth canal. The duration of labor is influenced by a variety of factors and can vary substantially among women, but contractions last 16 to 17 hours on average for firstborns. The duration of the first stage of active labor (from 5 cm dilated until full dilation) does not typically exceed 12 hours for first labors or 10 hours for subsequent labors. The second stage, from full dilation to birth, typically does not exceed 3 hours for first labors or 2 hours for subsequent ones (World Health Organization, 2018).

Birth represents a transition in a process of continuing development. The organism before and after birth does not usually deviate from the typical, genetically maturing schedule. Central nervous system function and motor behavior are not discretely altered by the birth process. Like fetuses, newborns are dependent in all ways on others. For example, newborns are unable to maintain their own body temperature, lacking both the insulating material (subcutaneous fat) and the functional neural capacity. At the same time, birth is a monumental event. With incredible suddenness, and for the first time, newborns are responsible for circulation and respiration. Moreover, vision, audition, smell, taste, and touch are new or radically different from prenatal life.

The narrowness of the birth canal leaves most newborns looking red and battered with misshapen heads, but these consequences are temporary. More significant are dangers during the birth process, for example, ones associated with oxygen deprivation (**anoxia**). Fetuses can experience anoxia for many reasons; some involve the fetus pinching, holding, or squeezing the umbilical cord (through which the mother supplies the fetus with oxygen). Whatever the cause, a baby who is deprived of oxygen for a very short amount of time is in little danger; however, deprivation for minutes or more may result in some brain damage because brain cells require continuous oxygenation to survive and function, and brain cells are not usually replaced when they die. Severe anoxia places newborns at risk for seizures, cerebral palsy, and impaired cognition. Second, anoxia builds up pressure in the blood system, and that pressure can lead to bleeding in cavities (**ventricles**) in the brain (**intraventricular hemorrhage**, or IVH); the ventricles produce and store cerebrospinal fluid (CSF), lack of which can injure the hippocampus, a site for memory (Aylward, 2005). Fortunately, the probability of anoxia is normally limited because fetal metabolic rate and temperature fall during delivery, reducing the need for oxygen. Gray skin color at birth (as recorded in an Apgar assessment, discussed later) can indicate anoxia. Other risks involve the fetuses' orientation in the birth canal. Babies are normally born headfirst, but sometimes they present feet- or buttocks-first (**breech**).

The pain of childbirth prompts some women to make use of pain management at some point during labor and delivery. Local anesthetic methods, such as the epidural block, are common (70–75% of women use an epidural block; MacMillan, 2023), and they are effective in reducing labor pain without adverse effects on the newborn. An epidural block is administered at the spine and reduces sensation in the lower extremities, allowing the mother to remain conscious but alleviating some or most childbirth pain. A downside of the epidural block is the possible loss of mobility, which makes it difficult for mothers to move around or to push during the final stages of delivery (Collis & Davis, 2010). Many fathers or other supportive partners often are present during delivery, and their presence can also help mothers cope with the pain. A happy side effect of mothers' use of pain management is a reduction in fathers' anxiety and stress during labor and delivery (Johansson et al., 2015).

Not all newborns are born naturally (through the vagina), for a number of reasons, including health of the mother, health of the fetus, or fetal position. Instead, they are delivered by a surgical procedure that involves cutting into the uterus to remove the newborn (called a **Cesarean section**, although historians reckon that Julius Caesar was not delivered this way; Dahlke & Chauhan, 2025). C-sections, as they are commonly called, accounted for approximately 32% of all births in the United States in 2021, up from 21% in 1997 (March of Dimes, 2021). Older women are more likely to have C-sections, as are women who prefer the predictability of a planned birth rather than waiting for labor to start naturally. C-sections, however, are not without risk of complications (it takes mothers longer to recover). Moreover, reasons for the first C-section may persist in subsequent pregnancies, making it likely that a woman will have multiple C-sections during her childbearing years; fewer than 15% of successive pregnancies result in a vaginal delivery following a C-section (March of Dimes, 2025).

PREMATURITY

The typical or full-term newborn is delivered about 40 weeks after the mother's last menstrual period (following 38 weeks' gestation). On average, the term newborn measures 20 in (51 cm) and weighs 6 to 9 lb (2,700 to 4,100 g). However, as of 2018, approximately 5–18% of babies worldwide are born too early (WHO, 2018). Newborns are considered preterm if born before 37 weeks' gestational age and considered of low birth weight if born under 5.5 lb (2,500 g). Gestational age and birth weight are highly correlated, as fetuses gain most of their weight during the last two months of pregnancy. In Figure 3.1,

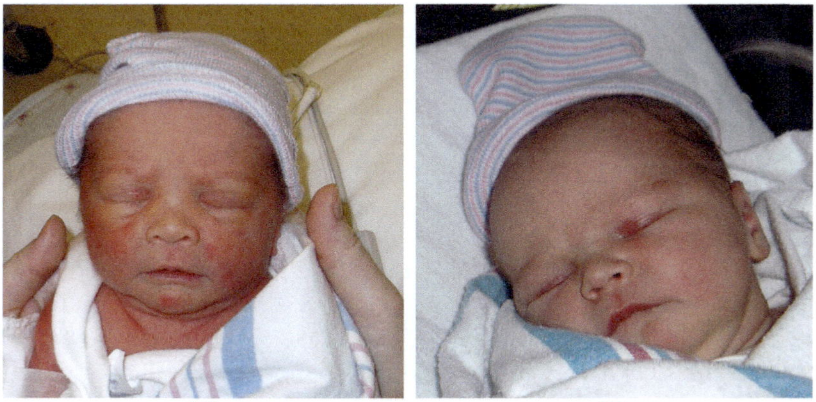

(a) (b)

FIGURE 3.1 Newborn brothers, one born at 34 weeks (a) and one born at 40 weeks (b). Despite his preterm birth and low birth weight, Newborn A was otherwise healthy and showed no long-term effects of prematurity.

Source: Courtesy of L. Cote.

notice the differences between these two brothers. Newborn A is lean compared to Newborn B. Also, Newborn A's newborn beanie is too large, and Newborn B's beanie barely fits.

Newborns may arrive preterm for a number of reasons. Abnormalities in the mother's reproductive system or general health might prevent her from carrying her pregnancy to term. Multiple births (e.g., twins) also place excessive metabolic and other demands on the mother (Hamer et al., 2025), and so multiple births tend to be preterm (Hezelgrave & Shennan, 2025). The mother's reproductive system might be immature or may not have had sufficient time to recover from a previous pregnancy; teen mothers and mothers over the age of 35 are at greater risk of delivering preterm babies (Cavazos-Rehg et al., 2015). As discussed earlier, conditions that adversely affect general maternal health – including drug use, poverty, malnutrition, inadequate medical care, and unhealthy lifestyles – are associated with preterm delivery.

Newborns who are marginally preterm face little danger. They might be hospitalized briefly for observation or to gain weight and are afterward discharged. A variety of medical complications can arise when the degree of prematurity is more marked, however. Newborns born at less than 32 weeks of gestational age often experience **respiratory distress syndrome** (RDS; Mosca et al., 2011). These newborns may lack **surfactin**, a soapy substance that coats the lungs and facilitates the exchange of oxygen from the air. To assist them in breathing, preterms are placed in incubators, where the concentration of oxygen is higher than in the normal environment. The actual concentration has to be titrated carefully to avoid producing an excess oxygen that damages the retinas (**retinopathy of prematurity**), risking permanent blindness (Deuber & Terhaar, 2011).

Very early preterms are at greater risk of health and developmental problems. They can develop a condition of chronic lung disease (**bronchopulmonary dysplasia**) identified by thickening and inflammation of the walls of the lung and a reduced airway, resulting in a significant decrease in the amount of oxygen for the newborn (Mosca et al., 2011). They are also at significant risk of brain complications, such as IVH. For a number of reasons, therefore, immature preterms may need close supervision in a hospital for the first weeks or months of life. Preterm low-birth-weight newborns have average hospital stays of 45–50 days, and between one-third and one-half experience one or more hospitalizations during the first three years of life (Behrman & Butler, 2007). Moreover, survival is not guaranteed: Despite modern technological advances in neonatal care, most babies born at 22 to 23 weeks' gestation fail to survive (Ishii et al., 2013).

In addition to health risks, preterms are also at a psychological risk. Very preterm, very low-birth-weight newborns can have lower IQs and developmental and learning disabilities (Kavšek & Bornstein, 2010; Muraskas et al., 2012; Rose et al., 2011). In the United States, prematurity and low birth weight are linked to socioeconomic disadvantage (Blumenshine, 2010; Venkatesan et al., 2023), and thus, many preterm low-birth-weight newborns are at medical *and* environmental risk. It is important that, in the absence of clear organic bases for abnormal development (e.g., blindness and brain damage), the degree to which preterms develop well or poorly reflects the caregiving environment they encounter after hospital discharge. Preterms who grow up in enriching, supportive homes do better, whereas those in less-resourced environments develop more poorly (Gattis, 2019).

Section Summary

Birth is a momentous event for families. After approximately 38 weeks' gestation, the uterus expels the fetus or the fetus is delivered via Cesarean section. From the fetal (now newborn) perspective, respiration, temperature, and nutrition change, but development continues to unfold as it did in the last few months of pregnancy, with refinement and growth. Some newborns arrive preterm, before 38 weeks, and they are at risk of complications such as intraventricular hemorrhaging, anoxia, or immature respiratory systems. Very preterm newborns face greater challenges, and many do not survive despite advances in neonatal care practices.

NEWBORN ASSESSMENT

At about 1 minute and 5 minutes after birth, newborns in most U.S. hospitals are given their first test. The **Apgar**, named after its originator, Virginia Apgar (1909–1974), rates newborns as 0, 1, or 2 on each of five dimensions, easy to remember because of the acronym: **a**ppearance, **p**ulse, **g**rimace, **a**ctivity, and **r**espiration (Apgar, 1953). The criteria for each score are listed in Table 3.1. Total scores of 3 and below are critically low and require medical attention, whereas total scores between 7 and 10 give evidence of a generally healthy newborn. The Apgar determines the need for intervention or documents normal functioning.

The Apgar is only one of several tests designed for newborns. It is probably the best known because it is administered right in the delivery room, but it is only a gross screening instrument. Other tests evaluate the status of newborns more thoroughly and systematically. For example, the **Dubowitz test** (Dubowitz & Dubowitz, 1981) is used to estimate gestational age. It scores newborns on a variety of neurological items (including posture and reflexes, simple, unlearned stimulus–response movement sequences common to all members of a species) and external characteristics (including skin quality and gross morphology). The **Neonatal Behavioral Assessment Scale** (NBAS; Brazelton et al., 1987) evaluates newborns' neurological functioning using 18 reflex items and newborns'

TABLE 3.1 Criteria and Scoring the Apgar Test

	A	*P*	*G*	*A*	*R*
Score	*Appearance (color)*	*Pulse (heart rate)*	*Grimace (reflex irritability)*	*Activity (muscle tone)*	*Respiration (respiratory effort)*
0	Blue, pale	Absent	No response	Limp	Absent
1	Body pink, extremities blue	Slow (below 100)	Grimace	Some flexion of extremities	Slow, irregular
2	Completely pink	Rapid (over 100)	Cry	Active motion	Good, strong cry

interactional repertoire on 27 indices of information processing, motoric capacities, ability to control state, and response to stress.

NEURAL DEVELOPMENT

One reason that teratogens can be so harmful is that significant brain development occurs in the early life period. Figure 3.2 shows a single **neuron**, including its components of **cell body**, **nucleus**, **dendrites**, and **axon**. Dendrites conduct information to the cell body, and axons transmit information away from the cell body by way of the **action potential**, the electrochemical exchange along the axon fiber. This fiber can be infinitesimally short or extremely long (up to 3–4 ft, approximately 1 m). Neurons communicate with each other by means of a chemical called a **neurotransmitter** across **synapses**, which are the gaps between neurons. The most common neurotransmitters are norepinephrine and acetylcholine, but more than 50 different neurotransmitters have been identified

The development of the CNS reflects highly complex processes (Stiles et al., 2015). The CNS originates as a cell layer on the outer surface of the embryo and is already visible 4 weeks after conception. Neurons continue to appear throughout the embryonic and fetal periods. After cells form (**neurogenesis**), they grow, migrate, and eventually associate with one another to form relatively stable interconnected networks.

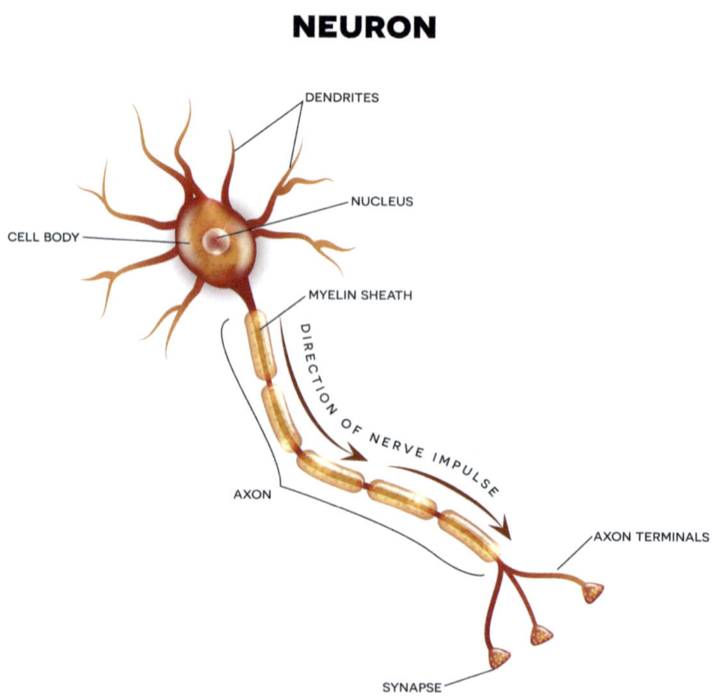

FIGURE 3.2 A single neuron showing the cell body and nucleus, dendritic fibers, and the axon, surrounded by a myelin sheath, and flow of the action potential (nerve impulse) toward the synapse.

The layers of the brain are generated from the inside out. As a result, cells constantly migrate, and they send their axons from one location to another. A fascinating aspect of neural development is that migration routes seem to be predetermined (Stiles et al., 2015). After their generation and migration, individual cells grow dendritic connections, which allow for communication between neurons. Dendrites and axons continue to grow, and dendrites continue to branch out through adulthood. Also, axons begin to be covered with **myelin**, a fatty substance that surrounds the axon and facilitates the speed of nerve conduction, rendering information transmission more efficient (Klingberg, 2008). Undeveloped neurons are naked fibers; developed ones are usually (although not always) wrapped in a sheath of myelin. With myelination, the velocity of neurotransmission in a cell more than triples, from a rate of less than 20 ft (6 m) per second to more than 60 ft (18 m) per second. The process of myelination loosely correlates with the development of function and provides a general index of maturation, although some functional activity still occurs in the absence of myelination. The visual and auditory cortices of the brain myelinate before birth, whereas higher brain centers, such as the prefrontal cortex, which integrates information, are not completely myelinated until puberty (Shaw et al., 2006).

The human brain grows as developing neurons aggregate into cell masses that soon give the brain its characteristic structure. The outer covering of the surfaces of the cerebral hemispheres (**cerebral cortex**) is folded into peaks (**gyri**) and grooves (**sulci**). In the human brain, the cortex is 0.16 in (less than 4 mm) thick and makes up 40% of the brain's mass. The cortex of a human fetus in the second trimester already reveals the sulci and gyri of its eventual adult form. The human brain has two hemispheres, is covered by a cortex, and has four sections (lobes). Different structures of the brain control different functions; this specialization in the cortex is illustrated in Figure 3.3. The **occipital lobe** registers and processes

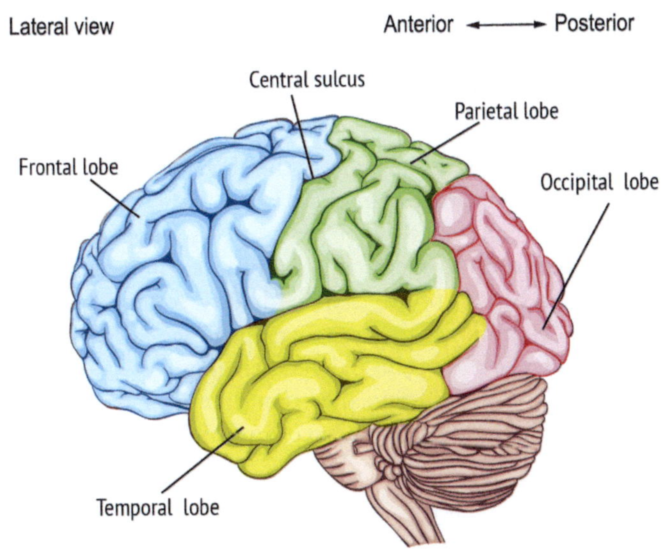

FIGURE 3.3 The human brain contains four cortical lobes on the left and right sides. In this image, the eyes are to the left (in other words, the frontal lobe is at the front of our head).

visual information. The **temporal lobe** governs auditory processes and language. The **parietal lobe** registers temperature, taste, and touch and governs motor movements. The **frontal lobe** is the center of higher-order cognition and controls voluntary movement and activities.

The two hemispheres and the brain stem contain three major substructures that develop in an orderly fashion (Johnson, 2011; Stiles et al., 2015). **Subcortical structures** that control state (such as the hypothalamus) and the arousal system emerge first. Indeed, the nuclei of the **reticular formation**, which govern sleep/wake cycles, are among the earliest to differentiate in the brain. Components of the **limbic system** and **basal ganglia**, which govern emotion, instinct, and posture, develop next. Finally, the cortex and **cortical association areas** concerned with awareness, attention, memory, language, and the integration of information emerge. The cortical regions are also among the last to myelinate and are influenced most by the individual's experience with the outside world. Developmental phases for these three major components of the nervous system overlap, and development in each component continues well past the first three years of life (Shaw et al., 2006). Because neural development is ongoing, essentially from conception to early adulthood, it is particularly vulnerable to external influences.

The brain is central to survival, so CNS development in prenatal and early postnatal life is far from fixed. Experimental work with animals such as monkeys indicates that disrupting the amount of input to one brain area relative to another area reduces the size of the target area. In addition, if a section of cortex is moved to a different part of the brain, the transplanted part adapts structurally and functionally to its new location (e.g., if moved to the visual cortex, cells from the auditory cortex become responsive to visual stimuli; Johnson, 2011).

Experiences affect CNS development in one of two ways (Greenough et al., 2002). **Experience-expectant processes** are common to all members of the species and evolved as neural preparation for incorporating general information from the environment efficiently and satisfactorily. For example, all infants, regardless of whether they can hear or not, begin to babble in the middle of the first year of life. Hearing infants continue to babble, and these early sounds emerge into words. Deaf infants stop babbling. Thus, both hearing and deaf infants are prepared for language development, but without the expected experience – exposure to language – the developmental process is stalled. By contrast, **experience-dependent processes** reflect brain change unique to individual experience. The neural basis of experience-dependent processes appears to involve the active formation of new synaptic connections that are a product of experience with particular individual events and thereby contribute to individuality. An example are newborns with **cataracts**. A cataract is a clouding of the lens; overall presence of light can be perceived, but fine-patterned stimuli, like the details of a face, cannot. Detailed visual input is critical for full development of the visual cortex, and when that does not happen, as in the case with cataracts, permanent neurological damage can result (Gandhi et al., 2017).

REFLEXES

Although newborns appear helpless, they are capable of a small number of integrated and organized – if limited – **reflexes**. A general characteristic of reflexes is their all-or-nothing quality; if elicited, they occur in full-blown form. Many reflexes are biologically meaningful in that they promote survival.

Reflexes are traditionally divided into three groups. **Approach reflexes** are concerned with intake, including breathing, rooting, sucking, and swallowing. One example is **rooting**. Rooting occurs in response to stimulation around the mouth. It involves tracking, searching, and head redirection toward the source of stimulation, and it typically concludes with sucking. Rooting is of major significance to newborns because it allows them to locate and ingest food (e.g., breast milk).

The second major group of reflexes is concerned with **avoidance**. This group includes coughing, sneezing, and blinking, as well as muscle withdrawal. These reflexes keep foreign substances or stimulation away from the body. Sneezing, for example, allows newborns to expel irritants from their airways.

The third group of reflexes, categorized under the nondescript term "other," does not have obvious functions. Reflexes, such as newborns closing their fingers when something touches their palm (**palmar grasp;** Figure 3.4a) and, when the bottom of the foot is stroked, the toes fanning out (**Babinski reflex**; Figure 3.4B) were likely important at an earlier point in human history, but they continue now without obvious function. For example, the **Moro reflex** is the tendency to swing the arms wide and bring them together again in the midline (as if around the body of a caregiver). This reflex is elicited by a loud sound or when newborns suddenly lose support and allows newborns to briefly support their own weight. These reflexes are still present in many nonhuman primate newborns, helping such creatures maintain proximity to their mothers by clinging to body hair. In the **placing reflex**, a newborn held in an upright position in front of a table or other object will raise a foot to try to step onto the object or will raise an arm automatically.

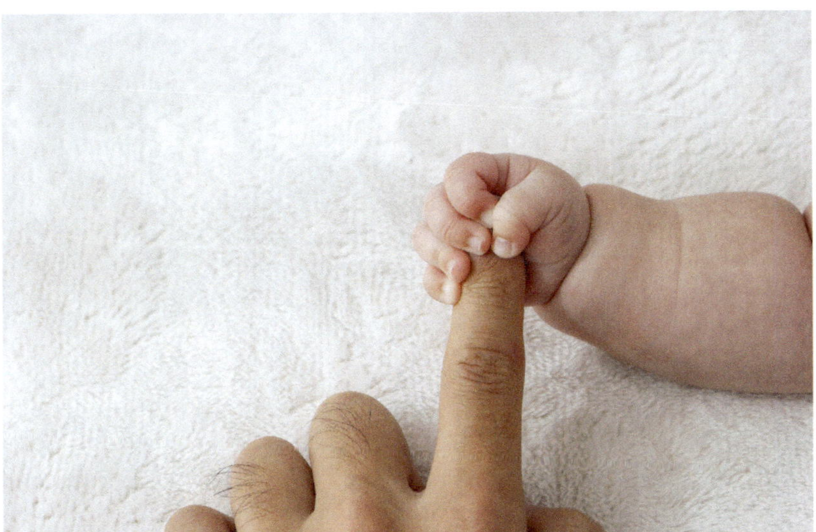

FIGURE 3.4 Several examples of newborn reflexes: (a) palmar grasp, (b) Babinski reflex, (c) Moro reflex, and (d) placing reflex (note raised leg behind the adult's arm).

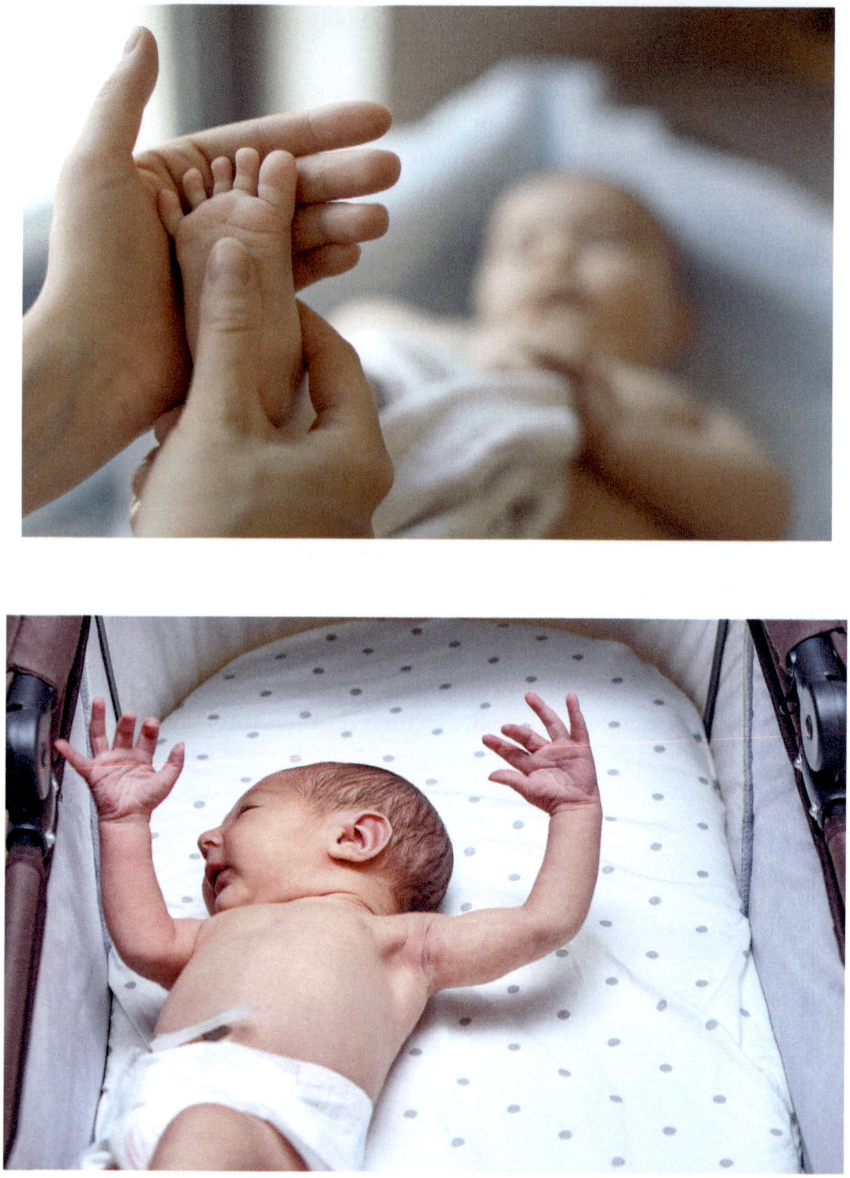

FIGURE 3.4 (Continued)

Most reflexes develop before birth and are only present for four to eight months postnatally. The regularity of reflex emergence, function, and disappearance provides pediatricians and neurologists with a means of assessing normal development. In consequence, reflexes are involved in every major neonatal examination and screening test. Figure 3.5 shows the time course of the emergence and disappearance of a variety of reflexes before and after birth.

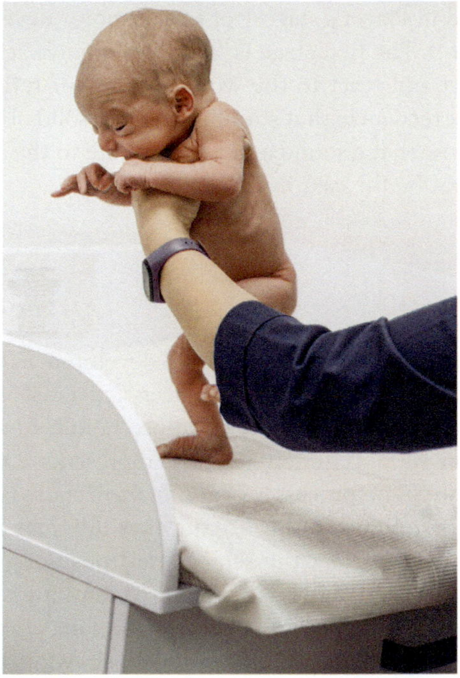

FIGURE 3.4 (Continued)

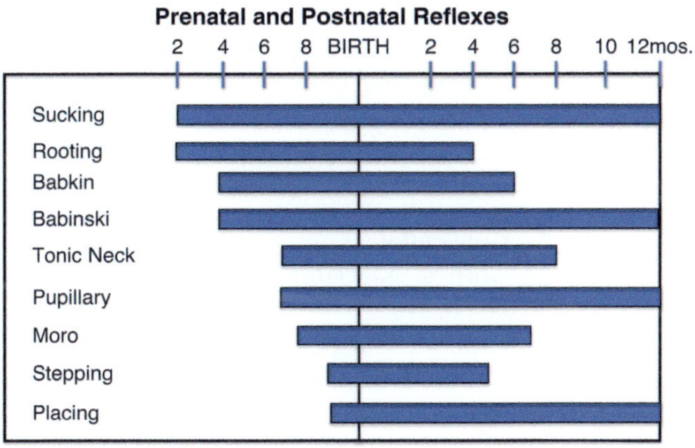

FIGURE 3.5 The appearance and disappearance of prenatal and postnatal reflexes. Some reflexes, such as sucking and rooting, appear very early in prenatal development, whereas others, such as stepping and placing, appear much later. Some reflexes, such as rooting and stepping, disappear early in postnatal development, whereas others, such as sucking and placing, persist well past the first year of life.

Source: Redrawn after Gottlieb (1971).

Reflexes are featured in Piaget's stage 1 of sensorimotor development, which we more fully discuss in Chapter 9. The first stage is "stage 1: reflexive schemes, birth to 1 month." At this stage, infants act and react to the world using their reflexes. Piaget believed that infants in stage 1 cannot recognize that stimuli belong to solid objects in the outside world. Thus, infants do not know that a sound and a sight relate to the same object (however, we will see that this may not be the case in Chapter 4).

CONCLUSIONS

Newborn nervous system, physical, and motor development reflects combinations of genetic and biological processes with experiences and environmental factors. In these domains of development, newborns show structure before function. Structures need to mature before they can support function. Birth represents a transition in a process of continuing development. Some processes begun *in utero* show continuity after this transition. Newborns in the first month of life are not that different from fetuses: Their sleep/wake cycles are similar; they prefer the same (fetal) position, with their legs folded up into their midriff (which many adults unconsciously continue to do when lying down on the side to sleep); sounds (e.g., mother's heartbeat or voice); and movements after birth (e.g., thumb-sucking) as before birth. Other processes show discontinuities in this stage of development, where bodily systems need to operate independently, new sensory experiences impinge, and there is more room to move. Most newborns arrive at term, but many today are born preterm, with varying potentialities for normal or atypical development. To gauge their health, newborns are assessed in a variety of ways soon after birth, and they are capable of a variety of revealing reflexes. Major accomplishments of the newborn stage involve healthy development of the nervous system and the brain.

KEY TERMS

Action potential
Anoxia
Apgar
Approach reflexes
Avoidance
Axon
Babinski reflex
Basal ganglia
Breech
Bronchopulmonary dysplasia
Cell body
Cerebral cortex
Cesarean section
Congenital
Cortical association areas
Dendrites
Experience-dependent processes
Experience-expectant processes
Frontal lobe
Gyri
Innate
Intraventricular hemorrhage (IVH)
Labor
Moro reflex
Myelin
Neonatal Behavioral Assessment Scale (NBAS)
Neurogenesis
Neuron
Neurotransmitters
Nucleus
Occipital lobe
Oxytocin
Palmar grasp
Parietal lobe
Placing reflex
Reflexes

Respiratory distress syndrome
Reticular formation
Retinopathy of prematurity
Rooting
Subcortical structures
Sulci
Surfactin
Synapses
Temporal lobe
Ventricles

SUGGESTED READINGS

Aral, N. (2020). *Handbook of prenatal, postnatal, and early childhood development*. Medical Information Science Reference/IGI Global.

Arterberry, M. E., & Bornstein, M. H. (2024). *Development in infancy* (6th ed.). Routledge/Taylor & Francis Group, Chapter 4.

French, T., & French, K. (2016). *Juniper: The girl who was born too soon*. Little, Brown Spark.

CHAPTER 4

Newborns

Perception and Thought

Perception and thought take place in successive stages of information processing. Our interactions with the world begin with our senses. Energy in the environment, such as light, sound, or chemical properties, impinge on and are sensed by our eyes, ears, tongue, or nose. Our brains then transform these sensations into more meaningful perceptions, such as blue, language, sweet, and peppermint. Later stages involve remembering and acting on these sensations and perceptions in even more elaborate and meaningful ways. In this chapter, we describe newborns' early perceiving and thinking capabilities.

PERCEPTION

The Five Senses

The senses begin to function before birth, and determining approximately when they begin to function is important for several reasons. First, knowing about the development of the sensory systems advances our understanding of the general relation between structure and function. Just because we have a structure does not mean it functions (e.g., newborns have legs but do not walk). Second, it is theoretically and practically important to learn how early brain development is influenced by sensory stimulation. Preterm babies can be born as many as 2 1/2 to 3 1/2 months before their expected due date, and so they are exposed to environmental stimulation from which they would normally be shielded. If sensory systems are not functional at this stage, preterm babies are protected. If specific sensory systems do function, however, preterm babies may be adversely affected by environmental stimulation, such as certain sights, sounds, smells, or invasive procedures (e.g., blood draws and feeding tubes) of the **neonatal intensive care unit** (NICU).

Two generalizations about the development of the sensory systems are well established. First, maturation within systems tends to occur peripherally (at the sense organ) before it occurs centrally (in the brain). For example, the eye differentiates structurally and reaches functional maturity before the visual cortex does (Johnson & Hannon, 2015). Second, across systems, different senses achieve structural and functional maturity at different times. Figure 4.1 shows the staggered development of three sensory systems – touching, hearing, and seeing.

Newborns are reasonably well prepared to sense and perceive the world almost as soon as extrauterine life begins. This preparedness is due to the fact that by the third trimester

DOI: 10.4324/9781003381709-5

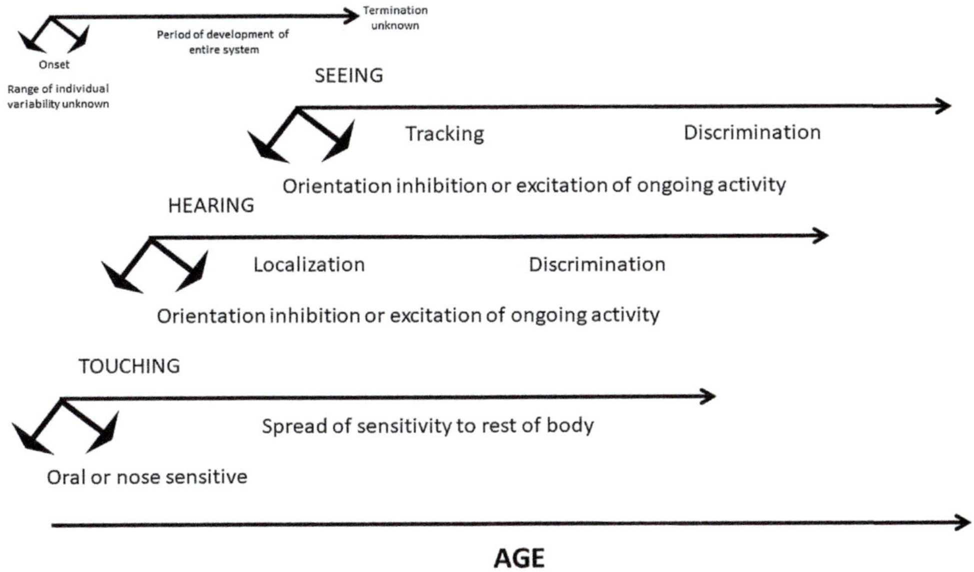

FIGURE 4.1 The order in which seeing, hearing, and touching begin to function.
Source: Redrawn after Gottlieb (1971).

of gestation, the eye and the visual system, the ear and the auditory system, the nose and the olfactory system, the tongue and the gustatory system, and the skin and the somesthetic system are essentially developed structurally, although their levels of functional competence lag behind (Johnson, 2011; Partanen & Virtala, 2017).

Attention

Much perceptual development in the early life period first depends on attention. As described in Box 4.1 on preference, what newborns orient to and look at provides a window into what they may perceive and then think about. Attention determines which information enters the brain, and as such attention is the gateway to perception, so attention is a significant mechanism by which newborns acquire knowledge about the world (Reynolds et al., 2013; Reynolds & Romano, 2016). Attention in the early life period also has social consequences (Kristen et al., 2011). Visual gaze is a basic unit of social exchange. Establishing eye-to-eye contact with newborns is rewarding to caregivers and sets in motion routines and rhythms of social interaction and play.

Newborns, infants, and children (like adults) are bombarded by sensory stimuli. An important general aspect of our functioning is that, even from birth, newborns both actively seek out and attend to information in their environment. Attention is generally associated with behavioral changes, such as orienting to a stimulus, and physiological changes, such as changes in heart rate, which can be measured. Figure 4.2 shows newborn heart rate before, during, and after paying attention to a visual image. Heart rate slows as newborns orient to the stimulus and visually inspect it (sustained attention). Heart rate begins to speed up as newborns disengage from the stimulus (pre-attention termination).

Box 4.1 *How Do We Know This?* Preference Methods

Babies do not hide their likes and dislikes, so to assess early sensitivity and capacity, researchers often record babies' expressed natural preferences. In the late 1950s, Robert Fantz argued that if babies look preferentially at one of two stimuli regardless of the spatial location of the two, their preference reveals a capacity to discriminate the two stimuli. This inference has developed into a procedure called preferential looking. It is pretty simple: Researchers show babies two displays (often images) and watch which one babies look at more. Across trials, the left and right positions of the displays change. If babies look at the same display independent of change in location, then they are showing that they prefer (and can see) that display. Although this example focuses on preferential *looking*, babies will also engage in preferential *reaching*, preferential *head turning*, and the like.

This method opened the door to hundreds of studies designed to capture the sensory and perceptual abilities of babies. However, the failure to demonstrate a preference is fundamentally ambiguous. For example, a baby might look to mother and stranger equally (showing no preference) but still be able to tell them apart and may very well prefer one to the other. As a result, researchers are cautious when interpreting the absence of a preference.

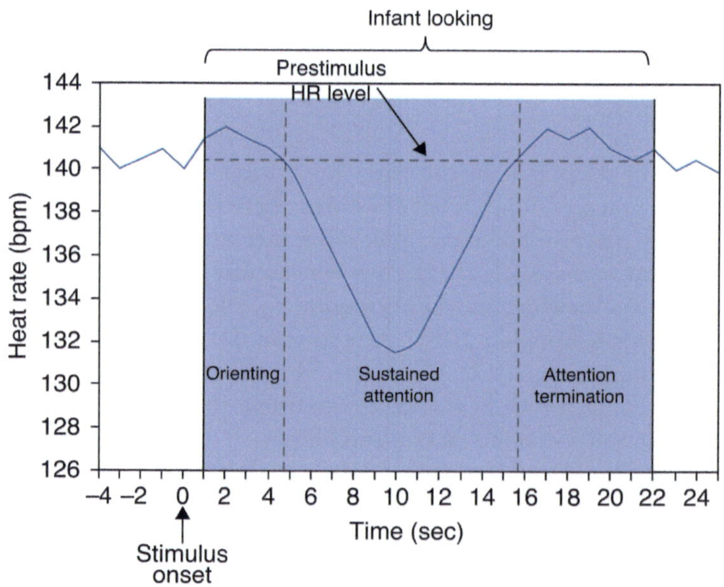

FIGURE 4.2 Heart rate (HR, in beats per minute) slows from its prestimulus resting level during sustained attention to a visual image and then speeds up after to return to its resting level.

Patterns of attention like this demonstrate that even newborns are discriminating observers. They select and, importantly, filter features of the environment and are not simply passive registrants of experience. A number of stimulus features selectively capture newborns' visual attention, including contour, contrast, and motion. An example early study showed this. Kessen and his colleagues (1970) photographed the reflection of a stimulus on the front of a newborn's eye. First, they learned that even day-old newborns actively seek visual stimulation and input, scanning the environment in a controlled and alert fashion to find things to inspect, even in the dark. Second, they learned that newborns focus most of their attention on the boundaries of figures, where the greatest amount of information is contained (e.g., along the contour of a triangle or at the vertices). Newborn looking strategies seem to guarantee that they will learn something about their visual environment.

Touching, Tasting, and Smelling

The **somesthetic system** regulates temperature, tactile, and positional information. Touch reflexes and vestibular circuitry (responsible for balance) develop early, and neuromotor organization in the brain stem and spinal cord produces fetal face and hand movements that suggest preadaptation for oral and manual grasp. In an early study, Spelt (1948) investigated tactile sensitivity *in utero* with fetuses ranging from 7 to 9 months of gestational age. He used a loud clapper to elicit fetal movement, pairing clapping with vibrotactile stimulation. After as few as 15 paired stimulations, fetuses moved regularly when the tactile stimulus was presented alone, indicating that the fetus felt the tactile stimulus and learned the pairing of the stimulus and the clapping sound. We learn from such research that newborns are well prepared to sense touch. Just consider how a soft touch or pat can soothe a distressed baby.

Newborns also discriminate among sensory qualities that signify different tastes and smells, and they even prefer certain tastes and smells to others. Taste buds form and are connected to taste nerves by about the 12th week of gestation (Mennella & Bobowski, 2015), resulting in newborns displaying characteristic facial expressions when sweet, sour, and bitter substances are placed on their tongues (Steiner, 1977; Steiner et al., 2001; see also Oster, 2005; Figure 4.3). A sweet substance evokes an expression of satisfaction, often accompanied by a slight smile and by sucking movements. A sour stimulus evokes lip pursing, often accompanied or followed by wrinkling the nose and blinking the eyes. A bitter fluid evokes an expression of dislike and disgust or rejection, often followed by spitting or even by the preparatory movements of vomiting (see Box 4.1 on adaptive responses in developmental research). These taste discriminations are organized at a primitive level of the brain, because Steiner also observed them in newborns who had no cortex. The magnitude of newborns' sweet and bitter reactions also varies with the intensity of the stimulus. The flavors of the foods that pregnant women eat are present in the amniotic fluid surrounding fetuses, and fetuses develop flavor preferences that last into childhood and adulthood (Trout & Wetzel-Effinger, 2012).

The sense of smell is less important to humans than to many other species, and this sensory modality has elicited less attention from developmental scientists than have vision or audition. Nonetheless, the olfactory system is highly developed at birth, and preferences for pleasant (e.g., bananas or chocolate) over unpleasant odors (e.g., rotten eggs) mirror

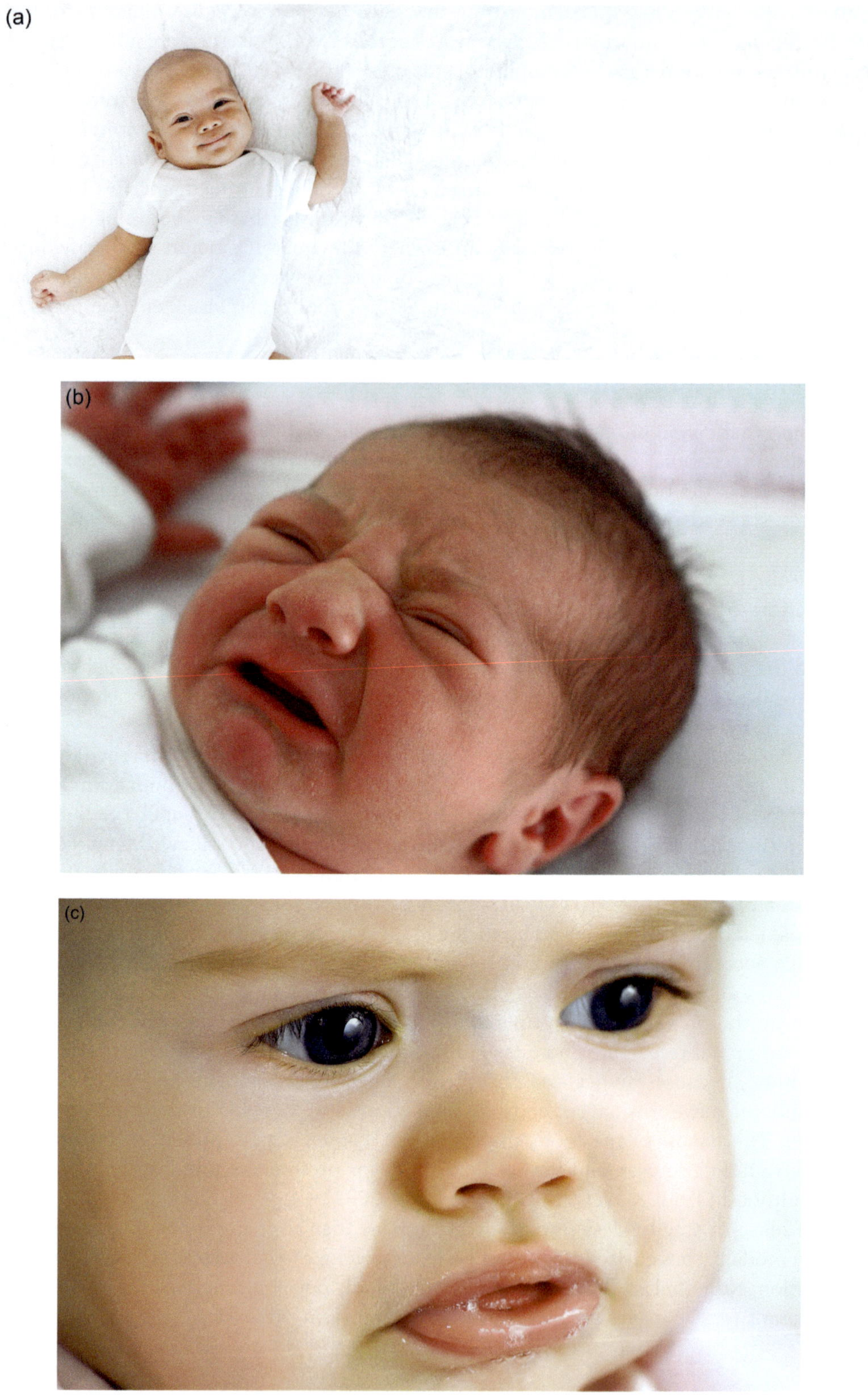

FIGURE 4.3 Newborns' facial responses to the tastes of sweet (a), sour (b), and bitter (c).

adult preferences. In early studies that paralleled his work on taste, Steiner (1977, 1979) observed newborns' facial expressions and reactions to odors placed on cotton swabs held beneath the newborns' nose. Newborns showed qualitatively different facial expressions to different food odors. Butter and banana odors elicited positive expressions; vanilla, either positive or indifferent expressions; a fishy odor, some rejection; and the odor of rotten eggs, unanimous rejection. Indeed, soon after birth, newborns discriminate among a variety of odors and use their sense of smell to associate odors to specific people or events (Goubet et al., 2002, 2007).

One odor appears to be particularly appealing to newborns and learned quickly: the scent of their mother (Marin et al., 2015). Porter (Cernoch & Porter, 1985; Porter et al., 1988) systematically compared olfactory recognition of mother, father, and stranger by breastfed and bottle-fed newborns only 12 to 18 days after birth. Newborns were exposed to pairs of gauze pads worn by these adults in the underarm area on the previous night, and newborns' duration of orienting to the pads was recorded. Only breastfeeding newborns oriented preferentially, and only to their own mother's scent, giving evidence that they discriminate their mother from other people on the basis of her unique scent. Newborns did not recognize their fathers preferentially, and bottle-fed newborns did not recognize their mothers, suggesting that breastfeeding newborns learn unique olfactory signatures. The chemical composition of breast fluids is similar to the chemical composition of amniotic fluid, and newborns may be pre-attuned to respond selectively to their mothers' unique olfactory cues (Porter & Winberg, 1999). But learning may also be involved. In naturally occurring circumstances (namely, breastfeeding) the odor is, of course, that of their mother, but newborns can learn to prefer other odors during feeding (Allam et al., 2006). Likely, the ability to recognize mothers very early in life by olfactory information alone plays an important part in early mother–newborn relationships.

Like touch, taste and smell may reach structural maturity and functional competence early in development. For these systems, however, birth is a significant event that introduces these senses to a much greater variety of stimulation. Postnatally, odor stimuli become gaseous and are carried by air rather than liquid. Touch, taste, and smell play key roles in the newborn stage, including all-important decisions about what is nourishing and what is not.

Hearing

Auditory perception provides newborns with important information about their new world. People, objects, and events make different sounds, such as speech versus cracking glass versus raindrops, so sounds provide important information about all three as well as information about where each is located in relation to the body (**auditory location**). Needless to say, auditory perception plays a central role in communication (**speech perception**) and thought.

The ear develops very early in gestation. By the end of the first month after conception, the part of the inner ear responsible for sensing sound (**cochlea**) is anatomically distinct. During the last trimester of pregnancy, fetuses can hear sounds outside of the uterus, including a mother's heartbeat, her voice, and loud sounds, such as a car horn honking. At birth, the auditory nerve is essentially mature (Johnson & Hannon, 2015), and it is an everyday observation that newborns respond to sounds. Make a sudden loud noise and newborns will startle. Newborns even respond selectively to sound frequencies that occur within the range of the human voice, setting the stage for their preferring those whose voices sound like what newborns may have heard before birth (Johnson & Hannon, 2015; Sulpizio et al., 2018).

How loud does a sound have to be for newborns to hear it? For adults, the amount of energy that defines the **auditory threshold** varies with the pitch (frequency) of the sound: Both low (below 1,000 Hz) and high (above 10,000 Hz) frequencies require more energy to register than frequencies in between. Newborns appear to hear low-pitch sounds more poorly and high-pitch sounds better than adults do. Developmental improvements with age vary with sound frequency, with infants coming close to adult levels by 6 months for high frequencies and by 10 years for other frequency ranges (Johnson & Hannon, 2015).

Newborns are prepared to perceive sounds because they already have heard sounds *in utero*, including speech. Consequently, newborns recognize sounds and spoken passages of stories which were read to them while in the womb (DeCasper & Spence, 1986). Newborns also prefer human speech over nonsense sounds (Newman & Hussain, 2006; Vouloumanos et al., 2010), and they are responsive to music (Palazzi et al., 2021).

Sensitivity to sound and the direction from which it is coming enables perceivers to find people or objects or events around them. Consider what you do when you hear a noise behind you. Most likely, you turn your head and/or body to look at it. Thus, our auditory system plays an essential role in spatial localization. Because our ears are located on either side of our head, most sounds arrive to the two ears at different times (an exception would be if the sound source were directly in front of or behind us). We use this even small difference in timing to locate the sound and thus make an appropriate eye, head, or bodily movement to learn more about its source. An early study of auditory localization involved making a clicking sound to one side of the head of a newborn who was less than 10 minutes old. When the newborn made a response (on many presentations, she did not do anything), she moved her eyes in the direction of the sound (Wertheimer, 1961).

Seeing

At birth, vision is poorer than the other sensory systems. The eye and the retina develop rapidly in the first and second trimesters, although the development of fine retinal structures and the neural pathways supporting vision continue to develop well into postnatal life (Johnson & Hannon, 2015). Of course, vision, unlike audition, for example, is limited prenatally because fetuses can hear sounds from outside the womb (from their mother's heartbeat to their father's voice to the beep of a car's horn outside the house) but have little or no visual experience. Newborns can see, but not unexpectedly, newborns' ability to see fine detail (**acuity**) is limited, and thus, newborns cannot see well most people or objects or events beyond 18 in (45 cm) away (Arterberry & Kellman, 2016). Even at distances of less than 18 in, newborns only see best regions of high contrast. As such, newborns are often described as "legally blind."

The preferential looking technique has been used to study how well newborns see fine detail (**visual acuity**). Capitalizing on the observation that newborns prefer to look at heterogeneous (e.g., striped) rather than homogeneous (e.g., solid) patterns, Fantz et al. (1962) showed them pairs of patterns, one always gray and the other black-and-white stripes that varied systematically in width. Using the preferential looking procedure (Box 4.1), the stripe width that failed to evoke a preference (longer-looking) was taken as the boundary of newborns' ability to tell stripes from solid gray. Figure 4.4 shows a newborn being tested for visual acuity, and Figure 4.5 provides a concrete idea of just how well newborns actually see compared to infants and adults. Newborns see high-contrast displays (like a black-and-white bull's-eye) better than displays made of shades of gray, and they attend more to moving targets than stationary ones (as infant Leo looked at the ceiling fan in his room).

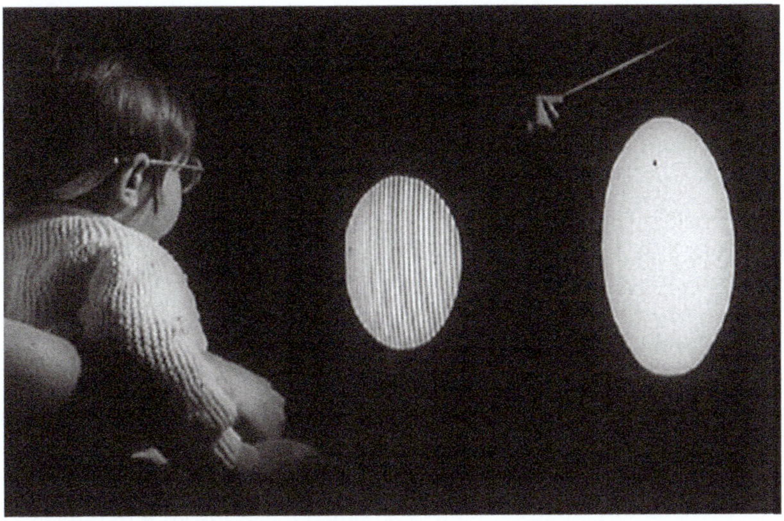

FIGURE 4.4 A preferential test of visual acuity.

Source: Courtesy of J. Atkinson and O. Braddock.

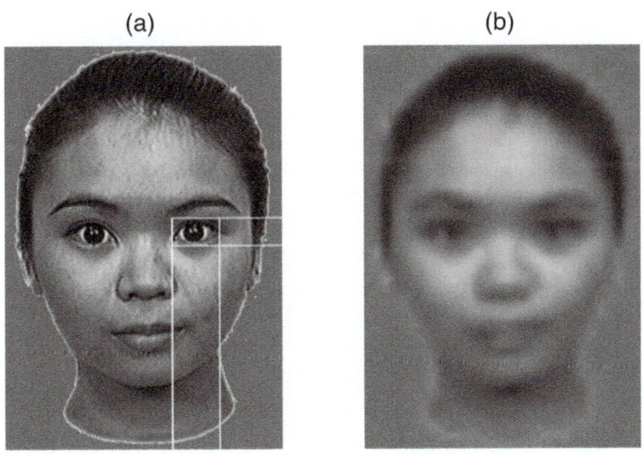

FIGURE 4.5 The face stimuli used by Farroni and colleagues (2002) in a study of newborns' perception of faces with direct and averted eye gaze. These faces show how the stimuli might appear to adults (a) and a newborn (b).

Faces appear to be special in newborn perception; this attraction is founded on an innate species-specific predisposition to attend specifically to faces mediated by brain structures present at birth (Johnson, 2025) and based on the fact that faces have visual properties, like high contrast and symmetry that attract newborns' attention (Simion & DiGiorgio, 2015). When two-dimensional stimuli in a schematic face pattern, a scrambled face pattern, and a blank stimulus (Figure 4.6) are moved slowly in an arc-like path in front of them, newborns look at and track the schematic face pattern more than the scrambled face pattern, and the scrambled face pattern more than the blank stimulus, suggesting an inborn preference for face-like stimuli (Johnson, 2025). These faces do not look much like human faces, yet newborns discriminate them and show a preference for the one that most resembles a normal face.

Visual perception does not develop in a vacuum. There is a sensitive period during which the visual system needs to experience patterned light. Taking advantage of a natural experiment (see Box 4.2), Mondloch and colleagues (2013) examined the impact of experience on the development of visual functioning by studying newborns with a dense cataract in one or both eyes. Recall that a cataract is a clouding of the lens; the overall presence of light can be perceived, but fine patterns cannot. Some newborns are treated for cataracts in the first 10 days of life by the insertion of new lenses. For others, treatment might come later, but typically within the first year. Tests of visual acuity administered within 10 minutes of initial insertion of new lenses revealed an ability common to all newborns. Remarkably, follow-up tests revealed modest but very reliable improvement in visual acuity after just 1 hour of visual input, and for infants receiving new lenses late in the first year of life, the pace of acuity improvement was fast. Yet years later, those who had cataracts in both eyes at birth showed some specific nuanced impaired perceptions (Mondloch et al., 2013). For example, these children had difficulty recognizing faces from different points of view and discriminating individual faces differing in the spacing of internal features. Yet other areas were spared: These children were able to discriminate faces based on overall external contour or a specific internal feature and to recognize eye gaze and facial emotional

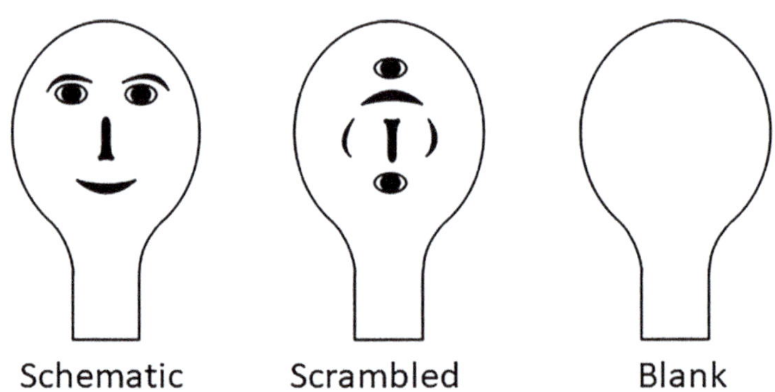

FIGURE 4.6 Examples of schematic (*left*) and scrambled (*center*) faces. The scrambled face has all the same features as the schematic face – only they are rearranged. The blank face (*right*) is a control stimulus that lacks internal features, but its shape preserves the overall outline of a head.

Source: Redrawn after Johnson et al. (1991).

expressions. The fact that some abilities are spared and others affected suggests that specific brain regions underlie these perceptions and that they are differentially impacted or there is more plasticity in some parts of the brain than other parts.

Box 4.2 *How Do We Know This?* True Versus Natural Experiments

True Experiments

Scientists from many disciplines conduct **true experiments**. In true experiments, participants are randomly assigned to treatment and control (no-treatment) groups, and efforts are made to ensure that the only difference between the groups is the treatment (or not). Thus, these experiments have a high level of control, and scientists can conclude that any differences between the groups can be attributed to the differing treatments of the groups. However, when working with humans, and especially with newborns, infants, and children, this level of control is difficult to achieve (except in interventions) and may be unethical. Moreover, not all questions can be addressed using true experiments, which is why scientists often turn to natural experiments.

Natural Experiments

Natural experiments allow scientists to ask questions that would be difficult or unethical to ask otherwise. For example, comparisons can be made between individuals who are not assigned randomly to different groups (as is the case in true experiments) but still experience different "treatments" in the course of growing up, such as deprivations of specific sorts or divergent experiences. It is obviously not possible or ethical to assign newborns, infants, and children randomly to deprived versus optimal experiences or to one or another culture, but we can learn from the fact that not all children have the same experiences or are reared in the same environments.

For example, identical (monozygotic, or MZ) twins share 100% of their genes, and fraternal (dizygotic, or DZ) twins share only 50% of their genes. MZ and DZ twins are siblings born at the same time, but some grow up in the same family in the same environment, whereas others grow up in different families in different environments. If heredity prevails, in one kind of natural experiment, MZ twins in the same family should be more alike than DZ twins in the same family in a particular structure or function. Dyslexia has a higher incidence rate in MZ twins compared to DZ twins (Erbeli et al., 2022). Another natural experiment of this ilk is to compare MZ twins reared in different families (as with the case of adoption) with MZ twins reared in the same family to determine the effect of varying experience for a presumably genetically identical structure or function (see, for example, the Minnesota Study of Twins Reared Apart; Bouchard et al., 1990). Other natural experiments compare biological and adoptive individuals being reared in the same family. Biological offspring share genes with their parents, whereas adoptive offspring do not (Rhea et al., 2013). So if some aspect of development is inherited, biological offspring should be more like their parents than adopted offspring would be like their parents.

Multimodal Perception

We have multiple perceptual systems, and we normally perceive people, objects, and events through two or more of them (**multimodal perception**). Different systems sometimes provide similar information. For example, by seeing and touching an object, we learn about its shape and texture. We see depth, and we also locate an object in space using sound. Other times, different systems provide different information. We put an object in our mouth and learn its shape, perhaps confirming what we perceived visually, but we also now gain information about its taste. Two questions arise about the origins of multimodal perception. One question pertains to the nature of multimodal perception: Are perceptions across modalities integrated at birth, or do multimodal perceptions develop over time? The second question pertains to the significance of being able to perceive multimodally: What does multimodal perception buy newborns?

Opinions differ about whether perception via different modalities is initially integrated and differentiates in development or that different modalities are initially fragmented and integrate in development. Integrationists propose that newborns' senses are unified at birth, in that newborns detect correspondences across modalities (a bright light and a loud sound are both intense, and newborns perceive only intensity), and that perceptual development consists of progressively distinguishing among sources and features of stimulation in the environment (separating out the sight and sound of intensity; Gibson, 1979). For example, Bower (1977, pp. 68–69) wrote, "A very young baby may not know whether he is hearing something or seeing something. . . . Very rapidly, [however,] newborns develop the ability to register . . . the modality of an input." In this view, newborns' earliest perceptions are not rooted in a particular modality, but rather, information is perceived as **amodal**, that is as belonging to no modality in particular. The contrasting school of thought argues that the processes involved in integrating information across modalities are complicated, that newborns are unable to integrate information from the different senses, and that the ability to coordinate input across the senses develops over the first year(s) of life through experience (Maurer et al., 2013).

Research tends to support the integrationist view: Newborns respond in a similar fashion to events that impinge on multiple sensory modalities. Newborns orient and look toward the location of a sound. As newborns attend to speaking people, they are learning about the auditory features of the language, in addition to visual features of speech, namely, the movement of the mouth (Tsang et al., 2018). Newborns also tactually recognize a textured surface seen previously when they were able to hold an object, showing some coordination between manual touch and vision at birth (Sann & Streri, 2008).

Why do newborns, who do not do much on their own, need multiple sources of information about their world? Perhaps this redundancy aids learning. The **intersensory redundancy hypothesis** (Bahrick & Lickliter, 2012) asserts the importance of multimodality for capturing attention, which then facilitates information processing, learning, and memory.

Section Summary

Newborns arrive with functioning senses. Their senses of touch, taste, and smell are well developed. Newborns also actively seek out information from the world that newly surrounds them, and they sense and prefer certain kinds of information. However, the senses come online in a staggered fashion, and vision is the least-developed sense at birth, as newborns are described as legally blind. Based on prenatal development, newborns are also prepared to perceive and acquire that information. For example, audition begins prenatally, and newborns may be especially sensitive to sounds in the frequency range of human speech because of their *in utero* experience. Each sensory system functions at birth, and newborns coordinate the senses. It is possible that newborns are not aware which sensory modality is providing which type of information, just that the person, object, or event exists and is having an impact on them.

THOUGHT

Cognition encompasses what is known, what is learned and remembered, and how information guides behavior. Given that newborns do not do much, it is hard to infer what they may be thinking or remembering. Thus, much of what we know about cognition in the early life period is based on research conducted beyond the newborn stage, with two big exceptions: **imitation** and **learning**. *Imitation* involves re-producing an observed action, and *learning* means acquiring and internalizing information.

Imitation

Can newborns imitate? Meltzoff and Moore (1977) observed 12- to 21-day-olds' responses to an adult modelling a mouth movement – tongue protrusion, mouth opening, and lip pursing. The newborns imitated the actions (Figure 4.7). To imitate, newborns needed to

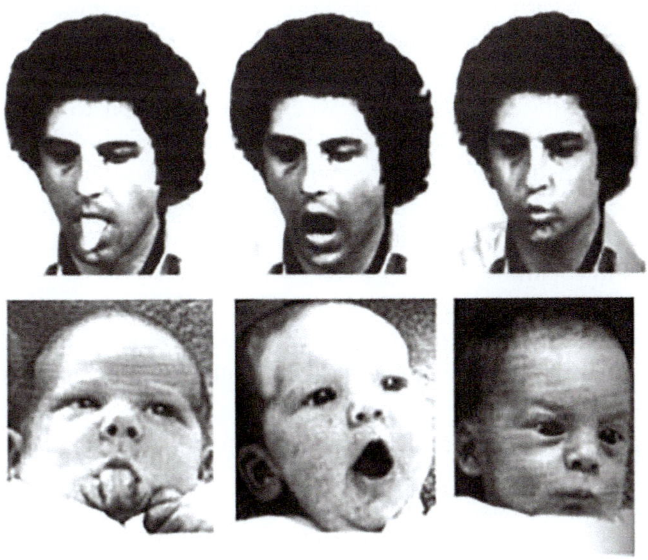

FIGURE 4.7 Two- to 3-week-olds imitating.

be able to perceive the action, know how to produce the action, and match the action they saw (the action made by the model) with one they feel (the action they are making themselves). This suite of actions was once deemed beyond the intentional abilities of newborns.

Since this study appeared, the reliability and interpretation of early imitation have proved controversial (Davis et al., 2021; Ray & Heyes, 2011). For example, Oostenbroek and colleagues (2016) tested imitation in 1-, 3-, 6-, and 9-week-olds and found no evidence of imitation before 6 weeks. It seems that for every report of newborn imitation, a failure to replicate may be found. On the basis of an extensive review of this literature, Davis and colleagues (2021) concluded that newborns *may* imitate under some conditions, but they were unable to describe precisely what those conditions are. Moreover, Davis and colleagues (2021) noted that some research groups consistently find imitation, whereas others consistently do not, suggesting that other factors may be at play. Although science is often uncertain, from our view, any valid and replicable demonstration of imitation is enough to support a claim, as newborns can imitate.

If indeed newborns imitate early in life, the next question is *how* they do it. As mentioned earlier, to imitate, newborns need to match a seen action (like someone sticking out their tongue) with a felt action (they themselves sticking out their tongue). How newborns make this correspondence could be due to the fact that neurons exist in the brain that are specialized to respond when a person observes another person making an action, typically with an object (**mirror neurons**; Del Giudice et al., 2009; Marshall & Meltzoff, 2014). The neurons in the brain that fire when a person is observing an action are the same neurons that fire when the person is actually doing the action. Mirror neurons help translate observed actions into one's own actions, and watching others' actions, as newborns would do in imitation contexts, may help tune the perception–action system to prepare newborns to make the actions themselves (Gallese & Rochat, 2013).

If newborns imitate early in life, a final question is *why* they imitate. There are several possibilities. According to Meltzoff and Marshall (2018), imitation is the starting point for newborns learning about their social worlds. As they develop, newborns can remember actions across longer time periods (e.g., 1 week), use imitation to identify people with whom they have previously interacted (are you the person who did "this" before?), and are more interested in people who imitate them, suggesting bases for bidirectional interactions. In short, newborns may come into the world prepared to interact with those around them, and their early imitative capacities set the stage for mature social interactions that have a foundation in cognition.

As newborns become infants and children, imitation becomes a powerful source for learning (observational learning). Two other types of learning that newborns engage in from the beginning of life are classical conditioning and operant conditioning.

Classical Conditioning

Classical conditioning capitalizes on the existence of stimulus–response relations built into the organism. This type of learning is often introduced with the famous example of Pavlov's dog (Clark, 2004). Dogs naturally salivate at the appearance of food, and when a sound is introduced with the appearance of food, dogs eventually salivate when they hear just the sound. In classical conditioning, the food is called the **unconditioned stimulus** (UCS, because it elicits a response, salivation, in the absence of any learning or conditioning), and the response, salivation, is the **unconditioned response** (UCR). In classical conditioning, a **conditioned stimulus** (CS), a stimulus that is initially neutral (the sound) and does not elicit the response (salivation), is paired with a UCS (sound and food together). After repeated pairings, the CS takes on properties of the UCS and elicits a **conditioned response** (CR) like the UCR, so the dog salivates when it hears the sound. This result is learning by association.

Several newborn reflexes (UCRs) lend themselves to classical conditioning, allowing newborns to make use of what they have learned. Fifer and colleagues (2010), for example, conditioned eye blink responses (CR) in newborns to a tone (CS) that was paired with an air puff (UCS) directed at the newborns' eyelid. Newborns in an experimental group, in which the tone was a reliable predictor of an air puff, made increasingly more anticipatory eye blinks than newborns in a control group, in which the tones and puffs were presented at random. The ability to learn is an important component for helping newborns adapt to their new and highly stimulating postnatal environment (Reeb-Sutherland et al., 2011). A second example of classical conditioning shows how some early associations can lead to comfort. Goubet and colleagues (2007) exposed newborns to a vanilla scent on a scarf worn by their mothers. When newborns later experienced a stressful medical procedure, they calmed when they could smell the vanilla scent during the procedure compared to newborns who had not experienced the scented scarf. Experienced newborns presumably associated the scent (CS) with their mothers (UCS), which in turn calmed them (CR). The odor of breast milk shows similar calming effects (Badiee et al., 2013).

Operant Conditioning

Operant conditioning involves associations between one's own action and the consequence of that action (Pelaez & Monlux, 2017). Actions that are rewarded (**reinforced**) are more likely to be repeated in the future, whereas actions that are discouraged (**punished**) are less likely to be repeated. The major difference between operant conditioning and classical conditioning is that, in classical conditioning, a previously neutral signal comes to elicit a response through association, whereas in operant conditioning, the probability of appearance of a naturally occurring response is increased by reinforcement and decreased by punishment that happen *after* the response.

Like classical conditioning, operant conditioning is a fundamental process of learning that is present at birth. Vouloumanos and Werker (2007) provided an example of operant conditioning in 1- to 4-day-old newborns using human speech and complex nonspeech stimuli as contingent reinforcers of sucking. The experimenters first measured newborns' baseline rates of sucking, and they then determined the average interval between newborns' spontaneous bursts of sucking. Next, they presented the newborns with the speech and nonspeech stimuli on alternate trials. Newborns could maintain the stimulus if they sucked at a rate that was 80% faster than their baseline. Most newborns in the study sucked more to hear real human speech as compared to complex nonspeech, demonstrating that speech is an effective reward. As the newborns were as young as 1 day of age, the results also suggest that newborns come into the world with a bias for listening to human speech.

Limiting Conditions on Learning

Even when necessary cognitive capacities are present and the learning task is well designed, many factors influence the course of learning in newborns. Two conditions that might limit learning are prominent. One is behavioral state. Observation learning requires that newborns be alert long enough to perceive a signal and to respond to it appropriately. Long ago, Papoušek and Bernstein (1969) demonstrated that state moderates the extent newborns could learn through conditioning. They found that learning took place most readily during periods of quiet alertness; not surprisingly, less learning took place when newborns were either drowsy or crying. The association used in learning is another limiting condition. It was once assumed that any stimulus–response association could be learned. This is not the case; rather, there are natural constraints on learning. Ethologists (Hinde & Stevenson-Hinde, 1973) and learning theorists (Seligman, 1970) have argued that certain associations are "prepared" in that they are biologically more appropriate than others and so are learned more readily. Blass and colleagues (1984) claimed that their success in classically conditioning newborns in the first days of life reflected their choice of an association between a natural mode of parent–baby communication (facial touch) and a desirable nutrient reinforcer (sugar). Certain stimuli and responses appear to go together naturally, and it is easier to learn to associate such naturally co-occurring contingencies. Finally, the fact that newborns can learn does not guarantee that they always make use of all these learning strategies in their daily life.

Section Summary

Newborns can learn in a variety of ways, including imitation or observational learning and classical and operant conditioning. These are examples of early cognitive abilities, which may also foster social connections. For learning to occur, newborns best be in a quiet, alert state.

CONCLUSIONS

Sensing, perceiving, and thinking may be rudimentary and limited in the newborn stage of development, but all seem to be present and functioning. Attention is a gateway to this cascade of information processing. All five senses – touch, taste, smell, sound, and sight – feed infant cognition separately and together. Newborns are capable of elementary and perhaps specialized kinds of cognizing, including imitation and learning, that is observational, classical, and operant conditioning.

KEY TERMS

Acuity
Amodal
Auditory location
Auditory threshold
Classical conditioning
Cochlea
Conditioned response
Conditioned stimulus
Imitation

Intersensory redundancy hypothesis
Learning
Mirror neurons
Multimodal perception
Neonatal intensive care unit
Operant conditioning
Punished
Reinforced
Somesthetic system
Speech perception
Unconditioned response
Unconditioned stimulus
Visual acuity

SUGGESTED READINGS

Arterberry, M. E., & Kellman, P. J. (2016). *Development of perception in infancy: The cradle of knowledge revisited*. Oxford University Press.

Slaughter, V. (2020). Foundations of imitation. In J. Decety (Ed.), *The social brain: A developmental perspective* (pp. 89–106). MIT Press.

CHAPTER 5

Newborns

Emotions and Temperament

Soon after birth, newborns display a range of physiological and emotional states (e.g., sometimes distressed, sometimes quiet and alert) and begin to display a temperament (e.g., some enjoy stimulating environments, others quieter ones). In this chapter, we first discuss central features of newborn emotional expressiveness and, afterward, newborn temperament. **Emotions** are immediate responses to ongoing experiences and circumstances (Niedenthal & Ric, 2017; Walle et al., 2025). Emotional development has long fascinated researchers because emotions help shape encounters with the social and inanimate worlds. People commonly react emotionally to other people, objects, and events, and parents pay careful attention to their children's expressions of emotions in order to manage, pacify, accentuate, or redirect them effectively. In contrast, **temperament** reflects stable individual differences in behavioral functioning (Rothbart, 2011). Even within the first month of life, newborns display individual differences in their activity level, predominant mood, soothability, and emotional intensity as overt characteristics of their behavioral organization, and these characteristics are markers by which parents increasingly think about and describe their children. Individual differences in these characteristics constitute temperament. Thus, newborns might show an emotional reaction of momentary fussiness owing to a change in routine or an unfamiliar person suddenly intruding on their personal space, but when fussiness constitutes a newborn's more persistent style, it is viewed as an ongoing attribute (rather than as attributable to some immediate circumstances) and thus as an aspect of temperament.

Emotions and temperament differ in other ways as well. Short-term fluctuations in emotional states are seldom thought to have long-term implications in development, but attributes of temperament are considered meaningful precisely because they are thought to be predictive, with temperament even viewed as a foundation for personality (Chen & Schmidt, 2015; Tang et al., 2020). Of course, mature personality is more than just temperament; it also includes the cumulative effects of social experience, self-referent belief systems, knowledge structures, values, and goals. Many of those processes have not developed or become consolidated in the early life period. To the extent that we can see the adult-to-be in the newborn, infant, or child, we see the personality-to-be in temperament. In a related way, the study of temperament raises questions about how peoples' enduring individuality influences their own development. As temperament affects cognition, social interaction, behavioral problems, and other domains of development, understanding temperament enlarges our understanding of the many roles temperament plays across the balance of the lifespan.

DOI: 10.4324/9781003381709-6

However different, emotions and temperament also share some common features. Facets of temperament – such as variations in predominant mood, difficulty, and proneness to fear or to smiling and laughter – often have an emotional quality. Emotions and temperament also have similar implications for adults. Parents and other caregivers devote considerable energy to identifying, adapting to, and channeling the temperaments of their offspring, just as they try to interpret, respond to, and manage their emotional states. Furthermore, emotions and temperament play critical roles in early relationships. Reading newborns', infants', or children's emotional cues enables interaction partners to engage appropriately. A sensitive parent, by definition, responds differently to a crying versus a smiling newborn, infant, or child and will become more and more adept at responding to those cues as their relationship develops. However, newborns, infants, and children differ in the extent to which they cue their interaction partners. Loud crying newborns may be just as distressed as ones who whimper and avert their eyes, making it harder for their relationship partner to respond appropriately. In addition, some newborns are more easily soothed and adaptable than others. Thus, interaction behaviors, such as bouncing, toward one newborn may not be successful toward another. Finally, parents bring their own predilections to the parent–newborn relationship. Their mental state and life circumstances affect their interactions. Despite their eagerness to be parents, depression, anxiety, and other forms of stress impact their ability to be quality interaction partners.

EMOTIONS

The study of emotions poses fundamental questions for the measurement and interpretation of children's behavior. How are emotions defined? How do we know about others' emotions? Do facial or bodily expressions, for example, reliably reflect underlying emotions? Does a smile always mean the newborn is happy? This section of the chapter considers these questions, starting with definitions of emotion from two prominent theoretical perspectives. The structural perspective emphasizes the components of emotions and emotional expressions, such as physiological and neurological reactions, whereas the function perspective emphasizes the operation and purpose of emotions, such as to communicate states like pleasure or distress to caregivers.

The Structural Perspective on Emotions

Structural perspectives define emotions in terms of their component processes. Developmental scientists focus on identifying the range of emotions individuals experience at different ages depending on their underlying physiology, cognition, and social experiences. Lewis (2015), for example, proposed that emotions have five defining components: (1) **Emotion elicitors** are internal and external events that trigger biological changes; they are thought to constitute bases of emotion. (2) **Emotion receptors** in the brain make it easy to register and encode emotion-relevant events. (3) **Emotion states** are kinds of psychophysiological activity instigated when emotional receptors are activated. (4) **Emotional expressions** include facial, gestural, and other behaviors. (5) **Emotional experiences** emerge as interpretations and evaluations of perceived emotional states and expressions.

Structural theorists also attempt to identify and distinguish primary and secondary emotions, albeit with some disagreement and overlap. Izard (2007), for example, identified six **primary emotions**, which structural theories believe are deeply rooted in human biology and are either present in newborns or quickly emerge in the early life period: interest, joy, sadness, anger, disgust, and fear. Other theorists also list distress as a primary emotion which, with maturation and experience, is believed to differentiate into sadness, disgust, fear, and anger (Lewis, 2015). **Secondary (self-conscious) emotions** emerge later in the early life period with advances in mental development. Specifically, Lewis (2015) proposed that the secondary emotions of embarrassment, pride, guilt, shame, and envy could only emerge after children developed the capacities to think about and appraise themselves.

Structural views have advanced our understanding of emotions and emotional development by describing constituent processes involved in emotional experiences. For example, facial and bodily expressions of different emotions have led to the development of revealing methodologies for studying emotions. However, structuralists have been criticized for sometimes mistakenly portraying emotions as nothing more than by-products of these other biological, perceptual, or mental processes. Conceiving, and representing, emotions solely as outcomes of other developmental achievements diminishes looking at the ways in which emotions influence biological, perceptual, mental, and social experiences (Wolfe & Bell, 2023).

The Functional Perspective on Emotions

Theories from a **functional perspective** emphasize the parts emotions play in everyday experience, with special attention paid to their purposes and roles in ongoing transactions between individuals (including newborns) and their environments (Camras, 2022; Walle & Campos, 2012). Functional definitions of emotion derive, in part, from ethological theories that emphasize the adaptive purposes of emotion in human evolution. (**Ethology** is the scientific study of animal behavior.) According to this view, emotions affect and regulate relations between individuals (including newborns) and their contexts. For example, emotional events such as crying may be directly relevant to newborns' goals or objectives (e.g., relief of discomfort), and the emotional reactions (e.g., cessation of crying or commencement of crying) will vary depending on whether those goals are achieved (e.g., diaper changed or hunger satisfied). Moreover, some events (such as sudden loud noises or bad smells) trigger emotional responses like aversion that communicate alarm to caregivers. Emotional events may also induce affective resonance, which occurs when newborns take on others' emotions (such as when newborns in the NICU start crying in response to another newborn crying, a phenomenon called **emotional contagion**; Sagi & Hoffman, 1976).

In the functional perspective, emotions regulate interpersonal behavior as individuals respond socially to the emotions they read in others and so adjust their own emotional expressions. The approach of someone who is visibly angry (with clenched fists, a flushed face, and an irate facial expression) arouses different emotions and reactions than does the approach of someone who looks joyful or fearful. Emotions organize and motivate biologically and/or psychologically adaptive reactions to people, objects, and events. Joy is expressed when individuals conclude that significant objectives or goals have been attained, and these emotional experiences tend to energize them, reinforce their activity, encourage others to maintain the pleasurable interaction, and stimulate attempts at new challenges. Anger, by contrast, occurs when individuals perceive obstacles that prevent them from attaining their goals. Anger could motivate efforts to restore progress toward achieving the goal, changing the behavior of others, and/or cause an individual to seek revenge or retaliation.

Functional views of emotion avoid many of the criticisms of structural views. By regarding emotions as central organizing features of human experience, for example, functional theorists recognize that emotions are influenced by biology, perception, and cognition but are never simply by-products of those internal processes. Emphasis on the functions and purposes of emotions, rather than their structural constituents, has also energized interest in the notion that emotional development can precipitate other developmental processes. For example, showing interest in people, objects, or events in your surroundings can prompt acquiring knowledge about those people, objects, or events. Functional theorists argue that focusing on the roles of emotion in human behavior comes closer to understanding emotion's adaptive and maladaptive influences. Functional perspectives have been criticized, however, for not making clear precisely how emotions relate to individual differences. By defining emotions in relation to goals, and by relating emotional arousal to broadly defined adaptive functions, the functional perspective on emotion generalizes across individuals.

Taken together, the structural and functional perspectives on emotions provide a foundation for considering newborn, as well as infant and child, expression of emotions. They also articulate with newborn, infant, and child temperament.

Newborn Emotions

Because emotional reactions are associated with biologically and psychologically adaptive action tendencies, it is not surprising that newborns express emotions, often in response to survival-related experiences. As shown, newborns respond to sweet tastes with positive facial expressions, and to bitter tastes with negative expressions of disgust or distaste (Figure 4.3). Although newborns may be capable of only a limited range of discrete emotional expressions (fewer than in infants and children), they are thought to be able to express about half a dozen primary or basic emotions (Dondi et al., 2007).

Distress is a primary emotion that newborns express from birth, and they almost always communicate these feelings by crying (Lewis, 2015; Figure 5.1a). When newborns first experience joy has been debated; however, newborns spontaneously smile, most often during rapid eye movement (REM) sleep (Dondi et al., 2007; Figure 5.1b). Also, the earliest elicited smiles to another person (either a voice or a face) appear toward the end of the first month of life (Lewis, 2015). Interest is another early-appearing emotion. When interested, a newborn is likely to become still and orient to best see or hear the object of interest. Movements of the eyes and forehead tend to convey a demeanor of attention and concentration. Interest may also be accompanied by physiological changes, such as heart

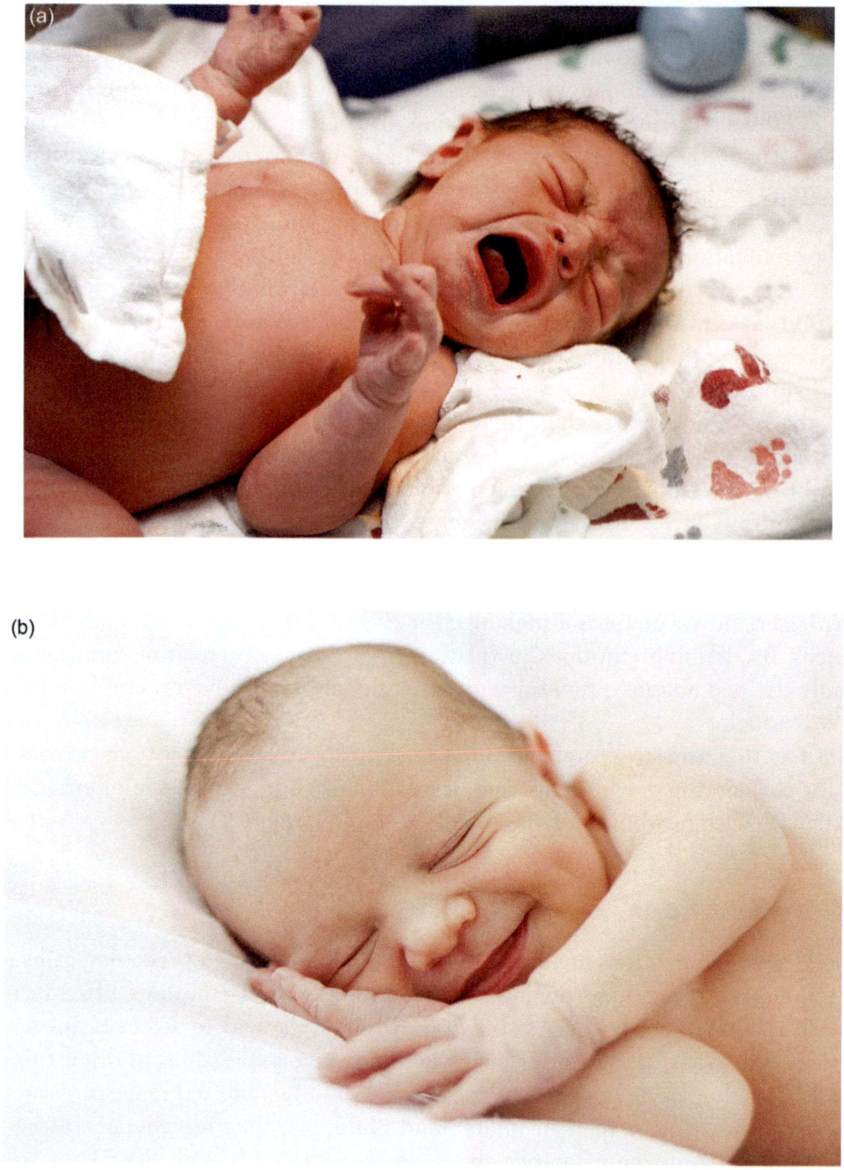

FIGURE 5.1 Newborns showing facial expressions signaling distress (a) and joy (b).

rate deceleration and increases in visual fixation, which are evolutionarily adaptive in that they function to activate orientation and behavior that help the newborn accrue critical information about the environment (Izard, 2007). For example, newborns in the first week of life show greater interest in looking at the human face than certain other visual stimuli, for example, a bull's-eye, which has clear adaptive value. Thus, newborns express at least three emotions – distress, interest, and joy.

When fear is present is unclear. Whereas infants as young as 6 weeks of age make defensive responses to stimuli that might lead to a fearful response in adults, such as the fast approach of an object, infants respond with a reflexive eye blink and not with a full-blown fearful expression. Also, infants looking over a drop-off, such as over the side of a bed, rarely display fear. Furthermore, Camras and colleagues (2007) noted that anger and fear are often interchangeable in certain contexts and that infants' expressions do not always match the level of physiological stress infants experience. Moreover, infants do not fear snakes or spiders, despite the fact that these two species have threatened humans throughout their evolutionary history (LoBue & Adolph, 2019).

Section Summary

Newborn emotional development is currently characterized by structuralist and functionalist perspectives, but shortcomings of each specific theory are balanced by the contributions each makes to explaining emotional development soon after birth – in terms of the biological heritage of the human species, learning and cognitive development, or the emotional climate of parent–newborn interaction. Each perspective helps explain small but important features of emotional development in infancy. Newborns might be capable of expressing several primary emotions, and current findings show convincingly that newborns express at least three – distress, interest, and joy.

TEMPERAMENT

Temperament emerges early in life, but temperament itself is an underlying construct and is only inferred from observable behaviors. For example, some individuals might be thought of as having an easy temperament if they were consistently sociable in interpersonal interactions: in smiling as a 2-month-old, in exploring other people as a 9-month-old, in animated exchanges as a 24-month-old, and in a range of complex social skills as a 16-year-old (Chen & Schmidt, 2015).

Temperament is characterized in terms of temporal and intensive features of individual behaviors (like the structural characteristics of emotions). **Temporal features** include the speed with which behaviors begin after stimulation (latency), how rapidly they escalate (rise time), how long they last (duration), and how slowly they go away (decay or recovery). **Intensive features** include how strongly behaviors express themselves (amplitude) and how sensitive they are to stimulation (threshold). As a concrete example, consider a procedure used to study crying in newborns (LaGasse et al., 2005). To record the cries of a newborn, a rubber band is snapped against the newborn's foot. Temporal features of the crying response would be how quickly the newborn cries after the rubber band snap and how long the cry continues after each snap. Intensive features pertain to the acoustics of the cry or properties of the snap, such as how loud or how hard the snap has to be in order to elicit a newborn's cry.

Temperament is a significant factor in how newborns, infants, and children are influenced by, and influence, their relationship partners. Scarr (1993) suggested that children evoke certain responses from others based on their attributes of temperament and that others' responses, in turn, affect children's development as in a transaction (Figure 1.5). Highly sociable newborns, infants, and children tend to elicit interest and play from adults, and that social stimulation benefits their development in many ways. Moreover, as newborns grow and develop, their temperament might lead them to prefer certain environments over others, especially settings that best suit their behavioral style.

In a different but related way, Wachs (2015) argued that newborns, infants, and children with different temperaments do not necessarily or only shape their environments but experience their environments differently depending on their temperament. Unexpected encounters with friendly but unfamiliar adults are experienced very differently by newborns who are sociable and positive in mood than by newborns who are low in adaptability and high in fear.

Newborns' primary caregivers shape the context in which newborn temperament develops. For example, in their daily interactions with their newborns, mothers can influence newborns' attentional styles and expressions of negativity (Bridgett et al., 2009, 2011). A sensitive parent might know to create a quiet environment for an easily distractible newborn to help the newborn focus. This way of thinking gives researchers rich insight into the ways individual characteristics in temperament interact with environmental demands to guide and shape developmental outcomes.

An important methodological implication of the behavioral basis of temperament is how temperament is measured. Although experimental paradigms have been developed to study temperament (Planalp et al., 2017), parent and observer reports of newborn, infant, and child behaviors are, by far, the most common (Rothbart, 2011; Box 5.1). Often, however, agreement between methods is only moderate (Bornstein et al., 1991; Spinelli et al., 2022).

Box 5.1 *How Do We Know This?* Interviews and Questionnaires

Various ways have been developed to measure temperament, including parent reports, observations of naturalistic behavior, and structured laboratory activities (Chen & Schmidt, 2015). Caregivers are likely to provide insightful reports of attributes of temperament based on their long-term and intimate experiences with their children. One parent report measure is the Infant Behavior Questionnaire – Revised (IBQ-R), developed originally by the American psychologist Mary Rothbart (Rothbart, 1981; Gartstein & Rothbart, 2003). It is widely used, valid, and reliable, and it has been translated into many languages and used across many cultures (Putnam et al., 2024). This 191-item report assesses dimensions of temperament via questions, such as "When playing quietly with one of his/her favorite toys, how often did the baby show pleasure?" (low-intensity pleasure), "How often during the last week did the baby startle to a sudden or loud noise?" (fear), and "Did the baby seem sad when the caregiver was gone for an unusually long period of time?" (sadness). Research has aimed to utilize the IBQ-R in studying temperament in newborns and infants longitudinally.

For example, Dias and colleagues (2021) used the IBQ-R to measure temperament at 2 weeks, and then at 3, 6, and 12 months. Enlisting a sample of 300 mothers, the researchers found that the IBQ-R is an effective measurement of temperament even in the first few weeks of life. Moreover, temperament measured in the IBQ-R remained stable.

That said, a concern about reliance on caregiver report measures of temperament are possible biases attributable to the reporter's subjective viewpoint, personality, or unique experiences. Perhaps mothers want their newborn to be seen in a positive light, depressed mothers may inaccurately interpret or report about their newborn, or mothers with more, as opposed to less, experience with newborns are more accurate reporters. Measurement instruments like the IBQ-R aim to overcome such biases in parent reports, for example, by asking about temperament in various situations and contexts (Gartstein & Rothbart, 2003).

The Styles Perspective on Temperament

Scientific interest in temperament has a long history. Thomas, Chess, and their colleagues stimulated interest in temperament when they began the New York Longitudinal Study (NYLS) in the 1950s (Klein, 2011). At that time, Thomas and Chess (1977) interviewed mothers extensively about their 2- to 3-month-old newborns. From those and later interviews, newborns were rated on several dimensions, including activity level, rhythmicity, attention span, and quality of mood (Table 5.1). In devising these dimensions, Thomas and Chess sought to delineate styles of newborns', infants', and children's emerging individuality (rather than what newborns, infants, and children did or why). In distinguishing temperament from motivations, abilities, or personality, Thomas and Chess viewed temperament as early emerging behavioral tendencies. In the end, Thomas and Chess settled on nine dimensions of temperament because these dimensions could be evaluated at all developmental stages and they appeared to be important dimensions of individuality that likely affect development going forward.

From their nine dimensions, Thomas and Chess then created a four-way typology of broader temperamental styles or profiles. **Easy** newborns, infants, and children were positive in mood, regular in bodily functions, and adaptable; they approached new situations positively and reacted with low or moderate intensity. Approximately 40% of the newborns, infants, and children in the NYLS were deemed easy. **Difficult** newborns, infants, and children, by contrast, were negative in mood, irregular, and slow to adapt; they withdrew from new situations and reacted with high intensity. They accounted for about 10% of the NYLS sample. **Slow-to-warm-up** newborns, infants, and children were negative in mood and took a long time to adapt; they withdrew from new situations, reacted with low to moderate intensity, and were low in activity. They constituted about 15% of the NYLS sample. The remaining newborns, infants, and children (about 35% of the NYLS sample) constituted **average** newborns, infants, and children and did not fit into the other three styles.

TABLE 5.1 Dimensions of Temperament Portrayed by Major Theorists

Thomas and Chess	*Buss and Plomin*	*Rothbart*
1 Activity level	1 Activity level	1 Negative emotionality (fear, sadness, frustration/irritability, falling reactivity)
2 Approach–withdrawal	2 Negative emotionality	2 Surgency/extraversion (approach, smiling/laughter, vocal reactivity, activity level, high-intensity pleasure, perceptual sensitivity)
3 Adaptability	3 Sociability	3 Orienting/regulation (low-intensity pleasure, cuddliness, duration of orienting, soothability)
4 Quality of mood		
5 Attention span and persistence		
6 Distractibility		
7 Rhythmicity (regularity)		
8 Intensity of reaction		
9 Threshold of responsiveness		

The Behavior Genetics Perspective on Temperament

Buss and Plomin (1984) approached the study of temperament from a behavioral genetics perspective. In other words, they viewed temperament as a set of inherited personality traits that appear early in postnatal life. Their conceptualization of temperament differs from Thomas and Chess's stylistic one in at least four ways. First, they did not seek to distinguish temperament from personality but instead regarded temperament as an early core of personality. As a result, Buss and Plomin included motivation and other characteristics in defining temperament that Thomas and Chess excluded from their definition. Second, Buss and Plomin viewed temperament as having exclusively genetic origins. This view is important because hereditary influences on behavioral style are presumed to be more stable than other influences. Third, Buss and Plomin emphasized that attributes of temperament remain highly stable throughout life and thus have enduring effects on personality development. Fourth, Buss and Plomin identified three dimensions of temperament, activity level, negative emotionality, and sociability (Table 5.1). Buss and Plomin settled on these three dimensions of temperament because they appear very early in life, are strongly inherited, and are sufficiently distinct to be characterized as independent of one another.

Biological and Psychological Factors in Temperament

Rothbart (2011) advanced a third perspective and defined temperament in terms of relatively stable, primarily biologically based individual differences in reactivity and self-regulation. **Reactivity** refers to the excitability or arousability of the newborn's, infant's, or child's response systems and is measured in terms of response parameters of time and intensity. **Self-regulation** refers to processes that modulate reactivity through approach or avoidance, inhibition, or attention. Rothbart argued that individual differences in these tendencies have genetic and/or constitutional origins, and they are based on specifiable neurophysiological, endocrinological, and behavioral processes.

Rothbart and her colleagues used reactivity and self-regulation to define three broad dimensions of temperament: negative emotionality, surgency/extraversion, and orienting/regulation (Table 5.1). These dimensions overlap in some ways with those of Thomas and Chess and Buss and Plomin, but they have some independent features as well. For example, Rothbart included individual differences in frustration and fear that resemble Buss and Plomin's emotionality dimension, but she also included positive emotionality, such as smiling and laughter, in her construction of temperament. Rothbart also viewed personality as a much broader construct than temperament, with temperament perhaps as the biological foundation.

Furthermore, Rothbart's conceptualization of temperament emphasized development. Temperament can be modified over time, because people, objects, and events can influence the expression and development of temperament and because temperament's biological response systems grow and mature. For example, with neuro-cortical maturation, such as the development of connections among brain regions, newborns gradually develop self-control over their reactivity in ways that affect the self-regulatory features of their temperament (Gao et al., 2009).

Benefits of the Multiple Perspectives on Temperament

It is clear from this discussion (and from an inspection of Table 5.1) that developmental theorists have conceptualized and studied newborn, infant, and child temperament in different ways. In science, different conceptualizations of a construct lead researchers to ask different types of questions. In temperament, such questions include (1) what the longer-term outcomes of different temperament characteristics are for later psychological health (taking a clinical perspective), (2) how experiences and genetics interact (taking a behavior genetics perspective), and (3) what other developments shape temperament (taking a biological and psychological perspective). As a result, much has been learned about temperament in newborns, infants, and children and its longer-term implications. For example, Thomas and Chess followed their sample at regular intervals into young adulthood to try to understand the temperamental origins of later behavioral disorders. Their findings suggest that early individuality of temperament can have long-term consequences, but it does not always determine later development. Individual adjustment is affected by the match between attributes of temperament and environmental demands (called **goodness of fit**), and as they mature, people may choose environmental circumstances that match their inherited behavioral characteristics (referred to as **niche picking**). For example, sociable people tend to make their environments more interactive; active people tend naturally to quicken the tempo of their lives.

In Rothbart's scheme, temperament also articulates with emotions. The growth of emotional responsiveness has implications for emotion-based dimensions of temperament, like smiling and laughter, distress to limitations (e.g., being told "no"), and fear. Partly for these reasons, Rothbart concluded that, although dimensions of temperament are more likely to be stable over time than are other aspects of behavioral individuality, stability is more likely within (such as within the first three years), rather than between (such as between the first three years and adolescence), periods of developmental change. In other words, stability is a contingent, rather than an absolute, feature of temperament that depends on environmental demands and on intrinsic maturational processes. Empirical investigation has confirmed that stability of temperament is indeed moderated by individual and maternal characteristics, such as age, gender, birth order, term status, and socioeconomic status (Bornstein et al., 2015, 2019a; Spinelli et al., 2022).

Section Summary

Temperament is defined by reciprocal influences of biology and environment. Contrary to simplistic views that good features of temperament lead to optimal developmental outcomes and bad features predict later behavioral problems, it appears that the outcomes of particular temperamental styles depend on several factors. These factors include biological endowment, demands of the environment, the sensitivity and adaptability of social partners, and the ways in which temperament itself guides individual choices of activities and interpretations of experiences.

CONCLUSIONS

Emotions are generally transient, whereas temperament is thought to be both stable and predictive of future personality. The structural perspective on emotions emphasizes component features of expressions that portray emotions. The functional perspective focuses on the purposes of emotions, including goals for signaling emotions. Both perspectives help explain emotions, including their development and their purpose. In some ways, emotions are independent of temperament; in other ways, emotions articulate with temperament. Emotions are labile, and temperament can change over time (function), as underlying biological response systems grow and mature (structure). A change in temperament may be explained by interactions between biology (nature) and experience (nurture). For example, newborn temperament may be modified by parenting. Yet the same type of events can elicit the same emotions, and temperament is generally stable across development.

KEY TERMS

Average temperament
Difficult temperament
Easy temperament
Emotions
Emotion elicitors
Emotional experiences
Emotional expressions
Emotional contagion
Emotion receptors
Ethology
Functional perspective
Goodness of fit
Intensive features
Niche picking
Primary emotions
Reactivity
Secondary (self-conscious) emotions
Self-regulation
Slow-to-warm-up temperament
Structural perspective
Temperament
Temporal features

SUGGESTED READINGS

Barrett, K. C., & Campos, J. J. (1987). Perspectives on emotional development II: A functionalist approach to emotions. In J. D. Osofsky (Ed.), *Handbook of infant development* (2nd ed., pp. 555–578). Wiley.

Dunbar, A. S., Leerkes, E. M., Coard, S. I., Supple, A. J., & Calkins, S. (2017). An integrative conceptual model of parental racial/ethnic and emotion socialization and links to children's social-emotional development among African American parents. *Child Development Perspectives, 11*(1), 16–22.

Morales, S., & Fox, N. A. (2019). A neuroscience perspective on emotional development. In V. LoBue, K. Pérez-Edgar, & K. A. Buss (Eds.), *Handbook of emotional development* (pp. 57–81). Springer.

Rothbart, M. K., & Bates, J. E. (2006). Temperament. In W. Damon, R. Lerner, & N. Eisenberg (Eds.), *Handbook of child psychology, Vol. 3. Social, emotional, and personality development* (6th ed., pp. 99–166). Wiley.

CHAPTER 6

Newborns

Communication and Relationships

Newborns emerge into a social world. Starting from the first day of life, they are part of a network of people and have relationships with them that vary in quality and strength. For their part, new parents are eager to meet their little one, having imagined what their newborn will be like during pregnancy, what it will feel like to be a parent, and how their everyday lives will change. From moments after birth, newborns also participate actively in relationship building. They display emotions to others that communicate social interactions: A crying newborn seeks and engages a comforting partner, and a quiet, alert newborn signals readiness to interact. Newborns have interactive preferences stemming from their differences in temperament. Thus, emotions and temperament play roles in early communication and relationships.

COMMUNICATION

Communication consists of both comprehension and production. The beginning of communication is listening to language and attending to its features. By listening to language, newborns start to figure out which sounds are present in their language and how those sounds go together. The meaningful sounds which are building blocks of language are called **phonemes**. Each language is built on a subset of all possible sounds, and each language has rules for which sounds go together. For example, in English, the sounds "*n*" and "*k*" can occur together in a syllable, but only at the end of a word (*sink*), and only in that order ("*sikn*" or "*nkis*" are not possible words in English). Although rules of language are similar in many respects, there are also clear differences. For example, in Dutch, "*kn*" is a possible word onset – the Dutch word for "*knee*" (*knie*) is pronounced like the English, except that the Dutch pronounce the initial *k*. Newborns start to learn language by figuring out regularities among the sound patterns they hear. Many Asian languages have tones, which serve the same purpose – sounds to mark different meanings.

Newborns also need to figure out which elements of the continuous speech stream are words (**segmentation problem**). When we talk, we tend to run words together without pausing between words or otherwise indicating word boundaries. Reflect on a time when you heard someone speaking a language you did not know, like a non-dubbed foreign-language movie. You heard a continuous stream of sounds, and likely it was difficult to pick out the individual syllables or words. Newborns have a similar experience,

DOI: 10.4324/9781003381709-7

but with time they figure out ways to divide or segment the speech stream based on which sounds are allowed to follow or proceed each other. In addition to knowing which sound patterns are allowed, such as how "*nk*" can only appear at the end of words, word stress may also help newborns solve the segmentation problem. For example, in English, stressed syllables tend to be the first syllable in a word. Spontaneously grouping syllables that have this kind of statistical consistency could help newborns find words and, thus, facilitate word learning (Saffran, 2020). The road to producing real words is long and winding, but it begins early with perceiving sounds.

Speech Perception

Meaningful phonemes are distinguished along a dimension called **voicing**. Voiced sounds, like /b/ (pronounced "ba"), /k/, and /d/, are released at the same time or within approximately 30 milliseconds of the onset of vocal cord vibrations. That is, they have a voice onset time (VOT) of under 30 ms from when the sound is released. In case of voiceless sounds, such as /p/ (pronounced "pa"), /g/, and /t/, VOT is greater than 30 ms. Only voicing distinguishes several pairs of sounds, for example, /b/ and /p/, /k/ and /g/, and /d/ and /t/. Different people may produce these sounds in slightly different ways, yet adults rarely misidentify them because adults perceive differences in voicing more or less categorically. **Categorical perception** involves the propensity to treat as similar otherwise discriminable stimuli. In the example, if voicing commences any time within the first 30 ms, it is perceived as /b/. But as voicing crosses the 30 ms threshold, it is perceived as /p/.

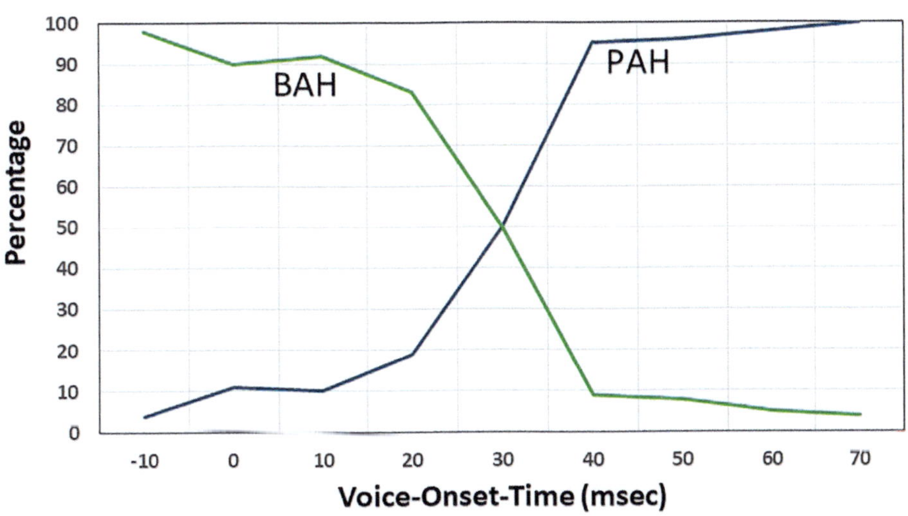

FIGURE 6.1 Percentage of responses as PAH versus BAH by adults as voice onset time (VOT) changes. The point at which the lines cross shows a sharp boundary between PAH and BAH even though the VOT varies continuously.

Many people have assumed that phenomena so consistent and significant as the categorical perception of speech sounds might have a biological foundation. An early test of this assumption was conducted by Eimas and colleagues (1971), who asked whether newborns perceive voicing categorically. Using an apparatus in which newborns' sucking above a certain rate turned on a sound, these investigators presented newborns with a voiced phoneme (/b/) until they habituated to it (see Box 6.1 to learn more about the habituation paradigm). Afterward, newborns were divided into three groups: One group heard a voiceless phoneme (/p/), a second group heard a physically different voiced phoneme from the same category (/b'/), and a third group continued to hear the habituation stimulus (/b/). The two new test stimuli (/p/ and /b'/) were equally different from the habituation stimulus (/b/) in terms of their relative onset times, but the two differed unequally in psychological terms (because adults categorize the two /b/ sounds and distinguish them from /p/). Newborns behaved as though they, too, perceived these speech sounds categorically: They distinguished between /b/ and /p/, but not between /b/ and /b'/. In other words, newborns have categorized sounds as either voiced or voiceless long before they themselves used language or even had extensive postnatal experience hearing language. This experiment showed that newborns not only discriminated speech contrasts involving voicing but also did so categorically. Because the study was conducted with newborns, the results were taken as evidence that categorical perception of some sounds is innate.

Although interpreted as supporting innateness, Eimas's experiment did not rule out a role for experience. The newborns who participated in the Eimas experiment were born into monolingual English-speaking families in which the voiced–voiceless distinction is common, as in "ba-by" versus "pa-pa." As we learned earlier, fetuses can hear and have

Box 6.1 *How Do We Know This?* Habituation, Novelty Responsiveness, and Violation of Expectation

Newborns typically look at a new stimulus, but if that stimulus remains available or is presented repeatedly, newborns' attention diminishes; that is they **habituate** (the habituation phase of an experiment is represented on the left side of Figure 6.2). The inference here is that newborns become bored with the habituation stimulus over time or repetition because they remember it. After habituation, newborns can be tested with the now-familiar stimulus (the one from habituation) and a new (novel) stimulus. If in this test phase newborns recognize the familiar stimulus, they should look at it less. Similarly, if newborns discriminate the new stimulus as being different, they should look at it more. The rebound in looking is called **novelty responsiveness**, the amount newborns attend to the novel stimulus relative to the familiar stimulus following habituation (the test phase of an experiment is represented on the right side of Figure 6.2). Another measure is how much looking recovers from the end of habituation to the test (**dishabituation**). These habituation test methods are commonly used with visual, auditory, and tactile stimuli.

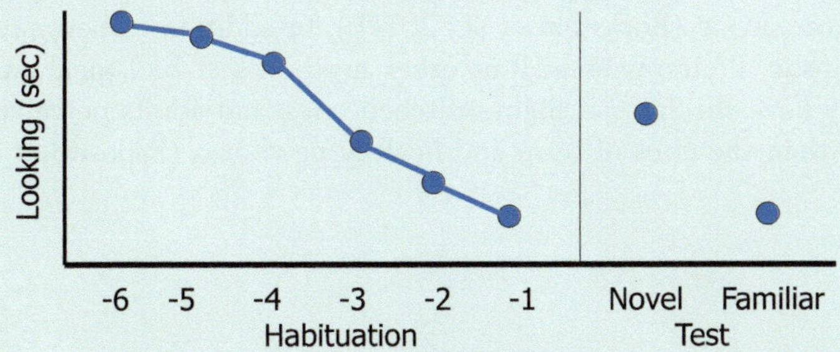

FIGURE 6.2 A schematic diagram of newborn, infant, or child looking during the habitation and test phases. The labels -6, -5, etc. indicate the trial number before the participant became bored. In the test phase, *novel* is a new stimulus and *familiar* is the same habituation stimulus, or very similar to it.

Source: Created by M. E. Arterberry.

Another procedure that relies on newborns' attention is **violation of expectation** (VOE). VOE procedures are also based on newborns looking longer to novel stimuli; however, in this case the test stimuli are events which are either expected or consistent (analogous to being familiar) or unexpected or inconsistent (analogous to being novel). Newborns in VOE studies do not necessarily need to be fully habituated. The key question is whether newborns find an unexpected test event attention-getting or not; newborns are often surprised by unexpected or inconsistent events.

Habituation, novelty responsiveness, and VOE have been used in countless research studies with newborns, infants, and children, but they are not perfect methods. For example, a habituated newborn is often temporarily unhappy due to boredom (and so may not complete the procedure). Also, just looking at a stimulus does not necessarily mean that it is perceived. Similarly, not attending more to a test stimulus does not mean that the newborn does not recognize its novelty.

experience with speech in the womb, and categorical perception could be induced or attuned even over the first days of life through postnatal experience.

Crying

Crying is a main type of verbal communication used by newborns. Different physiological states (hunger and sleepiness) are associated with different patterns of crying, and female adults, especially mothers, show different neural responses to cries versus emotionally neutral sounds (Rigo et al., 2019). Few adults can deny or disregard newborn cries; their cries compel us to respond, and in specific ways. For example, first-time mothers in 11 countries (Argentina, Belgium, Brazil, Cameroon, France, Kenya, Israel, Italy, Japan, South

Korea, and the United States) preferentially respond to their newborns' cries first by picking up and holding and by talking to their newborns, as opposed to displaying affection, distracting, or caregiving (Bornstein et al., 2017b). In addition to being communicative, cries are diagnostic. Preterms as well as other newborns at biological risk (such as for autism) usually have shriller and higher-pitched cries, and adults perceive their cries as more negative than the cries of term and healthy newborns (Esposito et al., 2013; Out et al., 2010).

Babbling

Newborns' cries inform parents and others about their state, but **babbling** is the infant's first significant non-distress communication. The development of pre-speech vocalizations emerges through a series of stages, with each stage adding a new set of vocalizations to newborns' repertoire of sounds. The first stage (0 to 2 months) is characterized mainly by vegetative sounds (sneezing and burping) which bear little resemblance to speech. In the second stage (2 to 3 months), **cooing** begins with vowels and consonants produced at the back of the mouth (e.g., /gu/, /ku/). Babbling typically accompanies excitation and motor activity. Babbling is significant because it comprises the first structured vocalizations, it sounds like fun, and it fills the eerie void between silence and crying so common in early life. Speech production develops from newborns' babbling at around 6 to 8 months of age to infants' one-word utterances at 10 to 12 months and eventually to children's two-word productions at 24 to 26 months of age.

The Russian linguist Roman Jakobson (1968) proposed the romantic view that, when they first begin to vocalize, newborns limit their articulations to a small set of contrasts. Some consonant sounds are produced primarily at the lips, called labials (/p/ and /b/); some are produced by positioning the tongue against the teeth, called dentals (/t/ and /d/); some are produced by placing the tongue at the ridge of the mouth just behind the teeth, called alveolars (/n/ and /l/); and some are sounded further back in the mouth nearer the throat, called velars (/k/ and /g/). Vowel sounds (/o/, /e/, and /a/) are articulated at roughly parallel points from the front to the back of the mouth. Jakobson argued that newborns' articulation of sounds follows a general developmental progression among consonants from the front to the back of the mouth and among vowels from the back to the front of the mouth. This means that in newborns, the earliest combinations ought to be front (labial /p/ and /m/ or dental /d/) consonants with back vowels (/a/). Thus, the highest-probability syllabic combinations in newborn speech tend to be those that connote important meanings very early in life – /pa/, /da/, and /ma/ – sounds that are used as parental kin terms in a vast majority of language communities. It appears that parents have directly adopted generic labels for themselves based on newborns' earliest vocal productions.

Section Summary

Newborns have already heard features of their language environment while *in utero*, and they soon process certain speech sounds categorically. These abilities set the stage for understanding and later producing spoken language. Crying is one main form of newborn communication; another is babbling. Both types of communication support newly developing social relationships in the family.

RELATIONSHIPS

Newborns' ability to imitate suggests that they enter the world ready to be social partners and develop relationships, but their overall repertoire of actions is limited. Newborns also have a small range of emotional expressions, and their main means of communication are crying and babbling. Because newborns vary in the extents to which they are soothed and willing to engage, parents do the heavy lifting for initiating and maintaining most newborn–caregiver interactions (Lavelli & Fogel, 2013). At this stage, parenting consists of a lot of trial and error in terms of reading newborns' signals and responding appropriately. The pattern has been called "errors and repairs," and it occurs roughly every 3 to 5 seconds during newborn–parent interaction (Sparrow, 2013). Under the best of circumstances, these early interactions are difficult; under less-optimal circumstances, such as when mothers experience anxiety or depression or families are experiencing other challenges, such as food or housing insecurity, parents can feel overwhelmed or defeated (see Box 6.2; Nath et al., 2019).

Box 6.2 *Application:* Helping Mothers With Postpartum Depression

Postpartum depression (PPD) affects approximately one in eight mothers (Centers for Disease Control, 2024). Many new mothers experience "baby blues" postpartum but tend to recover relatively quickly. In the case of PPD, however, symptoms tend to last much longer, severely impacting new mothers' relationship with their newborns and infants and their overall functioning. PPD most commonly occurs within 6 weeks after childbirth and can last many months or longer if left untreated (Mayo Clinic, 2022). According to Beck (2006), up to half of PPD in new mothers goes undiagnosed because some new mothers may be unwilling to reveal their feelings even to close family members, and some new mothers fail to receive a PPD diagnosis due to lack of attention to the issue by health-care providers. Despite the high prevalence of PPD, one study reported that 20% of mothers were not asked about depression by health-care providers during the prenatal period, and 12.5% were not asked about depression postpartum (Bauman et al., 2020).

PPD can negatively impact mothers' well-being, newborns' affect, as well as the mother–newborn relationship (Righetti-Veltema et al., 2002). Mothers experience feelings of loneliness and tiredness, even exhaustion; newborns present more functional disorders, such as eating and sleeping difficulties; and the mother–newborn relationship is characterized by less vocal and visual communications, less touching, and less smiling. Postpartum depression has been associated with decreases in the likelihood of exclusive breastfeeding, which both the American Academy of Pediatrics and the World Health Organization recommend for the first 6 months of life (Hasselmann et al., 2008; Silva et al., 2017; Slomian et al., 2019).

PPD in new mothers might affect multiple facets of development because of the strain PPD puts on the mother–newborn relationship. To address this issue, research has been done on interventions to mitigate the effects of PPD on both mothers and newborns. Therapy treatments, specifically cognitive behavioral therapy (CBT), help significantly reduce the symptoms of PPD and help improve mother–newborn relationships. One intervention, called "HUGS," targeted two key elements of this relationship: (1) maternal skills in communication, responsiveness, and observation and (2) distorted maternal internal representations of their newborn, such as having unrealistic expectations or attributing malevolent intents to the newborn. Thus, this brief intervention resulted in a greater positive effect on mother–newborn bonding compared to mothers who only received CBT treatment (Holt et al., 2021). This relationship-focused treatment, in combination with CBT, may be effective in mitigating the effects of PPD.

Despite the availability of effective interventions to treat PPD, many of those who struggle with it do not reach out for help due to stigma about mental illness. Unfortunately, PPD is not something that goes away on its own; treatment is often necessary to mitigate symptoms. Destigmatization of PPD, both socially and in the medical profession, is necessary for new mothers and their newborns to receive the help they need.

Feeding is an important context for early interactions. Newborns are held close to the parents' body, allowing for physical contact, and newborns are within an ideal range (approximately 18 in) for viewing parents' faces. Also, feeding is rhythmic, with sucking interspersed with pauses. This context anticipates the development of **turn taking**. When newborns pause their sucking, parents move the nipple, and when parents stop moving the nipple, newborns resume sucking. In addition, social games, such as peek-a-boo, begin to teach newborns about turn taking and the way interactions can be synchronized.

Many first interactions include physical touch. Parents engage in various types of touch, including static touch (touch without movement), affectionate or nurturing touch (stroking, caressing, rubbing, massage, patting, tapping), and playful or stimulating touch (poking, prodding, tickling, lifting, clapping; Mercuri et al., 2022). Two other types of touch are skin-to-skin contact and babywearing. Skin-to-skin contact, as the term suggests, involves parent and newborn touching each other without clothing (Figure 6.3a). This type of care is sometimes called **kangaroo care** because, after joeys are born, they spend an additional 9 months in close contact with their jill in her pouch. This type of care promotes development in preterms. For example, preterms in NICUs who received extensive skin-to-skin contact enjoyed more quiet sleep than those who did not receive such contact (Scher et al., 2009). **Babywearing** involves using a cloth material or commercial baby carrier to strap the newborn to the parents' body, often against the front torso (Williams & Turner, 2020; Figure 6.3b). This type of touch is done with at least one layer of clothing

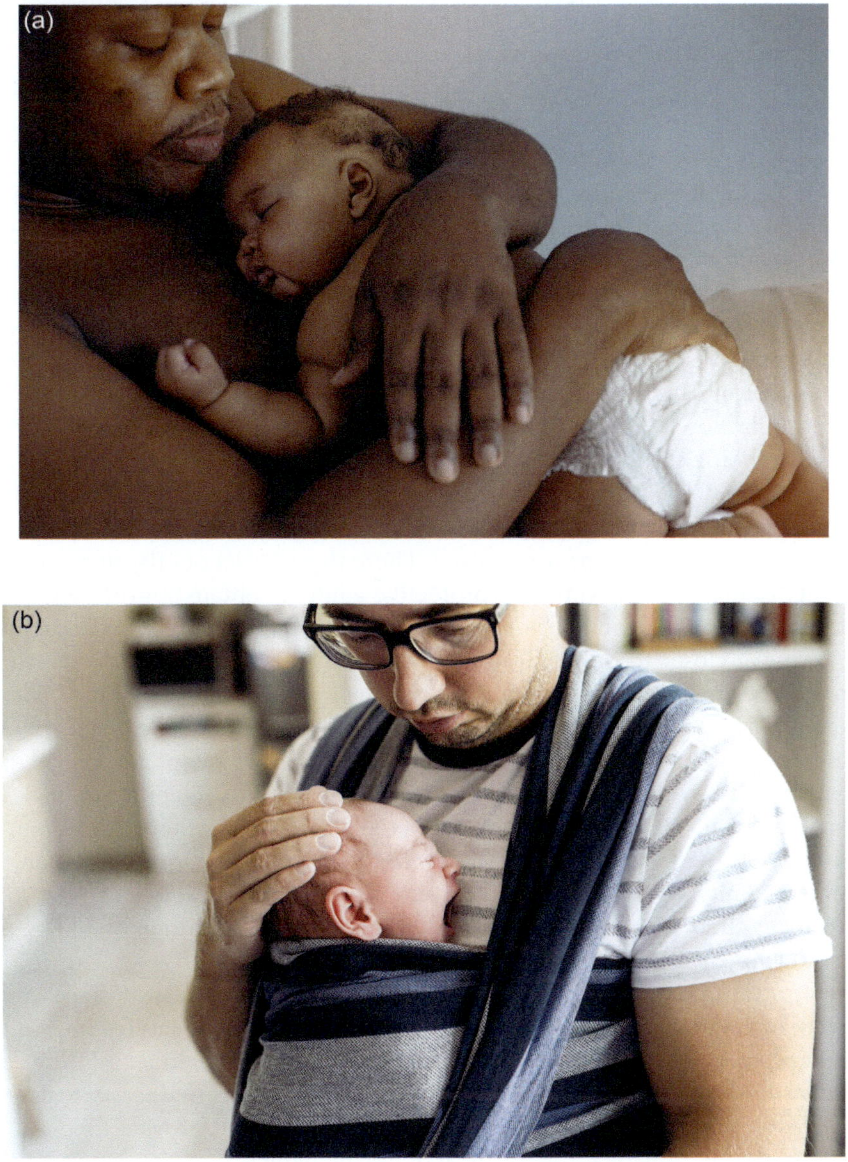

FIGURE 6.3 Two fathers engaging in newborn touch, one via skin-to-skin contact (a) and one via babywearing (b).

between the newborn and the parent, and thus (compared to skin-to-skin contact), it can be done in public spaces. The benefits of babywearing are many (Grisham et al., 2023). For example, parents and newborns can enjoy prolonged contact even though parents are engaged in other activities at the same time, because both hands are free. Moreover, parents are nearby and able to quickly respond to newborns' cues, such as signals for hunger.

Responsiveness, in turn, leads to less crying and sets the foundation for quality attachment between parents and their newborns (Williams, 2020).

Attachment

One consequence of early interactions between newborns and parents or other caregivers is the quality of their mutual attachment. **Attachments** are enduring emotional bonds that develop between offspring and their caregivers in the early life period. There are different types of attachments; one type, secure attachment, is described as optimal for healthy child development, and others, called avoidant or disorganized attachment, are nonoptimal, at least in a Western context.

The concept of attachment and how it develops was formulated by the British psychoanalyst John Bowlby (1969; Thompson et al., 2021). Bowlby was impressed by the capacity of ethological theorists to explain early emotional communications and the formation of social bonds in nonhuman species. One assumption of the ethological perspective is that the behavioral propensities of progeny and parents are best considered in the context in which the species evolved. There the survival of offspring depended on their ability to maintain proximity to protective adults to obtain nourishment, comfort, and security. Unlike the young of many other species, human newborns and infants are unable to move closer to or physically follow adults on their own for some time, and they are even incapable of clinging to adults to stay in contact. Instead, human newborns have to rely on signals of various sorts to entice adults to approach and stay near them. For these signals to be effective, adults must be predisposed to respond. A good example of such a signal is crying, which very effectively entices adults to approach, pick up, and talk to newborns to soothe them (Bornstein et al., 2017b; Esposito & Bornstein, 2019). As they grow older, infants and children develop a variety of other means to achieve and maintain proximity or contact, including independent locomotion, and they gradually come to focus their social bids on people with whom they are most familiar, thereby forming attachments.

At first, attachment researchers proposed that early social relationships developed exclusively with individuals responsible for newborns' basic care and feeding. In a study involving rhesus monkey newborns, however, Harlow and Zimmermann (1959) demonstrated that newborns formed attachments to cuddly terrycloth mother surrogates which did not provide food in preference to wire surrogates that did provide food. This study paved the way for Bowlby's theory of attachment, which emphasizes proximity and contact-seeking rather than nourishment and reduction of physical needs as a basis of attachment.

Bowlby (1969) described four phases in the development of progeny–parent attachments: (1) the newborn phase of indiscriminate social responsiveness (months 1 to 2), (2) discriminating sociability (months 2 to 7), (3) attachments (month 7 through the 2nd year), and (4) goal-corrected partnership (year 3 on). In this chapter on newborn relationships, we describe the first phase.

The first phase in attachment, **indiscriminate social responsiveness**, is marked by the development of a repertoire of signals. From the time of birth, the cry is a very effective signal at the newborn's disposal. Crying motivates adults to soothe newborns by picking them up and talking to them, and crying is the first-emerging example of a class of actions which Bowlby called **attachment behaviors**. The defining and common characteristic of these behaviors is that they ensure comfort and security by encouraging adults to approach, thus bringing offspring close to protective caregivers. Another potent attachment behavior enters the newborn's repertoire in the second month of life – smiling. Like crying, smiling is a signal that powerfully affects adult behavior. Smiles are effective because they are rewarding and encourage adults to stay nearby.

Thus, from birth newborns are capable of affecting the social environment around them, and adults respond to these behaviors and signals. A defining feature of this first phase of attachment, however, is that newborns are indiscriminate in their use of these proximity-promoting signals and in their social responsiveness. In other words, newborns are satisfied by whoever responds to their cries and smiles.

Section Summary

Early relationships are comprised of trial and error while caregivers and newborns figure out each other. Newborns try to communicate their needs, and caregivers try to determine how to meet them. *Attachments* are enduring emotional bonds that develop slowly over the first few years of life. There are four phases, the first of which is newborn indiscriminate attachment. In this stage, newborns signal their needs, often by crying, and adults attempt to meet those needs. This phase is called indiscriminate because newborns do not prefer a specific person to comfort them.

CONCLUSIONS

Newborns possess basic yet effective communication skills, such as crying and babbling. Even before birth, they hear elements of their language environment, enabling them to process certain speech sounds categorically soon after birth. These early abilities lay the foundation for understanding and producing spoken language. Crying and babbling serve as key forms of early communication, fostering social bonds within the family. Emotional attachments develop gradually over the early life period, beginning with newborns' indiscriminate attachment, so-called because newborns do not show a preference for any specific caregiver. During this stage, they signal their needs, often through crying, prompting adults to respond.

KEY TERMS

Attachment behaviors
Attachments
Babbling
Babywearing
Cooing
Dishabituation
Habituate
Indiscriminate social responsiveness
Kangaroo care
Novelty responsiveness
Segmentation problem
Turn-taking
Violation of expectation
Voicing

SUGGESTED READINGS

Grisham, L. M., Rankin, L., Maurer, J. A., Gephart, S. M., & Bell, A. F. (2023). Scoping review of biological and behavioral effects of babywearing on mothers and infants. *Journal of Obstetric, Gynecologic, and Neonatal Nursing, 52*, 191–201. https://doi.org/10.1016/j.jogn.2022.12.008

MacWhinney, B. (2015). Language development. In L. S. Liben, U. Muller, & R. M. Lerner (Eds.), *Handbook of child psychology and developmental science: Cognitive processes* (Vol. 2, 7th ed., pp. 296–338). Wiley.

Sroufe, L. A., Egeland, B., Carlson, E. A., & Collins, W. A. (2005). *The development of the person: The Minnesota study of risk and adaptation from birth to adulthood*. Guilford Press.

Werker, J. F., & Gervain, J. (2013). Speech perception in infancy: A foundation for language acquisition. In P. D. Zelazo (Ed.), *The Oxford handbook of developmental psychology, Vol. 1: Body and mind* (pp. 909–925). Oxford University Press.

CHAPTER 7

Newborns in Context

Newborns, infants, and children do not grow up in isolation but in nested environments, as captured in the bioecological systems model (Figure 1.6). Some environments are in close and constant proximity to newborns during their development (like their parents); others are increasingly distant from newborns but still influence their development (like their culture). In this chapter, we focus on some prominent contexts of newborn development and illustrate the many – some direct, others indirect – influences over newborn development.

Newborns are part of a family, but families can look very different for different newborns. In most families, parents typically play the major role in providing newborns' experiences. Parent–newborn relationships exist in broader contexts, such as the family and culture. For its part, the family shapes and is shaped by component relationships within it, as for example the relationship between the parents, and parents and family alike are shaped by the circumstances in which they live. These different contexts of development provide newborns with different experiences and thus contribute uniquely and cumulatively to development in the early life period.

FAMILIES

Whether a pregnancy is planned or not, expecting parents spend a lot of time getting ready to welcome a new person into their lives. Such planning may be instrumental in terms of creating a space for the baby, acquiring clothing and other supplies, and considering how one's life will change with the added demands of caring for a little one (see Box 7.1). Such planning is integral to forging positive relationships.

The arrival of a newborn is a monumental event for everyone in the family. At a biochemical level, hormones play a role in facilitating caregiving behavior in both mothers and fathers. For mothers, hormones activate key brain regions to increase their attraction to newborn cues, influence their affective state, and render them attentive and sensitive to their newborn's needs so that they can learn from their experiences and behave appropriately (Numan, 2006). The neuropeptide oxytocin (which stimulates labor) is also associated with cognitive, emotional, and behavioral aspects of bonding, such as empathy, closeness, and trust (Grewen et al., 2005). The effects of oxytocin are not limited to mothers: Higher levels of oxytocin are associated with sensitive paternal behaviors as well (Feldman, 2019). Fathers also show changes in testosterone levels after birth.

DOI: 10.4324/9781003381709-8

Box 7.1 *Application:* Investing in Newborns, Infants, and Children

"Baby fever" is a familiar concept, because having a baby comes with many emotional benefits. Babies bring a lot of joy, light, and excitement into a household. At the same time, babies are expensive. The Institute for Family Studies (2023) estimated that a middle-income family with a baby born in 2023 will spend roughly $310,605 for food, shelter, and other expenses necessary to rear that child through age 17 years.

Successfully rearing children also requires investment from society as a whole, including preschool programs, playgrounds, libraries, schools, and the like. However, investment in children pays dividends for families and for society. Heckman (2006, 2007, 2011), an American economist and Nobel laureate, conducted an analysis of the relative cost–benefit of early programming for pregnant mothers and young children compared to other social programs, such as increasing student–teacher ratios in schools and adult job training. His work was based on several facts of human development, including later abilities building on earlier abilities, sensitive periods in development, ongoing interactions between biology and experience, and the observation that children from lower-income families do not do as well in school, perform more poorly on achievement tests, and experience more difficulties in adulthood (joblessness, crime, and lower home ownership). Heckman found that interventions that start early and both target cognitive skill building and provide family support increase high school graduation rates, lower rates of teen pregnancy, aid in securing higher salaries, and help lower rates of use of public assistance. In terms of the return on investment, Heckman claimed that early intervention programs provided a better rate of return than programs targeting older children and adults. Whereas the investment in the newborn stage can seem daunting, it is well worth the cost for children to grow into healthy adults who benefit society.

Testosterone stimulates the development and maintenance of traits and behaviors that contribute to mating, including musculature, libido, aggressiveness, and courtship (Archer, 2006; Bribiescas, 2001). Following birth, a sign of successful mating, fathers who engage in daily newborn care have lower testosterone levels than fathers not involved in care (Gettler et al., 2011).

Families today are diverse: Some have two parents, one of each sex. Some have two parents both of the same sex. Some have only a mother or only a father (by choice or circumstance). Much of the research on families and their effects on development focuses on two-parent heterosexual couples, but research is revealing that many of the conclusions about parenting extend to same-sex couples (Ganong et al., 2015; Patterson, 2019).

Single parenting is different. There are multiple paths to single parenting, one being an unmarried woman giving birth to a newborn conceived either in a relationship or by donor insemination (Weinraub & Kaufman, 2019). Other common reasons for single parenting are divorce and the death of a partner. In the United States in 2024, there were approximately 11 million single-parent households, about 80% maintained by mothers and 20% by fathers. These households include approximately 26% of children under 18 years of age, or about 19 million children; in 1980, the percentage was 19%, and going back in 1965, 9%. To some degree, this situation reflects the social trend of fewer couples marrying. However, there is also greater social acceptance of single parenthood, and many more women are affluent and educated. As a result, more women elect to parent outside of a relationship. Single parenting is not limited to women either. Men, too, are single parents, gaining custody after a divorce or an out-of-wedlock birth, and adoption is another option to parenthood for some. Single parents can confront a number of obstacles, including financial hardship and lack of social support. Both these stressors affect all parents, but they can particularly challenge single parents (Weinraub & Kaufman, 2019).

Section Summary

Families come in all shapes and sizes, but their common main goal is to care for offspring. This responsibility is rewarding but stressful, and all members of the family need to adjust to the arrival of a new member and to one another's new responsibilities. Many families have multiple supports for caring for newborns, but some do not, especially single parents.

DIRECT EFFECTS OF PARENTING

Parenting has both direct and indirect effects on newborns', infants', and children's growth and well-being. Mothers and fathers directly influence the development of their newborns in many ways (Bornstein, 2019b). Parents contribute directly to the genetic (and epigenetic) makeup of their newborns and provide virtually all their newborns' experiences, including serving as their earliest and most immediate social partners. In the natural course of things, these two main sorts of direct influences are confounded: The parents who endow their newborns with their biology also structure their newborns' experiences. Can we disentangle heritable from experiential influences on development? Can we tell how the two mutually influence development? To study heritable and experiential direct effects, scholars have appealed to natural experiments (Box 4.2), such as twin and adoption studies, where these two effects can be disambiguated, at least to a degree.

Direct Effects – Heritability

Mothers and fathers directly contribute to the development of their newborns by passing on their genes, and scientists in the field of behavior genetics attempt to assess the separate contributions of genetics and environment to many individual characteristics, such as physical growth, intelligence, and personality. Two research paradigms – involving twins and adoptees, respectively – are commonly used in this field. Recall from Chapter 1 that twins born from the same egg and fertilized by a single sperm are **monozygotic** (identical), and they share 100% of their genetic inheritance; twins born from different eggs and fertilized by different sperm are **dizygotic** (fraternal), and they share approximately 50% of genetic inheritance, just as regular siblings do. Twin study designs involve comparing the extent to which certain traits are alike in (1) monozygotic twins reared together versus apart or (2) monozygotic versus dizygotic twins (Plomin et al., 2013; Silventoinen et al., 2019; Figure 7.1). If a trait is inherited, then identical twins, even when reared apart, should be more alike, just as identical twins should be more alike than fraternal twins. Researchers who study twins reared apart report surprising coincidences. For example, Segal noted:

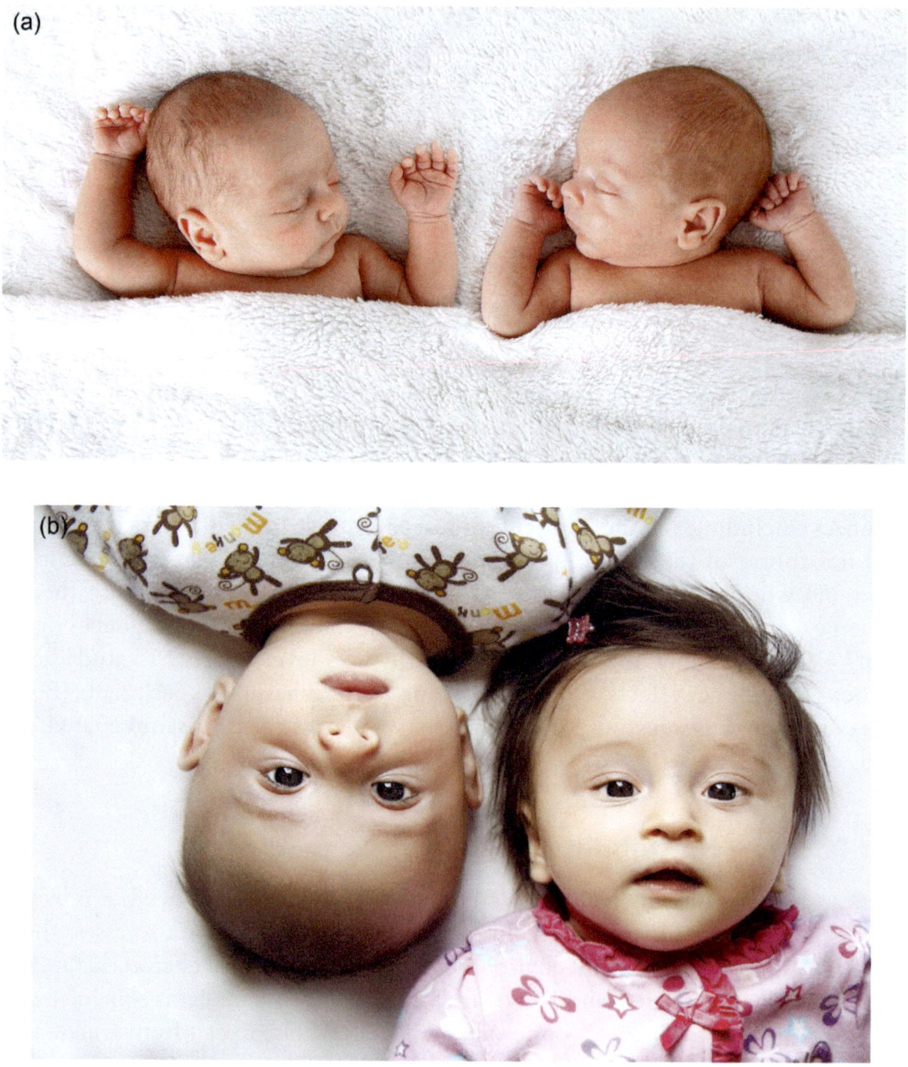

FIGURE 7.1 Monozygotic (a) and dizygotic (b) twins.

> [W]e studied these identical twins who were 32 when they met. They were both volunteer firemen, and they had similar full-time jobs: One installed chemical fire suppression systems, and the other installed burglar alarms. They both wore big belts, with big buckles and dangling keys, and always carried a knife.
>
> (Winerman, 2015)

At this juncture, we note that even twins who have identical genetics have different experiences during their 9-month gestation, and after birth they are often treated differently by parents, who wish them to be distinct individuals.

Behavior geneticists also use adoption designs to examine the degrees to which adopted newborns share traits with their adoptive versus biological parents, respectively (Leve et al., 2010; Tucker-Drob & Briley, 2014). If a trait is inherited, biological parents and their biological newborns should be more alike than adoptive parents and their adopted newborns would be.

Behavioral genetics studies support the contribution of genetic heritability for a surprising range of individual traits, but phenotypic characteristics and behavioral patterns that appear inborn and genetically pre-programmed are actually a function of complex interactions between the developing organism and the material and social environments in which the organism develops. Genes do not predetermine most development or outcomes. For example, **epigenesis**, the action of experience and environment on genetic expression, is operative across development. A simple example of epigenesis is demonstrated in the barnyard chicken's characteristic pecking at the earth for mealworms. This chicken behavior is so universal that the pecking seems innate, genetically programmed to appear shortly after hatching. Is it? Wallman (1979) housed newly hatched chicks individually inside plain white cardboard cylinders (ice cream containers) for their first few days of life. Just after they hatched, he placed white taffeta booties on half the chicks so that they could strut but could not see their claws; the rest went bare-clawed, as chickens normally do. After two days, both groups were presented with mealworms, standard chicken fare. The chicks shod in booties appeared baffled by the worms; many initially ran away, and few ate them. The chicks that had seen their claws, however, as if by instinct, immediately began pecking at the mealworms. Similar effects were seen when chickens' claws were painted black. Thus, pecking at mealworms may be instinctive for chickens; but it also depends on some kind of early visual experience, in this case chicks' seeing their claws. Visual exposure as minimal as seeing their own claws enabled the emergence of pecking behavior, which is essential to chicken survival. Because chickens are not normally reared in ice cream containers wearing taffeta booties, the key role of experience was hidden, and pecking behavior appeared to be instinctive. Consequently, even bird behaviors which superficially appear genetically hardwired actually depend on experience for their expression.

Direct Effects – Parenting Practices

Evidence for heritability does not negate or even diminish equally compelling evidence for direct (and indirect) effects of parenting on newborns. To cite an obvious example, shared genetics contributes to sibling similarity, but (as we all know) siblings are still very different, and siblings' different experiences contribute to making them distinct individuals.

Thus, even within the same family, parents (and others) create different environments for different newborns, infants, and children. This circumstance is an example of the effects of what are called nonshared environments. Developmental scientists distinguish between shared and nonshared environmental sources of experience. **Shared environments**, such as nutrition, household, and neighborhood, likely affect individuals similarly. **Nonshared environments**, which may be nonsystematic or systematic, act on individuals in the same situation or setting differently. Nonsystematic environments include accidents, illnesses, or other chance circumstances that influence one individual but not another and so contribute to individual differences. By contrast, systematic nonshared environment influences include gender differences, birth order, differential treatment by parents, and family or social factors.

Parenting is multidimensional, and so the parenting environments in which newborns grow and develop may be shared or nonshared (Bornstein et al., 2022c). **Nurturant caregiving** meets the biological, physical, and health requirements of newborns through such practices as feeding, thermoregulation, grooming, and clothing. **Physical caregiving** promotes newborns' gross and fine psychomotor balance and movement. **Social caregiving** includes visual, verbal, affective, and physical activities that engage newborns in interpersonal exchanges, express affection, and involve social play as well as regulate newborns' affect and emotions. **Didactic caregiving** consists of drawing newborns' attention to people, objects, and events in the environment as well as labelling and describing, demonstrating, and stimulating. **Material caregiving** provisions and organizes newborns' home and local environments, including the number, variety, and composition of inanimate objects available to newborns, level of ambient stimulation, limits on physical freedom, and overall physical features of newborns' experiences. **Language caregiving** constitutes verbal communications with newborns and supports all aspects of parenting and development; language is a major channel through which parents maintain contact with their newborns, interpret newborns' cues, respond to newborns, introduce newborns to experiences, and express affection to their newborns. These domains of caregiving are not mutually exclusive, and it is typical for two or more domains to occur simultaneously as, for example, when a parent reads (didactic caregiving) picture books (material caregiving) to a newborn while supporting the newborn in an upright position on their lap (physical caregiving) and wrapping their arms around the newborn (social caregiving). Specific forms of parenting at specific times shape specific aspects of newborn development in specific ways – the **specificity principle** (Bornstein, 2019b). It is also the case that newborns shape their experiences with parents just as they are shaped by those experiences, illustrating transaction (Bornstein, 2009; Sameroff, 2009, 2014; Figure 1.5).

Because mothers have traditionally assumed primary, if not exclusive, responsibility for newborn caregiving, theorists and researchers have been more concerned with mothering compared to fathering. A preponderance of research and theory has been influenced by cultural assumptions about the centrality of the mother–newborn relationship and the impact of mother-provided early experiences on later development. Yet fathers interact with and care for their newborns, infants, and children as well, and modern changes in family structure and functioning have led fathers to become more involved with their newborns. In some ways mothers and fathers engage in the same range of caregiving behaviors, but in other ways fathers' and mothers' emphases in interaction with newborns are quite distinctive (Parke & Cookston, 2019; Volling & Cabrera, 2019; Figure 7.2). In many cultures, for example, nurturant and social caregiving are dominant features of mothering, whereas didactics and material caregiving fall to fathers. Moreover, mothers and fathers spend different amounts of time with their newborns. Even in families where mothers work and at times fathers are primary caregivers, the amount of time fathers spend with their newborns is less than for mothers. Mothers and fathers hold equally positive

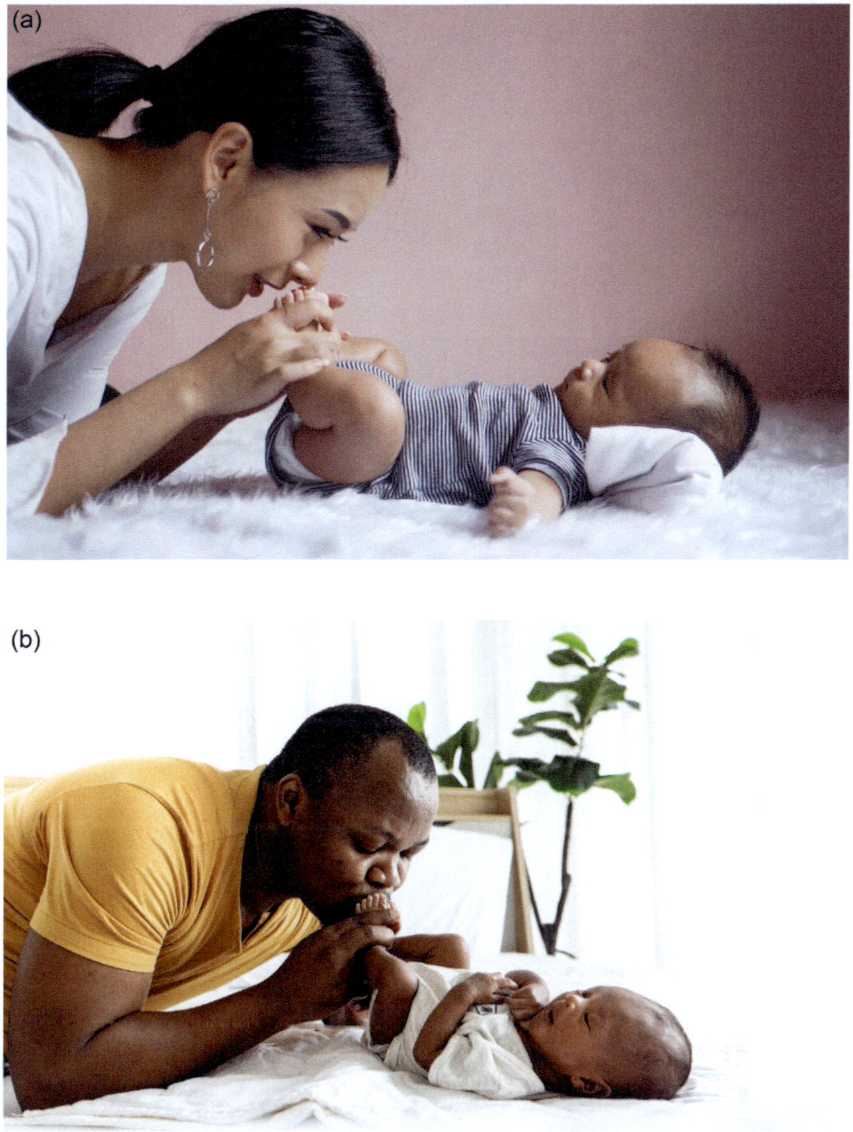

FIGURE 7.2 Similarities in mothers (a) and fathers (b) in caring for their newborns, and differences between mothers (c) and fathers (d) in play.

(c)

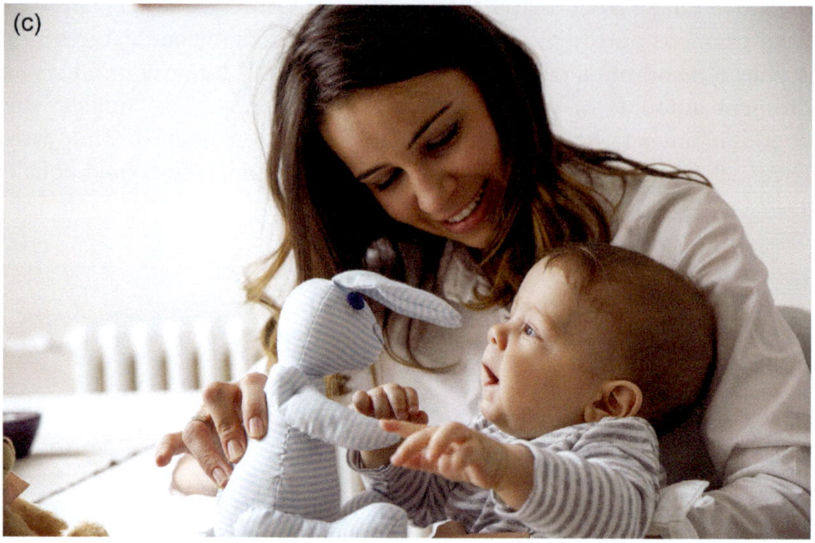

(d)

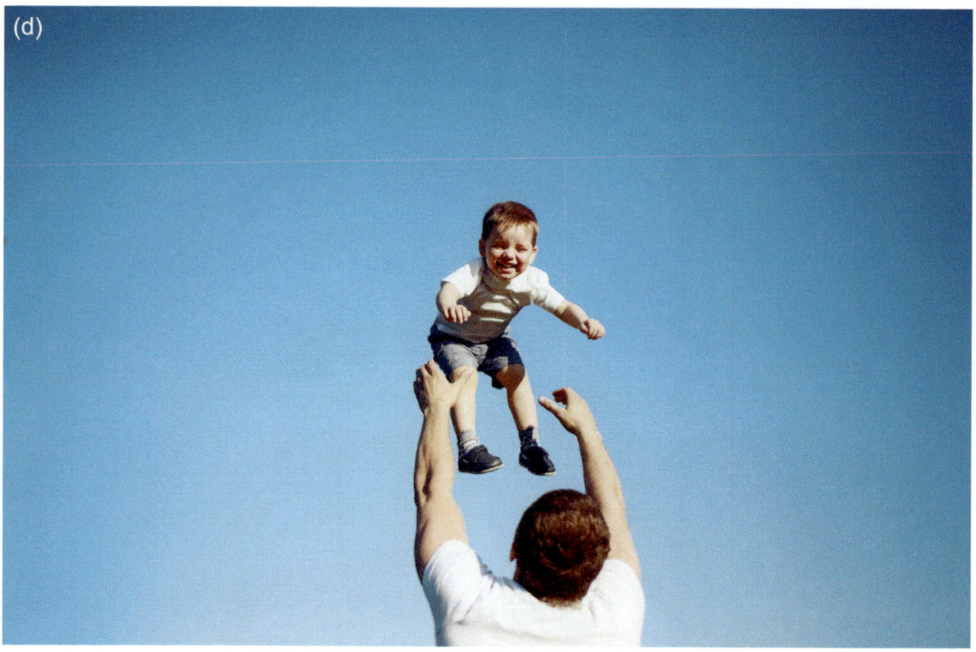

FIGURE 7.2 (Continued)

perceptions of their 3-day-old newborns; however, by a short time later at 1 month of age, mothers tend to rate their sons less positively than their daughters and fathers tend to rate their daughters less positively than their sons (Hernández-Martínez et al., 2011). By then, girls and boys have been placed in gender-distinctive contexts, like furnishing girls' and boys' rooms distinctively (MacPhee & Prendergast, 2019). Thus, parents do many gender-related things even in the newborn stage of life – well before their children could express gender-typed preferences themselves.

Section Summary

Parents' direct effects on newborns begin with their genetic endowment, but their immediate, differentiated, and nuanced direct-effect interactions with their newborns are equally determinative. To identify the relative contributions of parent-provided genes and experiences, researchers employ twin and adoption study designs. Mothers may be newborns' principal caregivers, but fathers assume many responsibilities for newborn care; and maternal and paternal care is similar in some ways but different in others. Parenting is not unidirectional; newborns also play a role in how they are parented.

PROXIMAL INDIRECT EFFECTS ON PARENTING

Newborns enter a social environment filled with people, of which parents are primary. How parents approach the responsibilities and tasks of parenting varies depending on the characteristics of their newborn, such as the newborn's sex and temperament, as well as on many characteristics of parents themselves. In this section we discuss four such indirect effects on parenting: parents' age, stress, family composition, and relationships with one another. Still other factors, distal to parents, influence parenting, such as parents' ethnicity, socioeconomic status, and culture, and they are discussed in the following section.

Age

Mothers' age impacts parenting. Caring for a newborn is physically challenging, and older first-time mothers might cope less well with its many demands. However, mothers over 35 years of age at the time of the birth of their first newborn do not systematically differ in their parenting from mothers aged 20–34 years (Guedes & Canavarro, 2015). By contrast, younger mothers, especially adolescents, generally have less knowledge about parenting, hold less-desirable child-rearing attitudes, and harbor less-realistic expectations about newborn, infant, and child development than older mothers. Moreover, younger mothers tend to be less sensitive, appropriate, and responsive to their newborns (Bornstein, Putnick, et al., 2012; Weinraub & Kaufman, 2019). Parenting differences between younger and older mothers in Western cultures could be due, in part, to differences in brain development or educational achievement or both. Adolescents who become parents have not yet completely matured in terms of their brain development (Mills et al., 2021) and associated cognitive readiness or executive functions (Korzeniowski et al., 2021; Whitman et al., 2001), and teen parenthood is often associated with having attended low-quality schools, school failure, early withdrawal from school, and diminished educational aspirations, resulting in reduced financial stability. All these factors cumulate in poorer-quality teen parenting compared to that of older mothers (Easterbrooks et al., 2019), and all contribute to more stress in child-rearing.

Stress

Stress is physical, mental, or emotional strain or tension that undermines normal physiological equilibrium. Stress can be general, or it can be specific to parenting (Crnic & Coburn, 2019). For example, stress often accompanies the transition to parenthood on account of parenting's new and varied responsibilities, and some newborn, infant, and child characteristics (such as fussiness) can incite stress. Straitened economic circumstances can also be a debilitating source of stress that undermines the quality of parents' caregiving directly, the nature of their relationship with each other, and the quality of each other's parenting. Conditions related to poverty and economic hardship are often the focus of arguments between parents that set the wrong tone and detract from each parent's ability to provide optimal newborn care. Mutual support and family composition can offset stress. For example, in a study of European American families living in the Appalachian region of West Virginia (known for high rates of rural poverty), Bornstein and Putnick (2012) found that mothers' parenting was improved by being married and having the father present in the home. In this situation, father involvement served to buffer life stresses and other difficulties common to communities where financial and other resource strains are common.

Parity and Family Composition

Being a first newborn in a family is one thing, but being the second- or much later-born in a family is another, and for parents, energy, resources, and time are all finite. Thus, later-born newborns can be expected to experience a lesser share of those parenting assets. As every second child knows, the number of their childhood photographs pales relative to the number for their older brother or sister. In other words, parity (the number of children a parent has) affects parental caregiving. An extreme example is families with multiple births. Multiple newborns of the same age present unique challenges to parents, and the situation provides a unique social context for development (Feinberg et al., 2019; Planalp et al., 2019).

Parents' Relationship With Each Other

Parenting is also a reflection of the status of parents' other relationships within the family, including with each other. Parents are more attentive and sensitive to their newborns when their coparenting relationship is warm and supportive (McHale & Sirotkin, 2019). Parents influence newborns through direct interactions with them and by parents' influences on each other. These many influences follow complex paths and networks (Kerig, 2019; McHale & Sirotkin, 2019). For example, paternal influences on newborn development may be indirectly mediated through the father's relation to or impact on the mother. In other words, even if the mother has the major direct influence on development in a traditional family (in which the mother stays at home to care for and socialize her newborn, infant, or child while the father works outside the home), the father may have important indirect influences on account of the financial resources he provides or the caregiving duties and responsibilities he assumes complementary to maternal caregiving (Parke & Cookston, 2019). Mothers can also control fathers' access to their newborns through **maternal gatekeeping**, which may minimize the influence fathers have on their newborns' development (Schoppe-Sullivan & Aytaç-DiCarlo, 2025). Maternal supportiveness has a greater effect on paternal behavior than paternal supportiveness has on maternal behavior, suggesting that fathers are more susceptible than mothers to indirect influences on their interactions with newborns (Sobelweski & King, 2005). It might be that conventional social expectations give fathers greater leeway to choose whether and how to be involved in their newborns' lives (Parke & Cookston, 2019). By contrast, mothers are expected to be committed and involved, regardless of their psychological state.

Section Summary

Numerous factors indirectly contribute to quality of parenting newborns. Prominent ones include parent age, level of stress, parity, and parents' relationship with each other, because families are a system.

DISTAL INDIRECT EFFECTS ON PARENTING

In the bioecological systems perspective presented in Chapter 1 (Figure 1.6), parents, and so parenting newborns, are embedded in multiple larger systems. We illustrate how three such contexts distal to parents – socioeconomic status, ethnicity, and culture – impinge on parenting newborns.

Socioeconomic Status

Socioeconomic status (social standing or class) is indexed by quantitative factors having to do with parents' educational achievement, financial income, and occupational prestige (Bornstein & Bradley, 2003). Socioeconomic status is known to shape parenting cognitions and practices, and differences in language used by middle-class and lower-class mothers with newborns (as well as with infants and children) are an example. Middle-class American mothers talk to their newborns in more sophisticated ways with richer vocabulary than lower-class mothers, even though newborns are far from talking themselves (Hoff & Laursen, 2019). Of course, extreme economic disadvantages affect development in ways that go well beyond maternal speech patterns, values, and expectations. When compared to newborns growing up in middle-class environments, newborns living in poverty experience lower levels of emotional and verbal responsiveness, fewer opportunities for variety in daily stimulation, fewer appropriate play materials, and more chaotic, disorganized, and unstructured environments (Maughan et al., 2018).

Upper-class cognitions and practices are often portrayed as more desirable and appropriate than those of lower class, even though the values of both upper-class and lower-class parents change over time. Maternal newborn feeding practices constitute a telling example. Bronfenbrenner (1961) observed that when the same values were held at different times by upper- and lower-class parents – say, the preference for bottle feeding or for breastfeeding – the preference was positively evaluated when held by upper-class parents and negatively evaluated when adopted by lower-class parents. Such positive and negative evaluations clearly say more about the times, researchers, and theorists than about parenting or health implications of feeding choices for newborns.

Ethnicity

Parents of newborns, even living in the same nation-state, can vary in their parenting cognitions and practices. For example, Tamis-LeMonda and Kahana-Kalman (2009) documented differences in parenting expectations among new mothers of different ethnicities in the United States within hours of the birth of their babies. New mothers were interviewed on maternity wards about how they thought things will change in life and the family now that they have a baby, about their hopes and plans for their newborn and family over the next year, and about any concerns they have right now about their child or family. Mothers' responses to these open-ended questions were coded as addressing four general categories – child development, parenting, family, and resources. African American and Dominican American mothers were most concerned about resources, and many comments pertained to rearing their children in a better environment. Chinese American mothers focused the most on child development, especially their child's future education. Mexican American mothers spoke most about family. Even from the start of their children's lives, mothers of different ethnicities hold contrasting ideas about what is important and what they want for their children.

Culture

Convention of the roles mothers and fathers play in parenting is one example of a cultural influence (Amir & Bornstein, 2025). Cultural influences over parenting cognitions and practices are pervasive and so reverberate in newborn development. First, cultures vary in the physical circumstances in which newborns may be found. Consider two newborns: One is born into a group of nomadic hunter-gatherers, living in temporary homes and spending much of each day in large multi-age groups, obtaining food (Jung & Fouts, 2011). The other is born into a modern Western culture, isolated at home with a single adult, whose food is purchased, and who comes into contact with many individuals, few of whom are seen frequently or show much interest in the newborn's welfare. Moreover, worldwide, many families have inadequate housing and other basic necessities, such as clean water and adequate sanitation, resulting in newborns' exposure to toxins, poor nutrition, illness, and shorter life expectancies (Bradley & Rothenberg, 2022). These circumstances make parenting extremely difficult, which has profound impacts on development in the early life period (Bizzego et al., 2021).

Second, cultures differ in ideology or worldview on parenting, such as where and when and with whom newborns sleep, the frequency with which newborns are cared for by other children or unrelated adults, and whether newborns' experiences are nurturing or restrictive. An example of the intersection of culture with parenting practices is deciding where newborns should sleep – alone in their own bed and/or room or co-sleeping with one or both parents. Newborns in Western industrialized countries are usually with their mothers when awake and alone when asleep. However, in many cultures around the world, newborns sleep bundled on their mothers' backs during the day and share a bed at night. In Japan, newborns are constantly within their mothers' reach, and co-sleeping and co-bathing from birth are conventional, normative, and widely practiced. Co-sleeping offers parents many benefits but may also be hazardous, and the jury is still out on the way to go. Newborn–parent co-sleeping alters newborns' sleep experience due to arousal levels, the frequency and duration of nursing, newborns' sleeping positions, and the number of maternal inspections (Barry, 2019; Marinelli et al., 2019). While co-sleeping, newborns regulate their respiration to their mothers, which may be a protective factor against sudden infant death syndrome (SIDS; McKenna & Gettler, 2016). However, in many Western cultures, a possible connection between co-sleeping and SIDS has resulted in recommendations against co-sleeping and for newborns to sleep on their backs and alone (American Academy of Pediatrics, 2024). The American Academy of Pediatrics also recommends room sharing for 6 to 12 months. Yet parent surveys show that despite recommendations not to sleep with their newborns, parents do, either intentionally or not (e.g., bringing the newborn to bed at night when they wake up for a feeding, feeding on a couch or in a chair and falling asleep with their child; Teti et al., 2016).

There's another (academic) reason the study of newborns in different cultural contexts has appealed to developmental and other scientists. When cultural groups are compared, culture and gene pool are naturally confounded, so it is difficult to determine whether observed differences in, say, temperament are due to differences in experience and environment (cultural customs, socialization, practices) or to variation in genetics and biology (ANS and CNS variation in different peoples). As a possible solution, researchers have studied structures and functions in newborns in different countries, hoping to uncover similarities or differences before much experience operates over development (Bornstein, 1989; Gartstein et al., 2015; Spinelli et al., 2022).

Section Summary

Socioeconomic status, ethnicity, and culture are prominent examples of distal indirect effects on parenting newborns and newborn development. Studying newborns across these social groups opens the opportunity to understand newborn structure, function, and development across a wide spectrum of circumstances. Parents in different social classes, ethnicities, and cultures differ in some cognitions and practices with respect to their newborns and are similar in others.

CONCLUSIONS

Newborns arrive and develop in multiple material and social ecologies, and thus we cannot understand newborn (or infant or child) development without knowing more about these several contexts and their sway over development. Families, regardless of their structure, share the primary goal of nurturing newborn offspring. While fulfilling, this role can be stressful, requiring all members to adapt to new dynamics. Families today come in many flavors, but all need substantial support systems to face and succeed at the personal and social challenges of rearing new life.

Within-family experiences may have major impacts during early life. Parents provide both direct and indirect effects on their newborns. Direct effects include their genetic endowment and how they parent. Indirect effects over parenting and newborn development include parent age, stress, parity, and the interparental relationship. Larger social and cultural contexts also shape newborn life. Family socioeconomic status, ethnicity, and culture exert direct and indirect influences on parents, parenting, and so on newborns.

KEY TERMS

Didactic caregiving
Dizygotic
Epigenesis
Language caregiving
Material caregiving
Maternal gatekeeping
Monozygotic
Nonshared environment
Nurturant caregiving
Physical caregiving
Shared environment
Social caregiving
Socioeconomic status
Specificity principle

SUGGESTED READINGS

Bornstein, M. H. (2019). Parenting infants. In M. H. Bornstein (Ed.), *Handbook of parenting: Children and parenting* (Vol. 1, 3rd ed., pp. 3–55). Routledge.

Cardenas, S. I., Morris, A. R., Marshall, N., Aviv, E. C., Marinez Garcia, M., Sellery, P., & Saxbe, D. E. (2022). Fathers matter from the start: The role of expectant fathers in child development. *Child Development Perspectives*, *16*, 54–59.

Evans, G. W., & Kim, P. (2013). Childhood poverty, chronic stress, self-regulation, and coping. *Child Development Perspectives*, *7*, 43–48.

Super, C. M., & Harkness, S. (2013). Culture and children's sleep. In A. R. Wolfson & H. E. Montgomery-Downs (Eds.), *The Oxford handbook of infant, child, and adolescent sleep and behavior* (pp. 81–98). Oxford University Press.

SECTION II

The Infant

4 Months to 17 Months

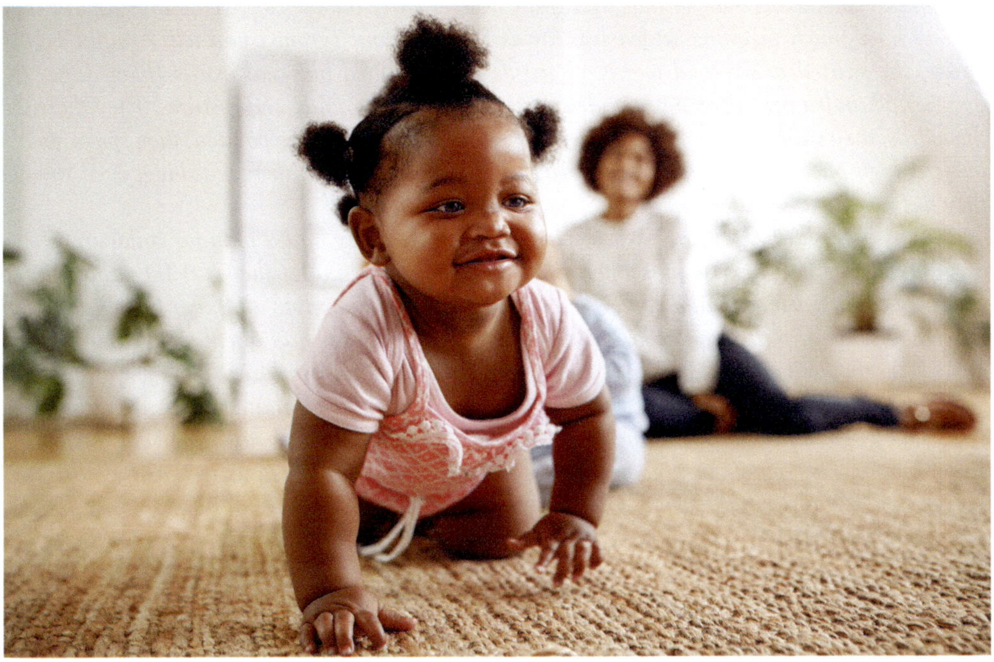

The newborn has been home for about three months now, adjusting to extrauterine life, just as the family is adjusting to a new (and demanding) member. This section of *Newborn to Infant to Child* describes growth and action (Chapter 8), perception and thought (Chapter 9), emotions and temperament (Chapter 10), communication and relationships (Chapter 11), and contexts of development (Chapter 12) between 4 and 17 months. The infant stage is a time of demonstrative change. In little over one year, infants make significant, impressive gains in all these spheres of development as they enchant and simultaneously challenge everyone around them. Let's meet parents Shandra and Tyrone and infant Rosa.

When Shandra and Tyrone married, they knew they wanted to start a family but soon after learned that some medical issues would prevent Shandra from becoming pregnant in a conventional way. So they spent a number of years exploring their options and saving their money in the event they decided to use an assisted reproduction technology like in vitro fertilization (IVF). During this time, they became foster parents and cared for a number of children in need

DOI: 10.4324/9781003381709-9

of a home. One child, Rosa, arrived at their home when she was only 1 month old, and Shandra and Tyrone knew they wanted baby Rosa to be part of their family forever. It was a very happy day when the adoption was completed!

During Rosa's first 17 months of life, Shandra and Tyrone marveled at how fast Rosa changed. Rosa came to them unable to roll over or lift her head, but soon she was sitting, crawling, and then walking. Rosa's "schedule" also became more predictable. She woke at about the same time during the night, napped about the same time during the day, and was hungry at the same times as well. Similarly, Rosa only cried in the early days, and soon she started to smile, showed surprise and fear, and even began laughing. Rosa explored her world, with her hands, her mouth, and her eyes. She seemed to want to know about everything, even if it could hurt (once touching a cactus plant in the living room). During this time, Rosa developed ways to communicate, using both sounds and gestures. Her early babbles were cute to hear, but they did not have much meaning, at least as far as Shandra and Tyrone could tell. Around 1 year of age, she started to say real words, or words that sounded like real words (like "daga" for doggie*). Shandra and Tyrone responded positively to these sounds and gestures: They repeated the words, they said "Yes!" or "I see," they looked in the direction she pointed, they spoke slowly using a high-pitched voice, and they engaged in conversations with turn-taking, even though they did not always understand what Rosa was saying.*

Because they had experience as foster parents, they already had a plan for childcare. Shondra and Tyrone had flexible jobs, often working at home even after the COVID pandemic, so that they could cover several days a week caring for Rosa themselves and later have her attend a neighborhood day-care center for the other days. Both parents had a few night commitments as well, so they relied on babysitters or neighbors who also had children. They felt that it was good for Rosa to be around other children her age or older, given that she was an only child. Rosa enjoys going "to school" now, but earlier she was anxious about being separated from either parent. Her reluctance to be separated was distressing for Rosa as well as Shondra and Tyrone, when Rosa showed strong preferences to keep near Shandra and Tyrone.

CHAPTER 8

Infants

Growth and Action

Anatomical, physiological, and psychological growth are all dramatic early in life, but development of the nervous system is particularly remarkable because of its infinite complexities and astonishing capacity to regulate and integrate information. The tremendous development before birth that continues into the first newborn months actually seems to accelerate during the infant stage of growth. Within 9 to 12 months after birth, the nervous system develops such that it supports a conscious infant capable of intelligent feelings, thoughts, and actions. Along with development of the central nervous system, the neurons and muscles that support motor movements mature, such that infants gain control over their head, arms, and legs. This control allows for intentional actions that infants put to good use by exploring their environments and moving toward people they prefer. This chapter considers multiple aspects of physical growth and the beginnings of intentional action in the infant in the contexts of the roles of biology and experience.

PRINCIPLES OF GROWTH

Three general principles of growth and action are exemplified in the study of anatomical development. The first general principle is **directionality** (Figure 8.1). Whether the subject of study is the growth of the body, complexity of function, or voluntary control, development follows several characteristic directions. One direction is that development proceeds **cephalocaudally**, that is, from "head to tail." For example, the visual system reaches anatomical maturity earlier than do the legs, and as a result, infants have voluntary visual control much earlier in life than walking. A second direction is that development proceeds **proximodistally**, that is from the center of the body outward. For example, infants acquire control over their neck and torso before their fingers. A third direction is that development typically proceeds in a **mass-to-specific** fashion, that is from large muscle groups to fine ones. For example, infants can move their arms intentionally before they are able to control fingering. The fourth direction is that development frequently involves **hierarchical integration**, that is simple skills develop separately and then become organized into more complex ones. For example, when reaching for an object, younger infants will move their arm toward the object and grasp it once the object touches the palm, whereas older infants will anticipate the grasp by modifying the shape of their hand during the arm movement.

DOI: 10.4324/9781003381709-10

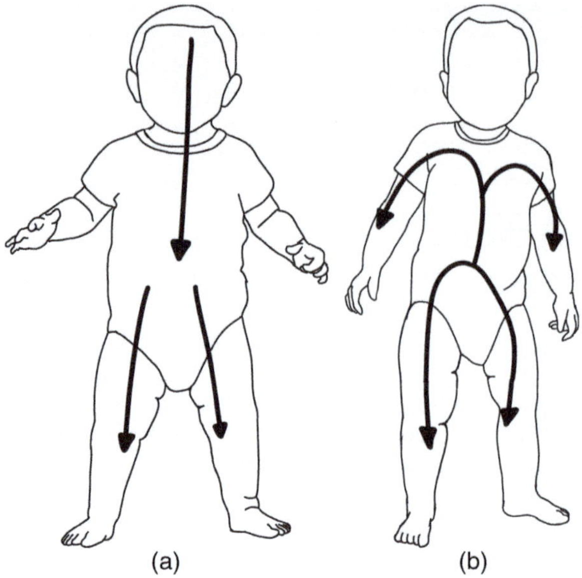

FIGURE 8.1 (a) Principles of development in infancy (b) Cephalocaudal (head to tail) a and proximodistal (center outward).

Source: Created by A. E. Arterberry.

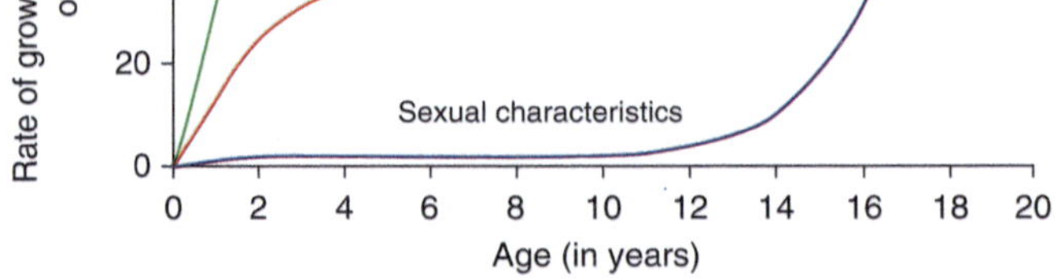

FIGURE 8.2 Different bodily systems grow toward maturity at different rates. In infancy, the nervous system is highly developed, body size is less developed, and secondary sexual characteristics are least developed of all.

The second general principle of growth and action is the **independence of systems**. Figure 8.2 displays rates of growth for three major systems, illustrating the point that different systems are in different states of maturity early in life and grow along different courses through the first year or two. By 2 years, for example, the nervous system has achieved more than one-half of its mature status, whereas physical characteristics of the body, such as size, have developed to less than one-third of their eventual mature level, and of course, secondary sexual characteristics have hardly developed at all.

The third general principle of growth and action concerns the interplay between norms and individual differences. Many physical, biological, and psychological characteristics are typically distributed in what is called a **statistically normal** fashion, that is the distribution of a given characteristic in the population forms a bell-shaped curve.

Consider the example of height. Very few adults are either 4 or 7 ft tall, many more are 5 and 6 ft tall, and most are in between. The average might represent the distribution of some structure or function, but the range and form of the distribution are critically informative about the structure or function as well. For example, the age at which infants first talk or walk has enormous psychological importance to them and to their caregivers and family ("Is she talking yet?," "Is he walking yet?"), but the age range for each of these and many other accomplishments is extraordinary, especially when considered as a proportion of the infant's age. Some infants say their first word at 9 months, others at 29 months; some infants first walk at 10 months, others at 18 months. All adults can generally talk and walk, suggesting that the exact onset of talking or walking might be less meaningful in the long run than anxious parents and relatives often think. **Norms** are the averages for a population and their distribution, but they are descriptions rather than explanations.

Variability reflects **individual differences**. Individual differences arise out of the unique combination of biology and experience, or the interaction of nature and nurture, over time. In addition, individual differences can follow several different courses in development. Consider three possibilities: (1) Different individuals might follow different rates of growth but eventually reach and stay at the same mature level; (2) different individuals may follow the same rate of growth but stop growing at different final levels; and (3) different individuals might follow different rates of growth and reach different final levels. These diverse developmental trajectories of growth can have many causes and consequences.

In the case of physical development, one cause for variation is nutrition. At birth as well as through the course of the early life period, newborns, infants, and children in high-resource circumstances tend to be healthier, heavier, and longer than those in low-resource circumstances. These differences could reflect genetic variation, but they are also the products of prenatal and postnatal nutrition and care and maternal health and education. By the end of the first year of postnatal life, the average U.S. infant weighs about 20 lb (9 kg) and is about 30 in long (76 cm). Infants in resource-poor countries are born with lower birth weights, and they are at risk for being underweight and underheight across the early life period (Aboagye et al., 2022).

Section Summary

Growth and action follow a small number of basic principles, including directionality, the independence of systems, and characterization in terms of norms and individual differences. Development does not proceed in the same way in all infants; rather, individual variation is expected in all structures and functions. Reasons for such differences may be genetic and biological or experiential and environmental, but likely the interaction of the two.

GROWTH OF THE NERVOUS SYSTEM

The nervous system is divided into autonomic and central components. When considering **autonomic nervous system (ANS)** development, we focus particularly on states of arousal as key indicators of function. When discussing **central nervous system (CNS)** development, we focus on different levels of neural and brain development.

Autonomic Nervous System

On first observation, young infants' activity appears to be spontaneous, disorganized, and sporadic. Infants seem to be constantly moving their eyes, hands, and feet without apparent purpose. Over longer periods, they appear to shift randomly and unpredictably from sleep to alertness (Rivkees & Hao, 2000). However, looks deceive, and infants are actually not so unpredictable. Close and consistent inspection reveals that newborns and infants are more or less regular in many ways and that their systems cycle in detectable patterns or rhythms. Many rhythms seem to be natural or **endogenous**, perhaps driven by molecular "pacemaker cells" in the brain. In short, apparent irregularity is only just that, apparent, and regularity underlies seeming irregularity (Figure 8.3).

Naturally occurring or spontaneous activities in infants are organized at fast, medium, and slow cycles or rhythms (Rivkees, 2003). Some activities occur regularly at high frequencies and cycle (appear and disappear or increase and decrease) perhaps once or more every second. Heartbeats, breathing, and sucking exemplify fast biological rhythms that maintain life, and kicking and rocking illustrate fast cycling behaviors. Other activities, such as involuntary body movements, cycle at medium rates, on the order of once every minute or two (Groome et al., 1999). As an example, consider sleep states. During the night, we pass through five different states (labelled 1–4 and REM, a period of dreaming that includes **rapid eye movements**). The full cycle takes about 90 to 110 minutes and then repeats throughout the night. Sleep is an example of a slow cycle. Other biological functions cycle at even slower frequencies, increasing and decreasing in periods of up to 24 hours, and they are governed by the **circadian clock**, an internally driven biochemical, physiological, and behavioral process that adjusts to environmental cues, such as light in the day versus dark in the night (Rivkees, 2003).

The coordination and integration of different cycles is a major accomplishment of neurological organization, and infant state is significant for many key reasons. First, state determines how infants present themselves, and whether and how infants respond to tactile,

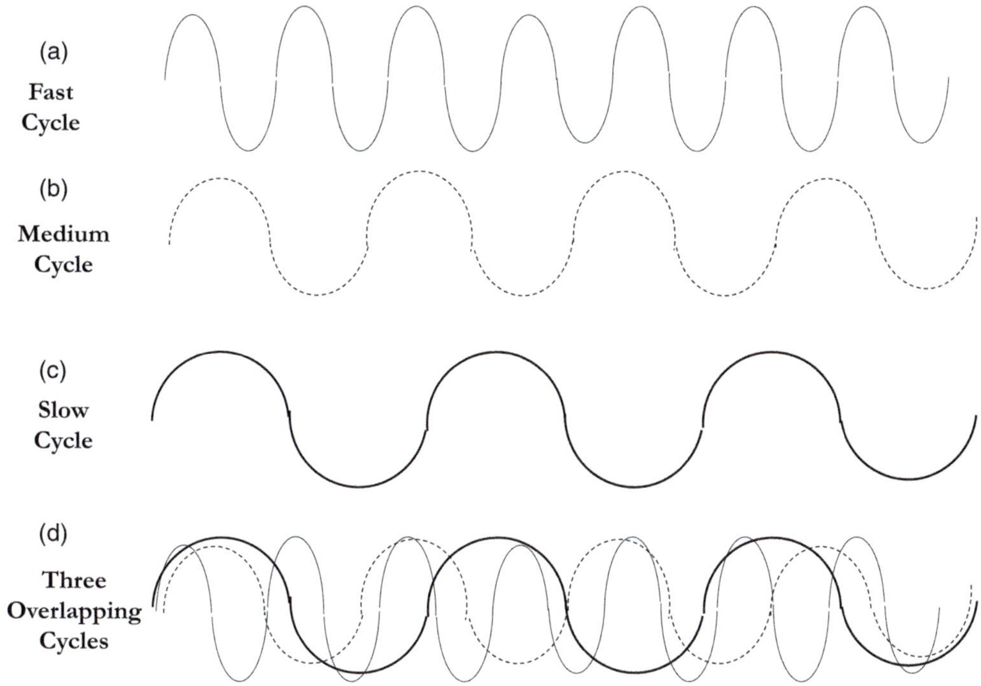

FIGURE 8.3 (a) Fast cycle. (b) Medium cycle. (c) Slow cycle. (d) Seeming chaos of the three overlapping cycles.

Source: Created by M. H. Bornstein.

visual, and auditory stimulation often depends on their state. In quiet alertness, for example, infants may attend to a voice. The same voice, however, may have no effect on the same infants when they are crying. Second, infant states influence adult behavior. Adults will rock and soothe distressed infants instead of trying to engage them in play or learning. Infants who are temperamentally fretful elicit different patterns of care than do infants who cry only infrequently. In this way, infants affect their own development by affecting how and how often others respond to them. Third, state regularity serves as a marker of nervous system integrity. Poor state regulation is common among infants born preterm, infants who have suffered significant perinatal complications (such as intraventricular hemorrhage or anoxia), and infants with congenital brain malformations. Also, poor state regulation in early infancy can indicate higher risk for SIDS (Myers et al., 2018). Finally, abnormal sleep state patterns can anticipate medical problems, such as epilepsy (Nunes & Costa da Costa, 2010).

Degrees of regularity in different structures and functions over time differ in infants, and these differences have developmental consequences. For example, the amounts of time infants spend in different states have implications for infant development in other domains, such as language and social interaction, because stages of the sleep–wake cycle cue adults to initiate caregiving and play. Thus, many sophisticated activities and achievements in the early life period have their roots in cycling structures and functions.

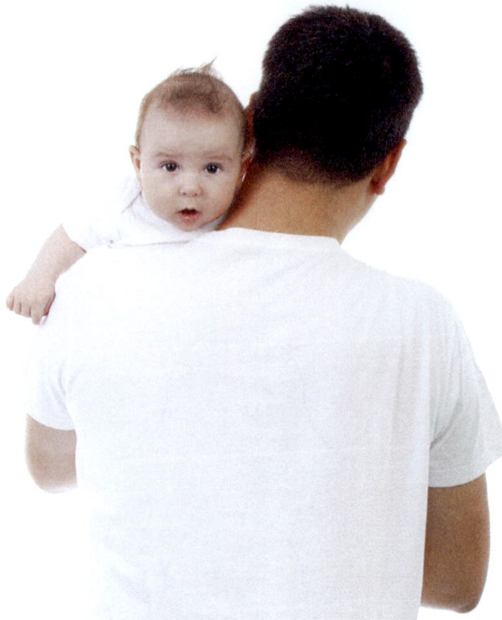

FIGURE 8.4 Infants placed upright are more alert than when cradled or lying down.

Behavior becomes more organized over time as internal neural control mechanisms develop. During the first two months, caregivers have a major impact on their infants' state of arousal. When infants are distressed, adults intervene to soothe them. Even when infants are drowsy, they become alert when held erect at an adult's shoulder (Figure 8.4). Thus, when young infants are alert and able to learn about the environment, they are often in the arms of their caregivers. Because the caregivers who are close by can be felt, smelled, heard, and seen when infants are alert, infants soon come to learn a great deal about their caregivers, and vice versa. Infants also rapidly learn to associate their caregiver's presence with alertness and the relief of distress (Thompson & Virmani, 2010). This association may be one of the earliest, and certainly one of the most dramatic, relationships for infants.

Central Nervous System

The CNS is largely concerned with information processing and mediating the organism's interactions with the environment. To adjust to complex changes from prenatal to postnatal life, the CNS develops in many ways and at many levels simultaneously. These include the neural level at the microscopic end of the spectrum and the overall structure of the brain at the macroscopic end of the spectrum.

Neurons. Neurons and their connections develop rapidly prenatally and after birth. Perhaps the two most important developments in the communication between cells involve biochemical neurotransmission and restructuring of neural organization. During infancy,

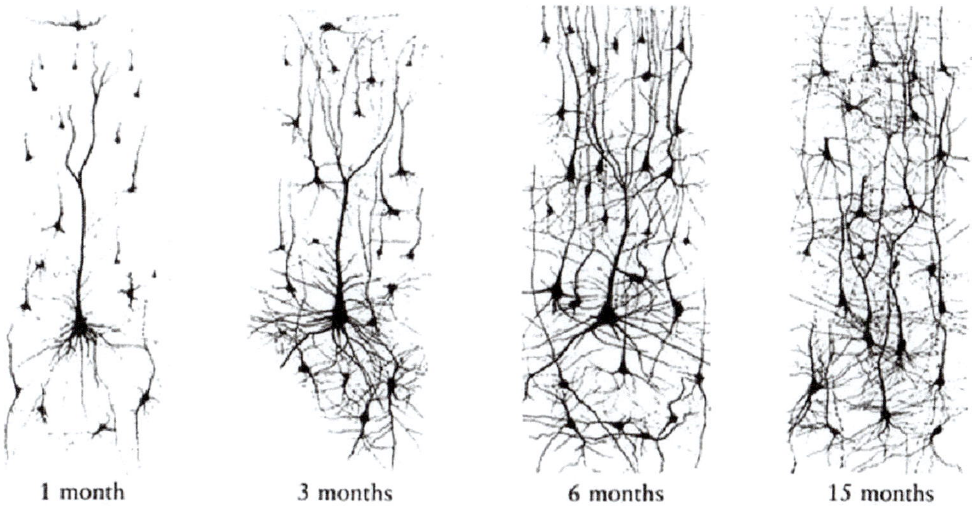

FIGURE 8.5 A schematic illustration showing how dendritic arborization of neurons increases from 1 to 15 months of age.

Source: Courtesy of Conel.

increasing dendritic complexity is reflected in the growth of spines or branches that enable connections between neighboring cells, a process called **arborization** (Figure 8.5). In the first two years of life, circuitry between neurons proceeds to the point where there are up to 10,000 connections per cell. Likewise, the number of **synapses**, connections between axons and dendrites which support communication between neurons, regularly increases in early life (a process called **synaptogenesis**), another indication of enhancing capacities for information transmission. During this time, specifically the first year of life, synapses are overproduced in many parts of the brain, with no part appearing to develop faster or slower than any other, and their appearance accounts for changes in function with age (Shonkoff & Phillips, 2000). In fact, more connections are made than are needed. As a result, the connections start to decrease, a process called **pruning**, resulting in increased specialization in some areas of the central nervous system (Figure 8.6). The result is an efficient and streamlined information transmission system.

Another development that improves neural function is **myelination**. Undeveloped neurons are bare fibers; developed ones are usually (though not always) wrapped in a sheath of a fatty substance that surrounds the axon and facilitates the speed of nerve conduction, rendering information transmission more efficient (Klingberg, 2008). Myelin also gives neurons their white appearance (called white matter). With myelination, the velocity of neurotransmission in a cell more than triples, from a rate of less than 20 ft (6 m) per second to more than 60 ft (18 m) per second. The process of myelination loosely correlates with the development of function and provides a general index of maturation, although some functional activity still occurs in the absence of myelination. The visual, auditory, and somesthetic cortex myelinate before birth, whereas higher brain centers,

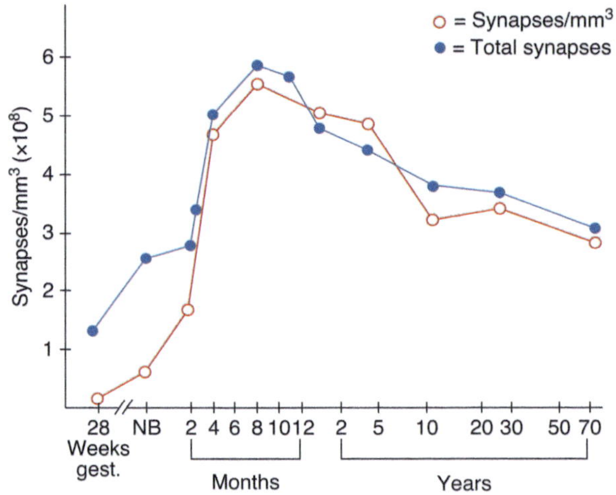

FIGURE 8.6 Total and density synapse counts in an area of the human brain (layer 3 of the middle frontal gyrus) as a function of age. Synapses increase rapidly through the first year of life and then decrease through puberty and into old age.

such as the prefrontal cortex, which integrates information, are not completely myelinated until puberty (Shaw et al., 2006).

These developmental processes have fundamental implications for successes of brain networks involved in social interactions, primarily face processing and eye gaze in infants (Stiles et al., 2015). Adults typically respond to faces in characteristic ways. For example, most adults recognize faces more quickly and accurately when faces are upright than when they are upside down. This preferential response suggests that in adults the face-processing network is finely tuned to upright faces. Because infants cannot verbally report what they see, event-related potentials (ERPs; Box 8.1) have been used to discover how infants perceive faces (Johnson, 2025). Between 4 and 12 months of age, infants come to respond differently to upright versus inverted faces. Significantly, neural regions that are activated by faces in adults are only partially activated by the same faces in infants. Thus, adult behavioral competence does not appear because new brain regions mature and come online; rather, relevant regions become more finely tuned and integrated for processing faces as a result of daily, repeated experience looking at faces (Stiles et al., 2015).

As infants interact with their environment, certain connections between neurons are preferentially activated and so gain a structural advantage. As a result, more routinely activated pathways become more readily, efficiently, and appropriately involved in function.

Brain Organization. The two hemispheres and the brain stem contain three major substructures that develop in an orderly fashion (Johnson, 2025; Stiles, 2008). **Subcortical structures** that control state (such as the hypothalamus) and the arousal system (for example, the **reticular formation**) emerge first. Indeed, the nuclei of the reticular formation, which govern sleep/wake cycles, are among the earliest to differentiate in the brain. Components of the **limbic system** and **basal ganglia**, which govern emotion, instinct, and

Box 8.1 *How Do We Know This?* EEG and ERPs

Researchers can glimpse how the brain is functioning by using electroencephalogram (EEG) techniques that measure electrical activity at the scalp produced by neurons deep in the brain. Averaging such electrical activity over repeated exposures to the same visual image (such as a face) yields a cortical event-related potential (ERP; Figure 8.7). ERPs can reveal how infants' processing compares to that of older children or adults, and ERPs can help index recognition memory (Mash et al., 2013).

A strength of the ERP technique is that it is sensitive to and reveals the time course and location of information processing by the brain, what region of the cortex is excited, what the magnitude (amplitude) of the response is, and how long (latency) it takes the brain to start responding or reach a peak amplitude. There are, however, challenges to using this methodology. Responses are individually weak and rapid; thus, many presentations of the same stimulus must be administered, and the responses averaged, before the ERP can be distinguished from the background of ongoing spontaneous brain activity (de Haan, 2015). Requiring infants to endure a large number of trials is difficult, and as a result, ERP studies are plagued by a high participant dropout rate (Stets et al., 2012).

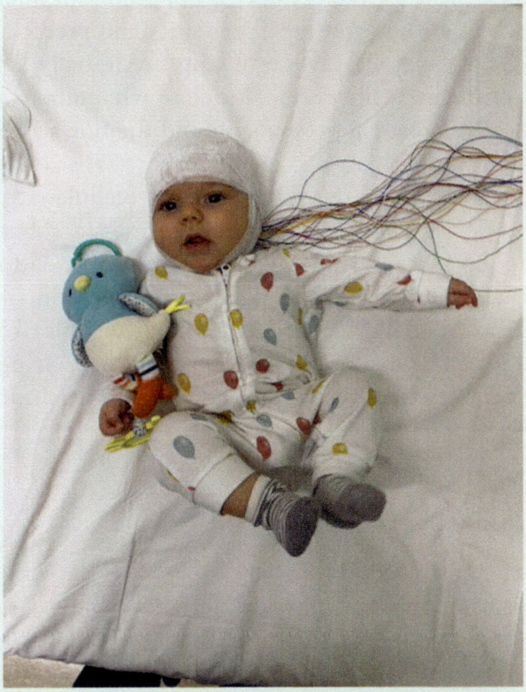

FIGURE 8.7 An infant wearing a cap with sensors that record electrical activity at the scalp.

Source: Courtesy of M. H. Bornstein.

posture, develop next. Last to emerge are the **cortex** and **cortical association areas**, concerned with awareness, attention, memory, and the integration of information. The cortical regions are also among the last to myelinate structurally and functionally are influenced most by experience with the outside world. The developmental phases for these three major components of the central nervous system overlap, and development in each continues well past infancy (Shaw et al., 2006).

The plasticity of nervous tissue (that is, its sensitivity) is also illustrated by restoration of function following CNS damage, due to illness, disease, or normal processes of aging. It has long been believed that the CNS was fixed at birth, such that any recovery of function following damage could only be mediated by the development of alternative neural pathways. However, neuroscience has since demonstrated that new cells or new cell processes can develop to repair damaged parts of the CNS or replace cells that have died (Burns & Verfaillie, 2015). Moreover, in some regions of the CNS, notably regions involved in learning and memory, neurogenesis persists into adulthood (Bergmann et al., 2015; Yuan et al., 2014).

Section Summary

The development of their autonomic nervous system enables infants to regulate state, such as sleep–wake cycles, whose predictability is important for infant learning and development and for caregivers, as they, too, need regularity and predictability to support adequate caregiving. States of quiet alertness in infants are initially rare and brief, but state changes noticeably over the early life period. Much of what infants learn about their own abilities as well as people, objects, and events around them is acquired during periods of quiet alertness and attentiveness.

In the central nervous system, intracellular and intercellular structures and functions change dramatically over the early life period as neurons are born, develop, and connect with one another so as to permit increasingly efficient and complex information transmission in the brain. During infancy, neurons generate an overabundance of connections to other neurons via dendrites and synapses. After this overproduction, pruning allows for specialization of certain brain regions, in part due to experience-expectant and experience-dependent processes. Alongside programmed specializations, malleability and compensation attest to neural plasticity in infancy.

MOTOR DEVELOPMENT

Motor development is as dramatic as physical growth. Table 8.1 shows Bayley's (1993) normative findings of monthly motor accomplishments of newborns and infants between birth and 16 months. Infants' abilities to coordinate their physical movements grow impressively during this relatively brief time period. Movements seem uncontrolled for the first few months, but coordination develops rapidly thereafter. Initially, newborns are unable to roll over from the position in which originally placed, but infants are increasingly mobile and deft, such that parents quickly learn that they must constantly monitor them.

TABLE 8.1 Representative Items From the Bayley Scales of Infant Development

Age Observed (Months)	*Psychomotor Development Index*
1	Thrusts arms in play
2	Holds head erect and steady for 15 seconds
3	Sits with support
4	Sits alone momentarily
5	Uses whole hand to grasp small pellet
6	Attempts to raise self to sit
7	Rotates trunk while sitting alone
8	Walks with help
9	Stands alone
10	Throws ball
11	Walks up stairs with help
12	Walks backward
14	Stands on left foot with help
16	Uses pads of fingertips to grasp pencil

The sequence and coordination of motor development depend on both maturation and experience. Certainly, motor development depends on the growth of limbs and muscles sufficiently strong and organized to act in a coordinated fashion. Two related neurological systems direct motor activity (including reflexes): The **pyramidal system** controls precise, rapid, and skilled movements of the extremities (such as walking), and the **extrapyramidal system** controls posture and coordination. The development of these systems enables infants to sit upright, move about, and manipulate objects. Motor development also unfolds as infants' bodies change. Infant weight triples on average in the first postnatal year, and infants' height increases about 10 in (25.4 cm) in this same time period. Moving a heavier and longer body requires ongoing adjustments as new motor skills come online and are refined (Adolph & Hospodar, 2025). Two significant achievements in the development of motor control in infancy are manipulation and locomotion.

Manipulation

Infants begin reaching between 4 and 5 months of age, but manual coordination is far from fully developed at that stage. Increasing control over the hands and arms provides for planning actions and opportunities to explore objects. For example, when anticipating contact with an object, infants plan the trajectory of their arm(s) and modify their hand shape, depending on the location and/or properties of the object (Chen et al., 2010; Gronqvist et al., 2011). By the middle of their first year, infants seem to reach for everything in sight and often bring what they touch to their mouths.

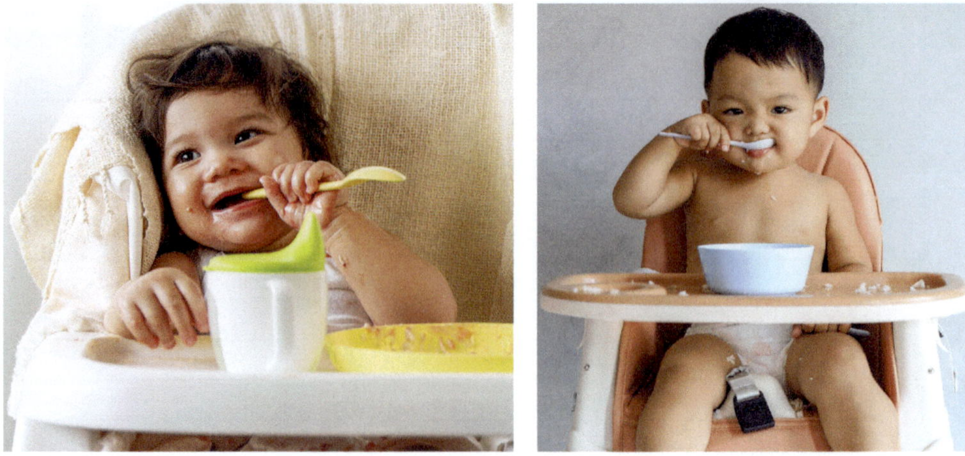

(a) (b)

FIGURE 8.8 Two infants feeding themselves with a spoon. In (a), the infant holds the spoon by the wrong end and is less likely to meet with success compared to the infant in (b).

Object exploration leads to learning about object properties. Infants learn about shape, substance, and other object properties through multimodal exploration (Needham, 2016; Soska et al., 2010). Even blind infants engage in manual exploration: They shake, bang, mouth, and finger objects similarly to sighted infants (Bradley-Johnson et al., 2004). Infants also learn about spatial relations via reaching. They know where objects are located in relation to their bodies, and they even know when they need to lean forward to make contact with an object (Yonas & Hartman, 1993). Infants as young as 8 months, who can barely sit upright by themselves, are also becoming adept at catching moving objects (von Hofsten, 1983).

Tool use, such as feeding oneself with a spoon, requires control over fine motor manipulation and thus emerges later than reaching (Adolph & Hospodar, 2025; Lockman & Kahrs, 2017). In addition to controlling their manual actions, infants must also learn the most efficient way to use tools. For example, there is a correct way to pick up a spoon to use it to eat (Keen, 2011). Holding the spoon such that the food end is toward the center of the body allows for easy access to the mouth. Moreover, control of movement, such as the speed or orientation of the bowl of the spoon, is important so that the contents are not lost (Figure 8.8).

Locomotion

Learning to locomote in infancy involves complex reciprocal relations among maturation, perception, and experience (Adolph & Hospodar, 2025). One example is the transition from crawling to walking. Kretch and Adolph (2013) investigated infants' judgments of different-sized drop-offs as crawlers and walkers. The drop-offs were either small steps or large cliffs. Experienced 12-month-old crawlers refused to go over the cliffs, but novice

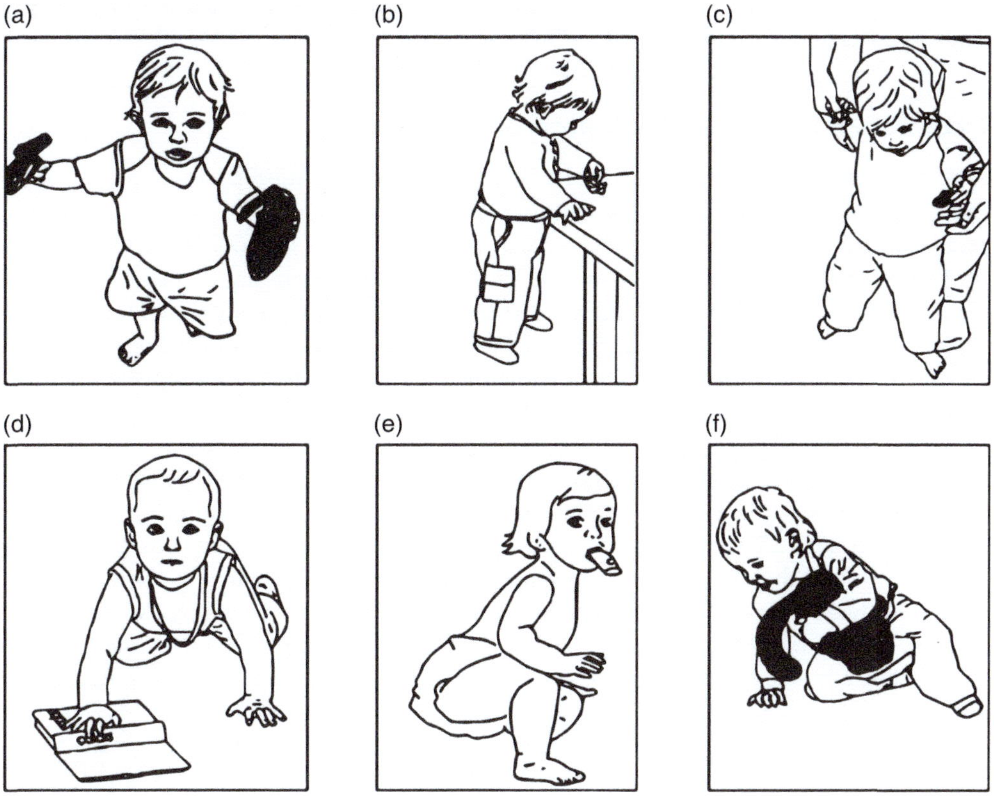

FIGURE 8.9 Different modes of carrying objects by crawlers and walkers.

12-month-old walkers stepped over the cliffs and needed to be rescued before falling. With their new mode of locomotion, infants need to reassess conditions for safe locomotion, particularly differences between which goals can be achieved by crawling and walking. Another example of the interplay among maturation, perception, and experience comes from infants' carrying objects while locomoting (Karasik et al., 2012). Either crawling or walking brings infants into contact with distant objects. Infants also like to share objects with other people, and thus they often carry objects while locomoting. Both crawlers and walkers engage in a number of strategies for carrying objects, as illustrated in Figure 8.9, and the more locomotor experience infants have, the more they carry objects while moving. Surprisingly, walkers fall *less* when carrying objects. Despite engaging in a more attention-demanding task (walking and carrying), balance control appears to improve compared to when not carrying objects.

Although achievements in locomotion (i.e., from crawling to walking) are expected as infants age, infants' abilities to negotiate challenging motor tasks, such as descending a sloped surface or moving through an opening, are not automatic but depend on the coordination of many systems. Infants take into account properties of the surfaces or openings, such as the degree of slant or width of a doorway, and explore different modes of locomotion before settling on a specific locomotive mode, such as crawling backward or turning their body sideways (Adolph & Hospodar, 2025). Experience also plays a large part in their development.

Experience Helps Shape Motor Development

A poster common in U.S. pediatricians' waiting and examination rooms displays motor milestones across the first years. Infants are expected to roll over at such and such an age, put a cube in a cup at such and such an age, begin to "cruise" by toddling while holding on to a support at such and such an age. These milestones date back to observations of Gesell (1945), who filmed and analyzed the motor development of New Haven (Connecticut) newborns, infants, and children over the first years of life. On the basis of his extensive and careful observations, Gesell then averaged these accomplishments and created a set of well-known guidelines of what normal motor development at different ages entailed.

Such a chart in another culture or country might look very different, however. Infants reared in different places often deviate from accepted norms for European Americans with respect to both the stages and the timing of motor development. Long ago observations revealed that Hopi infants began to walk alone late (Dennis & Dennis, 1940), Balinese infants followed a different set of stages on their way to walking (Mead & MacGregor, 1951), and African Ganda (in Uganda) and Wolof (in Senegal) infants tended to be more advanced in motor development than European American age norms (Ainsworth, 1967).

What is the source of these developmental differences? Delay in Hopi motor development apparently resulted from the traditional practice of having newborns and infants swaddled tightly on cradle boards (Dennis & Dennis, 1940). In contrast, the manner in which Balinese mothers habitually carried their infants appeared to promote their infants' unique motor performance (Mead & MacGregor, 1951). Likewise, advanced Ugandan motor abilities proved to be due to mothers granting their infants considerable physical freedom (Ainsworth, 1967). Thus, infants across cultures have different motor experiences, which result in different developmental trajectories (Adolph et al., 2010).

Caregiving practices affect the onset and trajectory of motor development. Some practices speed it up; others slow it down. Still others change the sequence of development. What these cultural comparisons reveal is that motor development is both variable and sensitive to experience. Even within a culture, caregivers may provide infants with differing experiences (Karasik & Robinson, 2022). Moreover, some cultural practices that appear to be different may not be that different after all. For example, Karasik and colleagues (2018, 2022) reported that in Tajikistan, infants are contained in cradles that limit movements of their arms and legs. These cradles can be used well into the second year of life, and infants may spend up to 15 hours per day in them. At first glance, this level of containment sounds much more than what U.S. infants typically experience. It turns out, however, that U.S. infants spend almost the same amount of time at 12 months contained as Tajik infants do. The difference is that U.S. infants have more variety in containers, including baby carriers that strap onto parents (Figure 6.3), high chairs (Figure 8.8), car seats, cribs (Figure 9.7), walkers, and playpens, and they spend less time in any one container than Tajik infants spend in their cradles. Notably, the two groups do not differ very much in terms of how much unrestricted time they have on the floor or ground.

So do differential experiences impact motor development? In a word, maybe. Like Hopi infants who spend time strapped to cradle boards, none of the Tajik 12-month-olds was walking, whereas all U.S. infants were. However, it is not clear that containment is the only limiting factor, given other vast differences between these Tajiks and Americans, including access to clean water, nutrition, and the like. Moreover, delayed locomotion may be an advantage in a context where there are dangers (e.g., open cisterns for collecting water) and where childproofing is not as easy to do as in a U.S. home (see Box 8.2 for more on infant injuries).

Even within-country comparisons show how experience – or opportunities – shape motor development. Infants walking naked compared to wearing diapers have more mature gait patterns and fall less (Cole et al., 2012), and infants who live in houses with stairs climb them earlier than those who do not (Berger et al., 2007). Thus, motor development unfolds in a specific infant living in a specific context at a specific time. Rather than focusing on normative milestones or emphasizing the emergence of certain skills, we stand to learn much more about the whys and hows of motor development through closer examination of varied infants, situations, and times (Karasik et al., 2022).

Box 8.2 *Application:* Preventing Injuries

According to the Centers for Disease Control and Prevention, in 2021, accidental injury was the fourth leading cause of death in infants under 1 year of age in the United States, following congenital malformations, low birth weight, and SIDS (Xu et al., 2022). To put this finding in perspective, in 2021, approximately 36 out of every 100,00 infants died from an injury before their first birthday. Falls were the most common type of accidents: Out of 461 incidents, the most common events leading to injuries were falling from furniture, being dropped by a caregiver, falling from baby products, and falling while crawling or walking (Cooray et al., 2022). Events leading up to these falls included infants rolling off objects or being left alone or unattended and caregivers falling asleep or tripping while holding infants. Being dropped or falling off furniture required more intensive medical treatment as a result of the injury (Mulligan et al., 2017).

Of course, all parents and caregivers want to do what they can to keep their infants safe. One relatively simple step caregivers can take to try to prevent infant injuries is to become more educated about dangers in the home (Cheraghi et al., 2014). Another common strategy is to "babyproof" the home (Pampers, 2023). Some actions in this regard include covering electrical outlets, putting in baby safety gates to prevent wandering into unsafe areas, securing furniture to prevent it from moving and falling over, being cautious of slippery floors, removing choking hazards, and storing batteries in a place where infants cannot reach them. More specific rooms, like the kitchen, bathroom, and living room, call for specific changes.

Connecting Motor Development to Other Domains

Systems theory maintains that development in one sphere of life will impact development in other spheres of life. Consistent with systems theory, motor development affects multiple aspects of physiological and psychological growth (Thelen, 2000, 2001). Motor development and infant state, particularly sleeping, are coordinated. As infants begin to master new motor skills, their nighttime sleep is disrupted. An intensive study of three infants across 12 to 20 months found that when a new motor skill first emerged (such as sitting up or crawling), infants woke up more at night (Berger & Moore, 2021). Despite variability in individual sleep patterns, this connection between skill onset and sleep disruption characterized a large number of motor milestones across the first 1 1/2 years of life. The interesting question is why. REM (active sleep) consolidates learning, and it is possible that when learning a new skill, REM sleep aids sensorimotor integration. One side effect of REM sleep is greater arousal, and so, in turn, an increased likelihood of infants waking up in the night. Even short naps consolidate new skills. Infants learning a new task, such as how to move through a tunnel, perform better at a later test if they napped for 30 minutes in between learning and test compared to infants who did not nap (Berger & Scher, 2017; DeMasi et al., 2021).

Development of the capacity to grasp an object with both hands, which involves the coordination of fine motor movements in each hand as well as two arms, two hands, and two eyes, makes possible the expression of intentional social- and object-related aspects of cognitive and interpersonal growth. Reaching and grasping enhance infants' appreciation of object properties, allow infants to engage socially with others through sharing objects, and heighten infants' sense of mastery. Crawling experience is associated with less negative affect and more flexible memory (Libertus & Needham, 2011; Whitney & Green, 2011). Nine-month-olds who crawl are able to recall a novel action when tested in a different context, whereas same-aged infants who do not crawl can recall the novel action when tested in the same context, but not when tested in a novel context (Herbert et al., 2007). Presumably, experience with self-locomotion provides infants with opportunities to retrieve information in a range of contexts, facilitating flexibility in recall. Moreover, object exploration and locomotion are likely reciprocally related. Crawling 11-month-olds who show interest in objects, carry objects, and share objects with others over distances are more likely to walk by 13 months than 11-month-olds who do not show such abilities (Karasik et al., 2012).

Motor development not only helps shape infants' perceptions of the world but also influences infant–parent interactions. Infants' first reaches, rolls, upright postures, or steps are occasions for parental pride and joy and for calling grandparents. These achievements also signal all sorts of cognitive and social changes at home, especially the new need to "childproof" the house. Change, as well as rate of change, is impressive. So is the average infant's physical energy. It is estimated that each hour the average toddler takes 1,200 steps, falls 16 times, and spends 30 minutes playing with objects (Adolph et al., 2012). Thus, each new motor skill that emerges prompts changes in other systems, such as state, and opens up new opportunities for infants to interact with the people, objects, and events.

Section Summary

With age, infants gain increasing control over their own movements, allowing for independent exploration of their world. Reaching allows infants to manipulate and view objects at the same time, and with increasing manual control, infants become more skilled tool users. Crawling and walking allow infants to carry objects and explore their larger environments. Moreover, infants now have greater control with regard to their proximity to caregivers and can initiate interactions by sharing objects. Motor development is biologically programmed but also shaped by experience and environment, as infants in different cultures have different experiences which affect the timing and nature of motor milestones. Finally, motor development connects to multiple other domains of development.

CONCLUSIONS

Growth and action follow basic principles, including directionality and the independence of systems, and are characterized in terms of norms and individual differences. Autonomic nervous system development enables state regulation, which in turn fosters improved and rewarding interactions with the material and social worlds. Central nervous system development proceeds at multiple levels from neuron to brain that augment information transmission. With age infants gain increasing control over their own actions, from manipulation to locomotion, allowing for independent exploration of their world as well as engagement with the social world. Growth and action are in degrees genetically and biologically programmed but also shaped by experience and environment, as infants in different cultures have different experiences, which affect the timing and nature of both. Finally, growth and action connect and interconnect across multiple domains of development.

KEY TERMS

Arborization
Autonomic nervous system (ANS)
Basal ganglia
Central nervous system (CNS)
Cephalocaudally
Circadian clock
Cortex
Cortical association areas
Directionality
Endogenous
Extrapyramidal system
Hierarchical integration
Independence of systems
Limbic system
Mass-to-specific
Myelination
Norms
Proximodistally
Pruning
Pyramidal system
Rapid eye movement
Reticular formation
Statistically normal
Subcortical structures
Synapses
Synaptogenesis

SUGGESTED READINGS

Adolph, K. E., & Hospodar, C. M. (2025). Motor development. In M. H. Bornstein & M. E. Lamb (Eds.), *Developmental science: An advanced textbook* (8th ed., pp. 234–269). Routledge.

De Haan, M., Dummonthiel, I., & Johnson, M. H. (2023). *Developmental cognitive neuroscience – an introduction* (5th ed.). Wiley-Blackwell.

Kahrs, B. A., & Lockman, J. J. (2014). Tool using. *Child Development Perspectives*, *8*, 231–236.

Tooley, U. A., Bassett, D. S., & Mackey, A. P. (2021). Environmental influences on the pace of brain development. *Nature Reviews Neuroscience*, *22*(6), 372–384.

CHAPTER 9

Infants

Perception and Thought

Perception constitutes the necessary first step in experiencing and interpreting the world. Yet perception is private. What is blue or loud or sweet to another person may not be the same blue or loud or sweet to you. To know what another person's perceptions are like, we can only make inferences from their reports or behaviors. Thought is similar. We may think we know what another person is thinking, but we are not really privy to what they are thinking unless they tell us. Sharing our perceptions and thoughts with others (and vice versa) is easily done via language. Because infants do not say much, at least initially, we cannot ask them about their perceptions and thoughts or expect an answer; rather, we must infer the tremendous gains infants make in perceiving and thinking from 4 to 17 months from their behaviors. In this chapter, we chronicle some highlights of what we now know about perceptual and mental development in infants.

PERCEPTION

Infancy is a time of impressive developments in perception. Visual perception is an example. As their visual acuity approaches adult levels (or 20/20, if an optician were to measure it), infants' visual world becomes increasingly rich and complex. It is in color, it is in three dimensions, and it is filled with people and objects and events. Here we highlight perceptual development in infancy of attributes (color and depth), form, people, and self.

Perception of Attributes

Color. In one of the first baby biographies (Box 9.1), Darwin speculated in the 1870s about the development of color vision in his son Doddy, but real progress toward understanding whether infants see color only began a century later. This delay in progress was due in part to a formidable challenge faced by scientists who study color vision – disambiguating hue from brightness. **Hue** (what we think of as color per se) and **brightness** (intensity) are two major components of color, but they vary together so that whenever the color of a stimulus changes, both its hue and brightness are changing. To tell if someone sees blue as different from green on the basis of what we usually think of as color (hue) alone, we must first equalize or otherwise account for any brightness differences in the two colors. Otherwise, they could be responding to a brightness, and not a hue, difference between

DOI: 10.4324/9781003381709-11

Box 9.1 *How Do We Know This?* Baby Biographies

Baby biographies comprised the first systematic observations of infants, and they were often written by famous people, like Charles Darwin. Darwin assembled for publication observations he made in the early 1840s of his firstborn son, William Erasmus, nicknamed Doddy (Conrad, 1998). It can be said that Darwin's publication of "A Biographical Sketch of an Infant" simultaneously in the German journal *Kosmos* and the influential English journal *Mind* in 1877 founded the study of infancy. Darwin, already famous for the *On the Origin of Species* (published in 1859), recounted sensory, intellectual, and emotional development in Doddy's first year. Scientific interest in infants blossomed after Darwin in part because scholars came to believe that adult human beings could be better understood with reference to their origins – in nature, in the species, and in childhood. Perhaps the greatest of the modern baby biographers was Jean Piaget, most of whose writing and theorizing about mental development in early life refers to observations of his own three young children, Jacqueline, Lucienne, and Laurent.

The strengths and weaknesses of baby biographies are worth noting. On the positive side, attention paid by important figures such as Darwin clearly excited more general interest in newborns, infants, and children and in their scientific study. These talented authors also proved to be exceptional and intuitive observers. On the negative side, baby biographers most frequently observed only single or a few children, usually their own. These children could hardly have been representative of the population of infants at large, and perhaps like their talented and thoughtful parents, they too were exceptional. Biographers were not concerned with comparison groups, and their observations were not always systematic. Furthermore, some baby biographers recorded their observations as they observed them, but many employed a retrospective methodology, trying to recall from hindsight what their child's early life was like. Baby biographers were also subject to bias in their observations: Frequently, these diarists held strong theoretical points of view and tended to write in ways that supported their theories.

On balance, baby biographies played an important role in founding the study of early childhood, and they provide an in-depth look at the development of individual children. However, this method limits generalization to understanding infancy, which is why it is not commonly used today and has been replaced with developmental science.

the colors. With adults, this is relatively easy to do because adults can first be asked to match two colored stimuli for brightness. In infants, however, the precise relation between brightness and color was not known for a long time, and infants cannot be asked to match brightnesses. As a consequence, understanding infant color vision needed to begin with studies of brightness perception and, on the basis of proper brightness controls, proceed to test infant discrimination, preference, and organization of color. Eventually, developmental scientists solved this problem. They unconfounded hue and brightness, and they showed that 3-month-olds could successfully discriminate blue, green, yellow, and red (Bornstein, 2015).

Adults do not merely see colors; they perceive the color spectrum as organized qualitatively into **categories of hue** (Bornstein, 2015). Although we certainly recognize blends in between, we distinguish blue, green, yellow, and red as qualitatively distinct. Bornstein and colleagues (1976a, 1976b) found that 4-month-old infants who were habituated to one color (say, a blue) readily noticed when light of a different color (green) was shown on a test trial afterward, but infants responded to a blue that was different from the habituation blue as though that new blue was the habituation blue (see Box 6.1 for a reminder about the habituation procedure). That is, infants perceived color categorically: They regarded two different blues as more similar than a blue and a green. Indeed, infants categorize the visible spectrum into relatively discrete hues of blue, green, yellow, and red in ways adults do. Moreover, infants seem to have similar aesthetic preferences to adults: Infants look significantly longer to hues that adults rate as more pleasant, like true red, blue, and green rather than rust, aquamarine, or sage (Skelton & Franklin, 2020).

Depth. Depth perception is important. We live in a three-dimensional world cluttered with objects and surfaces. Perceiving depth allows us to know where objects are in space, in turn allowing us to move toward or avoid them. Initial scientific study of infant depth perception started with the following observation:

> Human infants at the creeping and toddling stage are notoriously prone to falls from more or less high places. They must be kept from going over the brink by side panels on their cribs, gates on their stairways, and vigilance of adults. As their muscular coordination matures, they begin to avoid such accidents on their own. Common sense might suggest that the child learns to recognize falling-off places by experience – that is, by falling and hurting himself. But is experience really the teacher? Or is the ability to perceive and avoid a brink part of the child's original endowment?
>
> (Gibson & Walk, 1960, p. 64)

To address these questions, Gibson and Walk (1960) investigated depth perception in infants using a **visual cliff** (Figure 9.1; Rodkey, 2015). One side of the cliff shows the baby an illusory drop; the other side does not. Few infants between 6 and 14 months of age would crawl across the "deep" side when their mothers called them. These results suggested that depth perception must be present in infants as young as 6 months of age. By 6 months, however, infants may already have had plenty of experience perceiving depth. How early do infants perceive depth? One experiment monitored heart rate when pre-crawling 2-month-olds were exposed to shallow and deep sides of the visual cliff (Schwartz et al., 1973). These infants showed a decrease in heart rate when exposed to the deep side, indicating increased attention or interest (Box 9.2). Thus, infants give evidence that they perceive depth long before they crawl or walk. The wariness of drop-offs shown by older infants might result not from actual experience with falls but from the anxiety parents display when their infants approach a drop-off. Infants look to their parents and use their parents' emotional cues to interpret such ambiguous events, a development called **social referencing**.

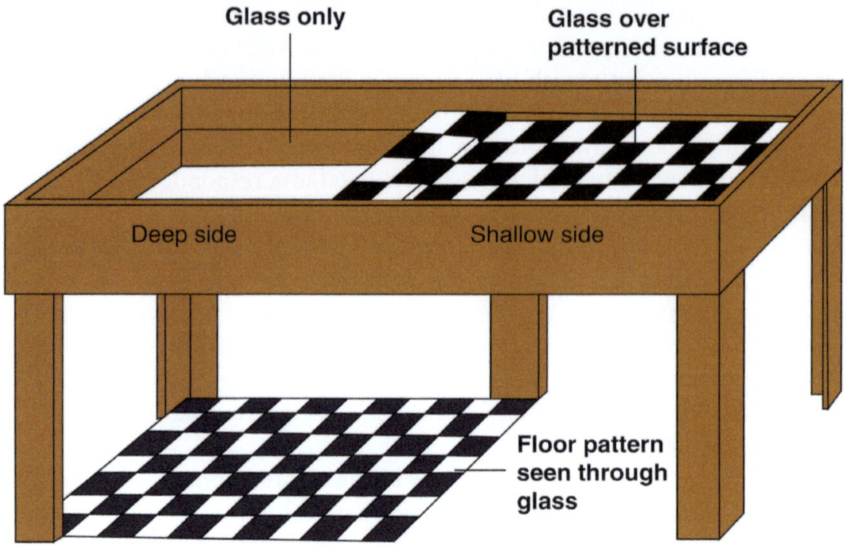

FIGURE 9.1 The visual cliff. Infants are placed on the center between the clear glass and patterned surface. Infants are observed regarding whether they are willing to cross the "deep" (clear glass) side.

Source: Redrawn from Gibson and Walk (1960).

Box 9.2 *How Do We Know This?* Physiological Measures

Heart rate and hormones index changes in the ANS that can be measured in the early life period. *Heart rate* is a sensitive and revealing index of infant capacity (Gao et al., 2022). Because heart rate does not depend on infant motor skills, such as reaching or crawling, and because it reflects infant state, heart rate researchers can tell whether infants are paying attention (Box 4.2) or becoming drowsy or fussy. *Hormones* are chemicals released by a cell or a gland in one part of the body that affects cells or glands in other parts of the body. An example hormone is cortisol, which is present in saliva and indicates response to stress (Szekely et al., 2025). Measures of heart rate and cortisol provide noninvasive and passive information about infants' responses to people, objects, and events around them.

Visual cliff experiments show that infants perceive depth, but they do not reveal what cues infants might be using when they perceive depth. Scientists who study depth perception have identified three such sets of cues. **Binocular cues** are based on the fact that we have two eyes, and our two eyes receive slightly different images of the visual world. To see for yourself, close one eye and look straight ahead; now, open that eye and close the other. The scene you see jumps a bit as you continue alternating opening and closing each eye. The difference between the two images is a cue for depth, called **binocular disparity**.

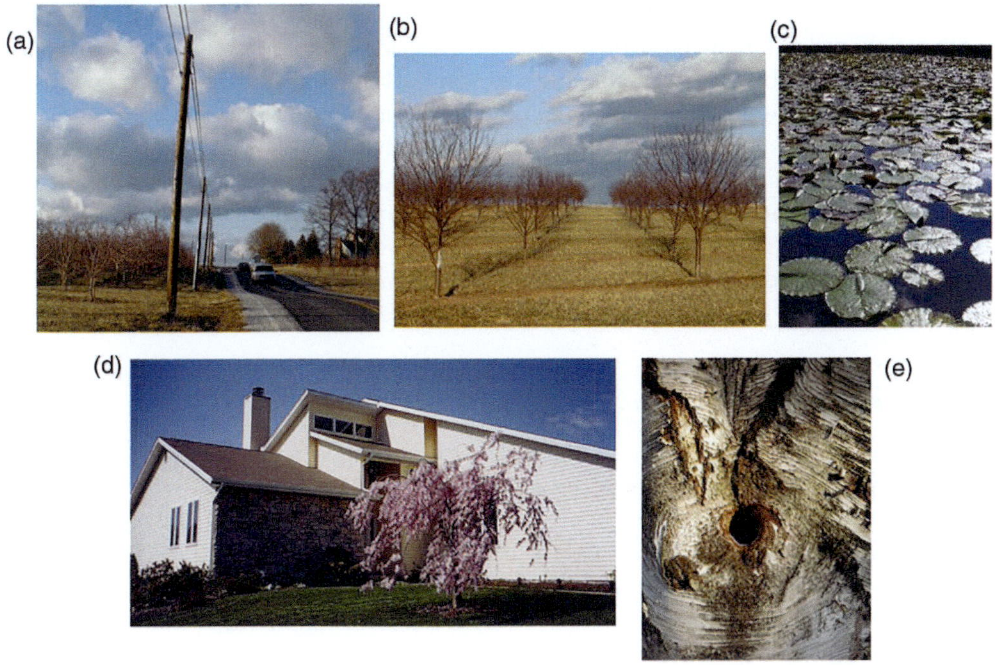

FIGURE 9.2 Examples of static-monocular depth cues, including familiar size (a), linear perspective (b), texture gradient (c), interposition (d), and shading (e).

Source: Courtesy of M. E. Arterberry.

Another cue is the convergence angle of the two eyes, or how much our eyes need to rotate toward each other to focus on an object. **Binocular convergence** appears to provide functional information about depth as early as 2 months of age, and binocular disparity sensitivity emerges around 4 months (Arterberry & Kellman, 2016).

Static monocular cues help us perceive depth as well (Figure 9.2). They are called monocular because these cues signal depth even when viewed with one eye. These cues are well-known and sometimes referred to as pictorial depth cues, because artists as far back as Leonardo da Vinci and Michaelangelo in the Renaissance used them to portray depth in a painting. One such pictorial cue is **familiar size**. If two like objects are known to be similar in size (e.g., the telephone poles in Figure 9.2a), having one appear smaller than the other in a two-dimensional space makes the smaller appear farther away. Another is pictorial cue in **linear perspective**: Two lines known to be parallel in real life (e.g., trees planted in rows in Figure 9.2b) are seen as moving away from the viewer (and so in depth) if they appear to converge. Other monocular cues to depth include **texture gradients**, which signal depth when the elements of the textured surface gradually reduce in size with distance (e.g., lily pads on a pond, as in Figure 9.2c); **interposition**, as when contours of one object partially block another object from view so that the first object is perceived to be closer than the second (e.g., a tree covering part of a house in Figure 9.2d); and **shading**, when areas of an object oriented away from a light source appear darker than areas oriented toward the light (e.g., a knot hole in the tree bark in Figure 9.2e). Infants become sensitive to these cues between 5 and 7 months of age (Arterberry & Kellman, 2016).

The world and the infants perceiving it are constantly in flux or moving, and movement information, called **kinetic** cues, provides a third set of cues to depth. One kinetic cue is **motion parallax**: Objects which are closer to you move across your field of vision faster than objects which are farther away. Infants appear to use this information about the relative motion of objects as early as 3 months of age (Nawrot & Nawrot, 2013). When you move through the environment, closer surfaces are also perceived to block more distant ones, a cue called **accretion-deletion of texture**. Such differences in the covering (deletion) and uncovering (accretion) of object surfaces provide information about the relative depth of objects, and infants respond to this information at 4 to 5 months of age (Bremner et al., 2012; Craton & Yonas, 1990).

Perception of Form

Objects like a simple cube have features, like edges and surfaces, but objects also have whole forms (the cube). Newborns can see object detail, like edges, but when do infants perceive whole forms? This question is interesting both practically and theoretically because some theorists (called Gestalt psychologists; Köhler, 1929, and Koffka, 1935) proposed that the perception of whole forms is innate, whereas others (called constructivists; Hebb, 1949, and Piaget, 1952) proposed that perception of whole forms is built up from perceptions of individual elements – lines, angles, and surfaces. Like the color question, the question of whole form perception has proven difficult to answer because almost any discrimination between two forms (say, a triangle and a circle) can be explained as a discrimination on the basis of some simple feature (such as an angle, from an arc, or different amounts of contour) without implicating the whole form. The clever use of **subjective contours** helped solve this problem. See Figures 9.3a and b. The black Pacman elements which are identical in (a) and (b) help the perceiver complete the edges and so see the illusory whole form square (a white square) in (a) but not in (b). At what age are infants able to perceive static subjective figures as whole forms? Some studies suggest they do so as early as 3 to 4 months, and others as late as 7 months (Kavšek, 2002; Kavšek & Braun, 2018).

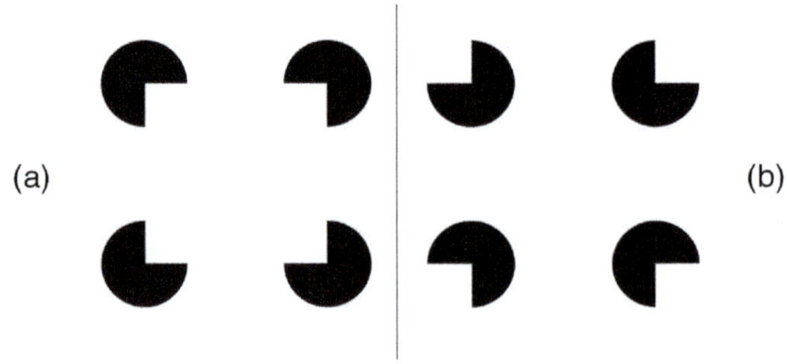

FIGURE 9.3 Pattern (a) is a static image that produces subjective contours, suggesting the whole form square. Pattern (b) made up of all the same elements, does not produce a static subject square.

Another challenge for perceiving form arises from perceiving form across different viewpoints and/or distances. The general term for this is **viewpoint invariance**, or understanding that an object viewed from different viewpoints is still the same object. Have a look your coffee mug. If you place it on your kitchen table and move to the other side of the table, it may look different. For example, the handle might not be visible, or if it is visible, the handle's shape might appear to be different from when you saw it before. However, you have no trouble recognizing your mug. You might use knowledge to help you recognize the mug. After all, you know that you just walked to the other side of the table. However, you could also be relying on principles of perception. Solid objects do not change even when our viewpoints of them change. Being able to recognize an object from different perspectives is an important step toward experiencing a stable perceptual environment, and at least by 5 months of age, infants perceive objects as the same object despite changes in their viewpoint (Mash et al., 2007).

Perception of People

Despite newborns' early start in face perception (Chapter 5), as infants grow and their acuity improves, so does their face perception. For example, the internal features of faces become more prominent on account of infants' ability to see finer detail (Turati et al., 2006). Moreover, 5-month-old infants can discriminate between a face with typical spacing of the eyes and mouth from a face with exaggerated spacing between those features, and they recognize faces across different emotional expressions (Bhatt et al., 2005; Bornstein & Arterberry, 2003). By 7 to 8 months, infants recognize the same face across different viewpoints (Kobayashi et al., 2011). Later in the first year of life, infants come to show better recognition of faces of their own race compared to faces of other races, likely based on their greater experience with same-race faces (Krasotkina et al., 2021).

People are not only unique objects in terms of how they look but also have distinctive motion patterns. The individual parts of the body, like the legs, arms, and torso, move in a coordinated way. In other words, they have **figural coherence**. A compelling example of figural coherence is the so-called point-light walker display, which specifies motions typical of human beings (Figure 9.4). All 11 elements are the same in 9.4a and 9.4b, and they all move in the same way, but when the elements are arranged as a person (as in 9.4a), adults and 6-month-old infants do not perceive these displays as unrelated randomly moving dots, nor do they focus on the motion paths of individual lights; rather, they observe such a dynamic light display as a person (Moore, 2012). Older infants even categorize motion patterns as specific to different emotions or different genders (Ogren et al., 2019; Tsang et al., 2018).

Perception of the Self

Proprioception is the sense we have of our own body in physical space. Information for proprioception comes from our vestibular system (in our inner ear) and receptors in our muscles and joints. Remaining upright and moving smoothly through space require

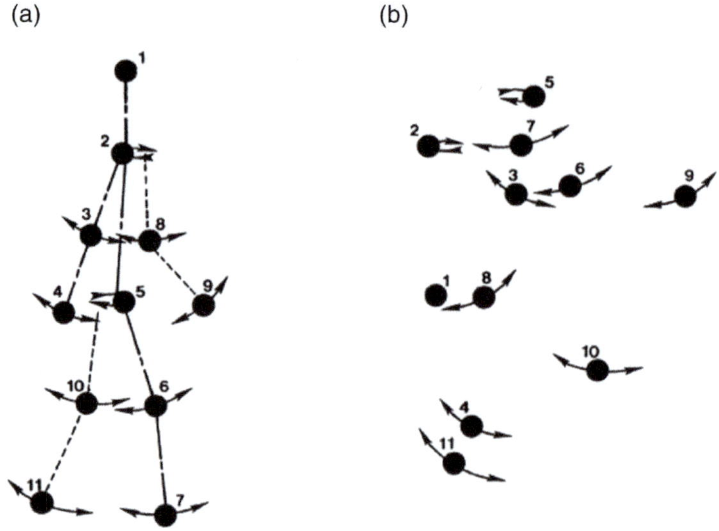

FIGURE 9.4 (a) An array of 11 point lights attached to the head and joints of a walking person. The motion vectors drawn through each point light represent the perceived relative motions within the figure. (b) An anomalous walker identical to (a), except that the relative locations of the point lights have been scrambled.

coordination of the visual and proprioceptive systems. Even before they are able to walk, infants seem to have an understanding of the visual consequences of their movements. A procedure to discover this involves showing infants a video image of their legs moving and an image of another child's legs or the mirror reversal of their own legs moving, which would be like *feeling* your left leg move but *seeing* your right leg move. Three- to 5-month-olds give evidence that they tell the difference between views of their leg movements that are congruent with their own actual movements from views that are incongruent with their actual movements (Schmuckler & Jewell, 2007).

Section Summary

The infant visual world is in color, and infants perceive color categorically. They also perceive their world in three dimensions. Infants are sensitive to different types of depth information at different ages: Motion-carried information about depth appears earliest, followed by binocular and static-monocular (pictorial) depth information. From an early age, infants perceive whole forms, even across different viewpoints, when they move, and even when the whole form is not fully visible, as in subjective contours and moving point lights. Infants are perceptually sensitive to characteristics of people and self, especially as they are sensitive to the coordination of what they see and what they feel when they make their own movements.

THOUGHT

Thinking in infancy encompasses what and how infants learn, what they know, and how what they learn and know guides their behavior. Thinking is broadly mental life, cognition, and intelligence. Consider for a moment what kind of mental life you might design for human infants. Certainly, you would not want to fix infants' intelligence in advance of any actual experience. It would be shortsighted and counterproductive to disregard likely effects of experience, because *intelligence* is fundamentally the ability to adapt successfully to the environment, which infants need to do. By the same token, however, you would not want to leave mental development wholly to experience. A big risk would be that developing cognition would only be shaped by particular, and likely limited, experiences, biasing some infants, possibly depriving others. In fact, both criteria appear to have been met in the evolution of infant cognition. Keeping these design criteria in mind, we now describe different ways of thinking about cognition in infancy. We begin with Piaget (who was mentioned at the start of this chapter) and the qualitative perspective on infant cognition. We then turn to a quantitative perspective on infant cognition, information processing, and memory.

Piaget's Theory

Between 1925 and 1932, Piaget watched closely as his own three children grew from infancy, taking note of the enormous intellectual progress each made during the first two years of life. Later, Piaget (1952) published *The Origins of Intelligence in Children,* a compilation of his observations and informal experiments.

To understand Piaget's theory, we need to appreciate that Piaget saw himself as a philosopher as much as a scientist and that he was formally trained as a biologist. He was initially motivated to study human children by a desire to resolve the debate about the origins of knowledge. Piaget was fascinated by the way in which the human mind comes to understand concepts like space, time, causality, and substance. He did not believe the strictly nativist idea that knowledge of these concepts was innate. At the same time, he also disagreed with the strictly empiricist view that all knowledge derived solely from experience. Rather, Piaget came up with a radically new solution to the philosophical problem of the origins of knowledge. Piaget asserted that infants construct an understanding of the world on the basis of their own activity and interactions in the world.

The Scheme

For Piaget, the basic element of infant knowledge is the **scheme**. The scheme is a hard concept to define concisely. Its meaning is, to some extent, captured in the notion that schemes are central nervous system structures that produce motor activities capable of processing information in the environment. Stated even more simply, schemes are ways of acting on the world. In newborns, schemes are more or less automatic motor activities, like reflexes, although not all reflexes (sneezes and coughs) are schemes. However, many automatic motor activities, like sucking, grasping, looking, hearing, and tasting, can be used to acquire or process information in the environment. Piaget considered looking and hearing to be actions – not simply the passive registration of sensory information. According to Piaget, knowledge begins to develop as the elaboration of simple reflex schemes present in the newborn.

Piaget's constructive notion of the scheme rests on the claim that knowledge begins with actions rather than sensations. However, Piaget argued that there must be a central mechanism for filtering out sensory inputs (i.e., we do not attend to every sensation that falls on our sense organs) and for assigning meaning to sensations. Schemes help infants give meaning to sensation. Behavioral schemes (physical activities) dominate infancy, but eventually, mental schemes, which are cognitive activities, come into play. Piaget emphasized that infant cognition is not static. Rather, infants create, respond to, and adjust to an ever-changing world; that is, infant mental development is self-modifying. To explain processes underlying this kind of development, he invoked the biological concept of adaptation but applied it to a psychological context.

Adaptation

Adaptation is the fundamental process whereby schemes are altered through experience. Adaptation itself consists of two complementary processes, assimilation and accommodation. Information processed according to an existing scheme is termed **assimilation**, and meaning is assigned to it on that basis. For example, the sucking scheme is initially applied to the breast or bottle, but when newborns mouth a finger and start sucking, they have assimilated the finger to the sucking scheme. For the moment, the finger has a single meaning or function – it is suckable. Individual sensations – taste, touch, vision, and so forth – that are simultaneously experienced have no meaning in themselves unless or until infants turn their schemes to them. According to Piaget, assimilation is a conservative process because infants do not change an existing way of acting on the world.

At times, however, an existing scheme cannot successfully assimilate new information. For example, infants may try to mouth a fist rather than a finger and, of course, will not succeed if attempts to do so are the same as attempts to mouth the finger (that is, by sucking through pursed lips). Two things could happen. One is that infants fail to assimilate the fist-to-suck event and simply move on to another activity. The other is that infants change the existing sucking scheme, perhaps by widening the mouth, so as to permit new information to be processed. Modification of an existing scheme to new information is termed **accommodation**. Importantly, in Piaget's view, the environment does not simply act on passive, receptive infants; rather, infants actively change to better respond to the environment.

Cognitive change through accommodation is slow. Newborns, infants, and children do not suddenly modify all schemes to accord with physical reality. The agreement between existing schemes and what may be novel in the environment must be sufficiently high that newborns, infants, and children know which schemes to modify. When there is agreement between reality and their schemes, a state of mental balance or equilibrium exists. Piaget was primarily interested in processes whereby mental equilibrium at more and more reality-based levels is attained.

With the concept of the scheme as a foundation, Piaget contended that knowledge begins with action and that acquiring knowledge depends on doing rather than observing passively (although we know that observational learning does often occur). Thus, Piaget was a constructivist in that he asserted that individuals actively construct their own development (as they do in a transaction). Piaget's influence is evident in our frequent stress in this book on the active role newborns, infants, and children play in shaping their own development (Arterberry & Kellman, 2016; Lerner, 2018).

Piaget's Sensorimotor Stages of Cognitive Development

As you may recall, stage 1, reflexive schemes, of Piaget's sensorimotor theory of cognitive development was introduced in Chapter 3. According to Piaget, newborns' mental development is minimal and very slow because newborns are unable to act on their own and thus are unable to shape their own development. Stages 2 through 5 of Piaget's theory emerge during the infant period of life.

Stage 2: Primary Circular Reactions. During stage 2, infants begin to coordinate schemes, but such inter-coordination still provides little information about the outside world. For example, 3-month-olds can coordinate their hands and mouths and may repetitively grasp and let things go, but they still appear to repeat these actions for their own sake rather than because they are learning how the outside world works. Piaget used the term **primary circular reactions** to describe infants' tendencies to repeat such chance discoveries involving the coordination of two actions. He called them circular reactions because they are repetitions of chance discoveries, and designated them primary because they are the earliest of a series of circular reactions to emerge. Another such coordination occurs when infants turn toward the source of sounds. According to Piaget, there is no evidence that infants expect to see something; rather, infants turn to activate looking and hearing schemes simultaneously.

Stage 3: Secondary Circular Reactions. In Stage 3, infants become aware of relations between their own behavior and the environment. For example, when infants accidentally produce environmental events, they may repeat them (like kicking their legs and seeing a mobile move) supposedly because they want to review their effects on the environment. Because infants produce actions repeatedly (as they did in stage 2), Piaget still termed them *circular reactions*, although he called stage 3 versions **secondary circular reactions**. Now, infants begin to notice and focus on events in the outside world, but infants still understand the world based on action, rather than on an appreciation of relations among objects. For example, if infants discover that kicking the side of the crib causes a mobile to move, they might continue to kick even when too far away to reach the side of the crib.

Stage 4: Coordination of Secondary Circular Reactions. By stage 4, infants coordinate secondary circular reactions. One circular reaction might be to reach for an object, and another might be to pull the placemat on which the object sits closer. Combining these actions would entail pulling a placemat closer and then reaching for the object sitting on the placemat. Infants have constructed some relations among environmental stimuli, now understanding that one object can be in front of or cover another. Consequently, infants are now able to remove a cover that is hiding an object. This action is something that should have been possible (in terms of motor abilities) far earlier if relations between the hidden object and the cover had been understood. However, infants still commit the **A-not-B error**. In the A-not-B task, an object is hidden at location A (as the infant watches while it is hidden), and then the infant searches for it. After several successful trials, the object is hidden at location B, again while the infant is watching. The most common response is the infant continues to search at A, not B. For Piaget, this shortcoming constituted strong evidence that perceptual information is not sufficient to account for cognitive understanding and behavior; rather, what infants remember and act on is their success with prior actions. The A-not-B error is a mistake infants make around 8 months or so. By this age, infants can retrieve an object that is fully covered, but they search incorrectly if the hiding location is changed.

Stage 5: Tertiary Circular Reactions. In stage 5, many infant schemes are accommodated to the world outside the infant, and many unexpected relations among objects are discovered. Hence the emergence of **tertiary circular reactions**, in which infants cause something to happen accidentally (as in secondary circular reactions) but then systematically and deliberately vary the manner in which the event is brought about. For example, infants might attempt to see whether milk leaks out of a bottle at different rates depending on the angle they hold the bottle and the force with which they shake it. These tertiary circular reactions help infants understand that their actions can produce novel ends. This achievement anticipates infants' capacity to engage in insightful problem-solving (without relying on trial and error) at times when they must employ novel means to achieve novel ends.

Infants in stage 5 still suffer limitations in understanding relations among objects. For example, they cannot conceive **invisible displacements**. In this situation, three cloths are lying on a table. If in one continuous movement an object is hidden in a hand and the hand moves under and then re-emerges from cloth A, and then moves under and re-emerges from cloth B, and then under cloth C, stage 5 infants can find the object only if they actually see the object being removed from and hidden behind each cloth. In other words, if the hider opens a hand between each pass under the cloth, infants can find the hidden object. However, if the hider's hand conceals the object being hidden, infants appear as if they have no idea where the object is or how to go about searching for it. Similarly, if the hider leaves the object at B but still moves a hand under C, infants search at C (called C-not-B; Figure 9.5). In short, stage 5 infants still have an incomplete understanding of possible relations between objects. According to Piaget, they cannot represent in their minds movements of objects that are not visible. Furthermore, although infants no longer make the A-not-B error when searching for hidden objects, their solution for new problems involves a slow process of trial and error. This result also gives evidence that infants use their knowledge of previous actions and do not rely on perceptual information (what is happening right in front of their eyes).

Piaget provided another example of faulty reasoning at stage 5. He described placing his daughter Jacqueline in a playpen with a cardboard rooster just outside it. (Playpens in those days had slats, like a crib, not the mesh screening used today in the typical "Pack and Play.") The rooster had to be tilted away from the child in order to be pulled between the slats of the playpen, and Jacqueline should have been able to see that the slats of the playpen would get in the way if she tried to pull the rooster in straight on. She tried to do this anyway. Moreover, although the rooster kept banging into the slats, Jacqueline did not try to adjust the orientation of the rooster. Only when the rooster fell from her hands

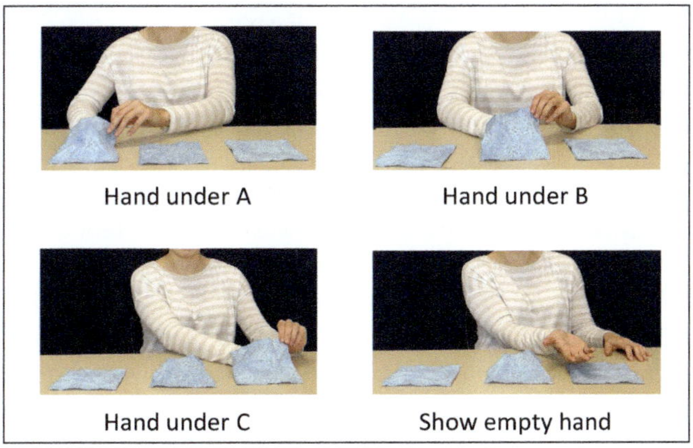

FIGURE 9.5 The C-not-B task tests infants' understanding of invisible displacement. The three cloths are referred to as A, B, and C (from left to right). The experimenter hides a ball in her hand and moves it under all three cloths. She leaves the ball at B in this example (note the bump) and shows the empty hand after passing under C.

Source: Provided by M. E. Arterberry, after Arterberry et al. (2018).

accidentally in the right orientation did she succeed in bringing the toy into the playpen. However, even this accidental success did not affect her behavior when her father once again placed the rooster outside her playpen. Only after Jacqueline started to drop the rooster deliberately, and to systematically vary its position in retrieving it, was she able to solve the problem. In this example, we see the importance of chance discoveries, the inattention to perceptual evidence, and deliberate variation of means only after chance success.

Mental Representation

Jacqueline's solution to retrieving the rooster anticipates a major development in mental life, **mental representation,** which refers to the ability to think about people, objects, and events even in their absence, and it is an important foundation of cognition. Piaget held that mental representations involve the internalization of motor activity. He theorized that the process of internalization unfolds slowly in time and does so for two reasons. First, motor activity initially does not closely match external reality but comes to match that reality over time and through exercising it. Second, motor activity might be internalized as thought or image or idea only if it is well rehearsed.

Information Processing and Memory

It is obviously important that infants attend to people, objects, and events in their environment to gain information about them, but it is also important that they be able to store, retrieve, and use that information later. Memory is vital to mental life. Memory representations underlie infants' awareness, experience, knowledge, and interpretation of the world. Memory is also multifaceted, and developmental scientists are interested in all dimensions of infant memory – in what infants can remember, in the nature of their memory representations, in the ways in which infants remember, and in how good infant memory is.

The information processing model of infant cognition focuses on how infants take in, store, and retrieve information, comparable to how a computer functions. One pair of processes of interest involves encoding and retrieval. **Encoding** specifies the transformation(s) of incoming information into memory. **Retrieval** specifies the search-and-find process(es) used to get information out of memory. The second pair of processes further differentiates retrieval into recognition and recall. To retrieve via **recognition** requires only to remember having previously experienced whatever is to be remembered, and contextual cues help with this type of memory. To retrieve via **recall** requires remembering a prior experience without the advantage of any cues.

How early in life do infants begin to remember? Does age affect memory processing? Does age influence forgetting? Perhaps the fact that so few of us remember anything about our own early life (before, say, the age of 2 years) provokes intense interest in such questions, although habituation and novelty responsiveness in newborns and infants strongly imply memory functions soon after birth (see Box 6.1). Indeed, the ability to remember may even go back to the prenatal period: Infants hear *in utero* and give evidence that after birth they remember what they heard (Pino, 2016).

Many physiological and behavioral components of memory change during the lifespan (Howe, 2015). Neuropsychological sites of memory (e.g., the hippocampus, thalamus, rhinal cortex, basal forebrain, and orbital prefrontal cortex) are still forming during the first year (Johnson, 2025). Some argue that there are two memory systems, one implicit or unconscious (non-declarative), as when children recognize their mother, and one explicit or conscious (declarative), as in remembering specific places. Implicit memory is believed to develop before explicit memory (Howe, 2015). Others argue that infants as young as 2 months of age encode, store, and retrieve information in ways similar to 18-month-olds and even adults, suggesting that memory processes are similar throughout development. Changes that occur over the course of development in this view are in amount or degree. In other words, a behavior becomes more efficient or refined, but it is fundamentally the same behavior.

Over the first 18 months of life, infant memory improves in several ways. They can encode information faster, retain information longer, and generalize better to different contexts and conditions. For example, a 4-month-old might recognize an object to which the infant had been familiarized up to a 10-second delay, a 6-month-old up to a 1-minute delay, and a 9-month-old up to a 10-minute delay. However, it is not simply that older infants remember more than younger infants. Factors that influence memory, such as study time and repetition, also change with age. Attention is a limiting factor in information processing at all ages, but with age infants focus more and more on relevant aspects of to-be-remembered people, objects, and events (Howe, 2015).

Repeated exposure to an event also affects later recall. To assess the effects of repeated presentation, Campanella and Rovee-Collier (2005) showed 3-month-old infants two puppets (A and B) paired together across 7 days. On day 8, infants saw a novel action with one of the puppets (B). Over the next 3 months, the infants saw puppet B (but not the modeled action) for approximately 30 seconds five more times. At 6 months of age, the infants were allowed to interact with puppet A, and they imitated the action they saw demonstrated with puppet B. This finding suggests that infants remembered the action done with puppet B, that seeing puppet B in the intervening months reminded infants of that novel action, and that infants associated the two puppets such that what was done with B could be done with A. Moreover, infants retained this information over 3 months!

Timing of the repeated experience is important as well. There appears to be a time window after experiencing an event during which the memory of the event is accessible (Hsu, 2010). If the event is re-experienced toward the end of this time window, it is likely to be remembered longer than if it is experienced at the beginning of the time window. Galluccio and Rovee-Collier (2006) tested the boundaries of this time window. Three-month-olds were trained with the mobile for 2 days (Box 9.3) and then given a session to reinstate memory – another training session with the mobile 1 day, 3 days, or 5 days later. Without reinstatement, infants remembered the mobile for 5 but not 6 days. Memory for the mobile was affected by the timing of the reinstatement. When reinstatement was 1 day after training, infants remembered the mobile for 6 days; when reinstatement was 3 days after training, infants remembered the mobile for 10 days; and when reinstatement was 5 days after training, infants remembered the mobile for 21 days. As infants age, the time windows become longer, yet reinstatement toward the end of the time window continues to be most effective for maintaining memories (Hsu, 2010).

Despite the preceding examples of impressive memory skills in young infants, we should not forget that infants forget more rapidly than adults. One factor that influences memory, or contributes to forgetting, is context (Howe, 2015). Context refers to aspects of the internal and external environments that are present during learning and processing information about an object. External context defines characteristics of the setting in which

Box 9.3 *How Do We Know This?* Operant Foot-Kick Procedure

One way developmental scientists have studied infant memory is using the operant foot-kick procedure. The procedure unfolds in three phases (see Figure 9.6). In phase 1, infants lie in a crib with a mobile overhead. A ribbon is attached to their leg, but their leg kicks do not cause the mobile to move (this phase serves as a baseline to measure spontaneous rates of foot kicking). In phase 2, the ribbon is connected to the mobile and infants' kicks cause the mobile to move; infants quickly learn the contingency between the two (or leg kick = mobile moves). This is the training phase. Phase 3 is the test. Like in phase 1, the infants' leg kicks do not cause the mobile to move; however, if infants remember that they could make the mobile move by kicking, then kicking during phase 3 should be higher than the baseline in phase 1. Using this paradigm, several questions can be asked about infant memory, such as how long infants can retain information, how different a new mobile can be to disrupt memory, and whether the context of learning matters.

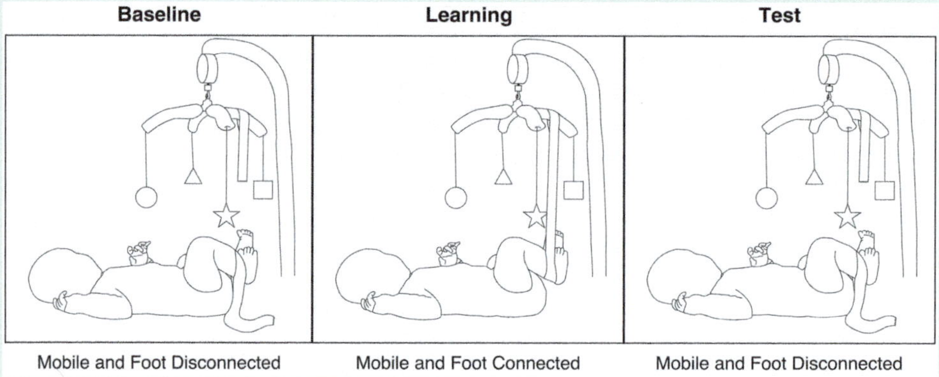

FIGURE 9.6 A setup for studying learning and memory using foot kicking.
Source: Created by A. E. Arterberry.

information about the person, object, or event is processed and encoded. Some attributes of context may be integral to information processing; others may be incidental. Nonetheless, both are important and influence how we sense, think, and remember information. For example, Rovee-Collier and Cuevas (2009) trained 3-month-olds to move a mobile by kicking. During learning, colorful bumpers (the context; Figure 9.7) lined the infants' cribs. Changes in the bumper did not affect retention of the contingency 1 day later, when the memory was fresh. However, after delays of 3, 5, and 7 days, retrieval was evident only when the bumper surrounding the crib during the retention test matched the bumper present during training. Older infants also show context effects. For example, 12- and 18-month-olds tolerate a change in room during visual assessments of memory, but 6- and 9-month-olds do not (Jones et al., 2011). Similarly, 12-month-olds tolerate changes in context with imitation tasks (Patel et al., 2013).

Rovee-Collier and Giles (2010, p. 203) suggested that "rapid forgetting is not a memory deficit but is an evolutionarily selected survival-related strategy." In their view, forgetting allows young infants to adapt to rapidly changing surroundings by forgetting unnecessary information and quickly learning new things. People, objects, and events that are frequently encountered (and thus are unchanging aspects of the infants' environment) are remembered due to study time, repetition, and context.

Section Summary

This section described two major schools of thought about mental life in infants. In his theory of sensorimotor intelligence, Piaget emphasized the importance of constructivism and motor activity in the development of knowledge. Piaget identified a series of stages in infant cognitive development. Fundamental to Piaget's theory are the scheme and the emergence of mental representation. Infant mental development is based on active engagement with the world, often employing trial and error to solve problems. The second

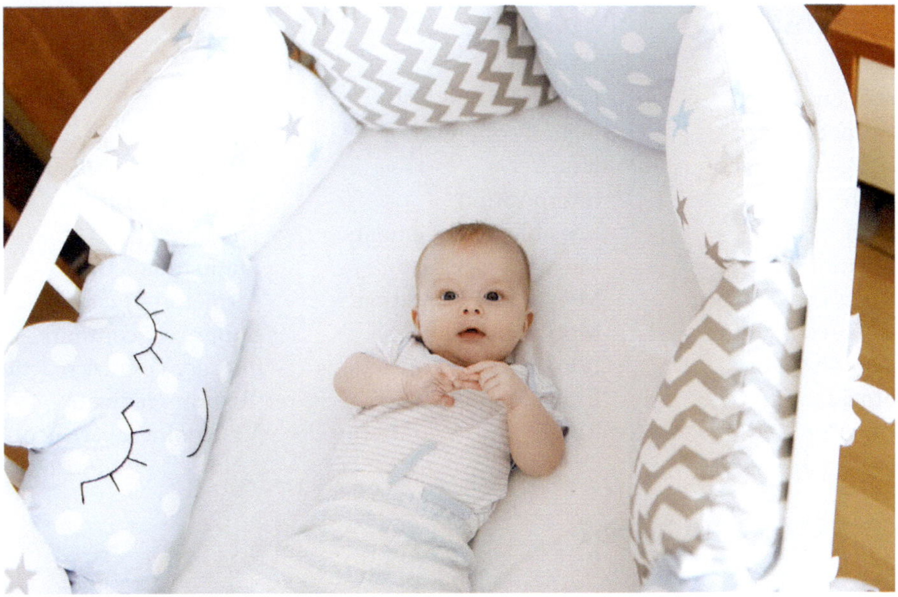

FIGURE 9.7 The colorful pillows along the edge of the crib are called bumpers. Bumpers provide context, and they can support retrieval of learned information after a delay. (By the way, the Centers for Disease Control and Prevention recommends that bumper pads be kept *out* of infants' normal sleep area; https://www.cdc.gov/reproductivehealth/features/baby-safe-sleep/index.html.)

school of thought related to information processing and memory. Infants have surprisingly sophisticated memory capacities. Common questions ask what skills or strategies infants use and how dimensions of memory define or limit infant memory. Encoding skills and short-term memory improve rapidly over the first year. As infants age, they demonstrate an ability to hold events in memory for longer time spans, and they require fewer cues and shorter periods of familiarization to recall past events. Infants appear to save some specific memories, and they can retrieve seemingly forgotten information if they are given a reminder. These memory abilities may be especially true for patterned, repeated events, such as those that occur in the context of parent interactions.

CONCLUSIONS

Infants see and process multiple dimensions of their visual world, like color and depth in space. They perceive details of forms as well as whole forms from an early age. They are perceptually sensitive to characteristics of people, including their selves. Two major schools of thought have developed to explain the mental life of infants. One is a qualitative theory advanced by Piaget, and it emphasizes stages, constructivism, and motor activity. The other is a quantitative information-processing theory that focuses on the skills or strategies infants use to remember as well as the dimensions of infant memory.

KEY TERMS

A-not-B error
Accommodation
Accretion-deletion of texture
Adaptation
Assimilation
Binocular convergence
Binocular cues
Binocular disparity
Brightness
Encoding
Familiar size
Figural coherence
Hue
Interposition
Invisible displacements
Linear perspective
Mental representation
Motion parallax
Primary circular reactions
Proprioception
Recall
Recognition
Retrieval
Secondary circular reactions
Sensory register
Shading
Static monocular (pictorial) cues
Subjective contours
Tertiary circular reactions
Texture gradients
Viewpoint invariance

SUGGESTED READINGS

Arterberry, M. E., & Kellman, P. J. (2016). *Development of perception in infancy: The cradle of knowledge revisited*. Oxford University Press.

Bornstein, M. H., Arterberry, M. E., & Mash, C. (2025). Perceptual development. In M. H. Bornstein & M. E. Lamb (Eds.), *Developmental science: An advanced textbook* (pp. 270–320). Routledge.

Flavell, J. H. (2020). *The developmental psychology of Jean Piaget*. Barakaldo Books.

CHAPTER 10

Infants

Emotions and Temperament

The gains made in growth, motor, perceptual, cognitive, and, as emotional development and temperament provide strong foundations for infants to engage with others around them. As we see too, infants between 4 and 17 months of age have complex emotional lives and demonstrative temperaments. Moreover, they communicate their feelings, which supports their social relationships, as we will learn in Chapter 11. Infants are not only influenced by the people in their environment but also influence those same people. The result is a strong enduring emotional bond called attachment. This two-part chapter first discusses emotions in infancy and then temperament.

EMOTIONS

Newborn emotions are largely circumscribed to three emotions: distress, possibly joy, and possibly fear. From 3 months onward, infants' emotional world expands. From distress, a primary emotion expressed from birth (Lewis, 2015), come sadness, disgust, fear, and anger by 6 months of age. For example, Lemerise and Dodge (2000) observed expressions of anger in infants as young as 3 to 4 months of age. Anger, rather than generalized distress, becomes increasingly typical in response to events that are unpleasant or restricting. For example, distress predominates the emotional responses of 2-month-olds to painful inoculations, but it is replaced by anger sometime after 12 months.

Sadness is another emotional expression, and it emerges in the infant period. Tronick (2007) observed that when mothers play with their 3-month-old infants and then suddenly become unresponsive (as in the still-face procedure; Box 10.1), infants show signs of withdrawal, wariness, and sadness in their facial and postural expressions. Infants react similarly if their social partner looks at a mobile phone rather than merely becoming unresponsive (Stockdale et al., 2020; Figure 10.1). Moreover, infants' responding with sadness to interruptions in social interactions is relatively stable from 3 to 9 months of age (Barbosa et al., 2018). This violation in the rules of interaction can be memorable. Bornstein and colleagues (2004a) found that infants tested in the still-face procedure at 5 months remembered the still-faced experimenter 15 months later, and they shunned looking at her.

DOI: 10.4324/9781003381709-12

Box 10.1 *How Do We Know This?* Measuring Emotions

Because babies cannot verbally express what they are feeling, emotion researchers rely on the emotional expressions babies make. Darwin (1872/1965) anticipated the current reliance of researchers on facial expressions of emotion when he noted that certain expressions are remarkably consistent across age and culture. Because the face has many muscles and can convey a broad range of expressions, and because we commonly use the face as our primary means of evaluating emotional experience, researchers have made extensive efforts to measure facial expressions of emotion in babies. Highly detailed, anatomically based measurement systems for coding specific muscle movements in the face have been developed. For example, Ekman's Facial Action Coding System (FACS; Cohn et al., 2007) illustrates how a broad range of specific and complex muscular movements in adults' faces can be discretely coded in a detailed but time-consuming procedure. Oster (2005) modified this system for babies (called Baby FACS), taking into account babies' unique facial configurations.

One powerful procedure for measuring emotionality is the still-face procedure. In the still-face procedure, adults, usually a parent, interact with their babies in a normal animated, interactive style for 1 minute. This interaction usually elicits joy. Next, adults assume a neutral facial expression and do not interact with their babies for 2 minutes. Babies differ in their response to this change in demeanor, but typically it is not a very pleasant experience for them. After making a few social bids, they often seem sad or confused; they avert their gaze and sometimes fret or cry. The session ends with 1 more minute of normal animated interaction, which hopefully relieves the stress babies experienced.

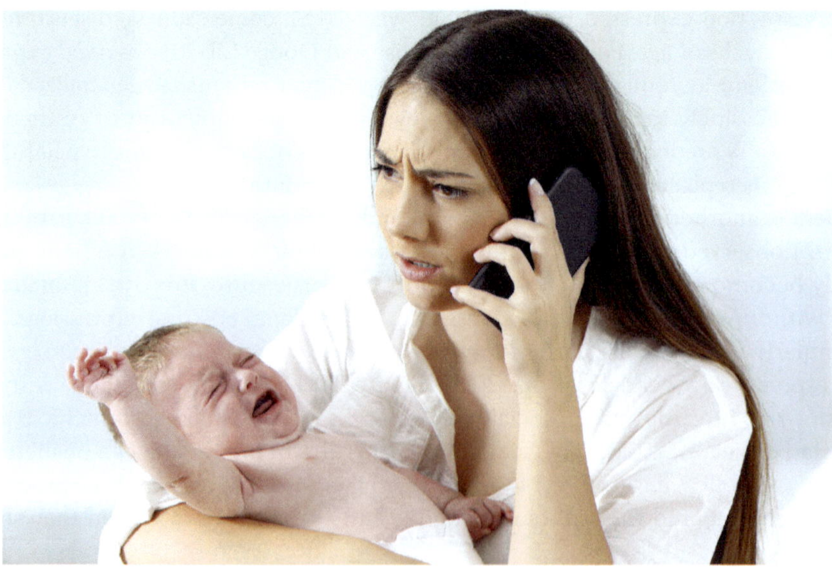

FIGURE 10.1 Infants often show distress when normal face-to-face interactions are disrupted.

Changes in Expressing Emotions With Age

As babies grow older, they become capable of expressing a wider range of emotions and become responsive to a growing variety of emotion-eliciting conditions. Advances in neurophysiological organization help inhibit primitive distress reactions and make it easier to express more complex emotions, such as anger. Other neurophysiological changes later in the first year also improve inhibition and self-regulation, especially of negative emotions (Leppanen, 2011). Cognitive changes further contribute to emotional growth by enabling babies to evaluate more complex situations. For example, toward the end of the first year, infants' reactions to strangers involve evaluation of the context (e.g., mothers' presence or absence), the setting (e.g., a comfortable and familiar environment or an unfamiliar one), the stranger's appearance (e.g., male or female, child or adult), and the stranger's behavior (e.g., approaching fast or slow, looming overhead or looking at eye level). These developments indicate that the growth of information-processing skills and reasoning processes (such as the capacity to anticipate events or to link means and ends) facilitates complex appraisals that underlie emotional reactions later in the first year. In other words, as infants' mental life dvelops in sophistication, their emotional life also becomes more sophisticated. Likewise, infants' growing verbal skills make possible alternative forms of emotional expression – through words rather than cries or clenched fists.

Infants' social experiences shape their emotional expressiveness. Mothers change their facial expressions an average of seven to nine times per minute during face-to-face play with their infants (Malatesta & Haviland, 1982; Malatesta et al., 1986). Mothers respond promptly to their infants' emotional expressions roughly 25% of the time, typically by imitating or responding positively to positive expressions (an example of positive reinforcement; Chapter 4) and ignoring negative expressions (an example of negative reinforcement; Chapter 4). Thus, contingent emotional responding of these sorts likely encourages the expression of positive emotions and mutes the expression of negative emotions.

Mothers become increasingly responsive to expressions of interest and decreasingly responsive to expressions of pain when their infants reach around 7 1/2 months of age (Malatesta et al., 1986). Not surprisingly, infants also change their expressive patterns at this time, showing more positive and fewer negative emotions, partly in response to their mothers' behaviors. Expressive behaviors of mothers and infants tend to be consistent over time, with substantial similarities between the two, suggesting that mothers may socialize and shape their infants' expressive styles from the early months of life (Granat et al., 2017).

In some extreme circumstances, parents can foster affective disturbances through similar socialization processes. For example, infants of depressed mothers tend to show depressed social behaviors (withdrawn, immobile, and nonresponsive) when interacting with their mothers (Bornstein et al., 2022b; Manian & Bornstein, 2009) and when interacting with strangers (Hane & Fox, 2006; Væver et al., 2020). These infants may have acquired such socioemotional styles on account of genetic similarity, through the psychological effects of the mothers' depression on them (e.g., learned helplessness, coping activities), by imitating their mothers' behavior, and/or by having fewer opportunities to develop social skills at home (Crnic & Lin, 2021; Mantis et al., 2019).

Darwin wrote that, when only 6 months old, his son Doddy may have expressed sympathy when his nurse pretended to cry. Pre-empathic capacities appear very early in a form of emotional contagion whereby babies spontaneously resonate with another's salient emotional expressions, most often observed in response to another's distress (Geangu et al., 2010, 2011). Such responses later become more genuinely empathic with the emergence of self–other differentiation and growth in the understanding of others' emotional expressions (Lewis, 2015). Instead of crying too, babies might try to soothe another baby by offering a toy or hug.

Perceiving Emotions of Others

Emotional competence involves reading as well as sending emotional signals, and many developmental scientists have studied babies' capacities to read the facial expressions of emotion in others. However, discriminating different facial expressions is not the same as understanding their meaning, and thus reading emotions requires important interpretive as well as perceptual capacities. As discussed in Chapter 4, visual acuity in early life is limited, possibly making it hard for newborns to distinguish among different facial features and expressive patterns. Yet at around 1 1/2 to 2 months of age, infants discriminate among different facial expressions of emotion; at 3 months they generalize emotional expressions among familiar faces (namely, their parents); and by 5 months they distinguish among and categorize variations in the intensity of some emotional expressions (Figure 10.2; Bornstein & Arterberry, 2003; Walker-Andrews et al., 2011). Discrimination and categorization of emotional expressions do not mean that infants understand the emotional meaning of these expressions. Infants may respond differently to different facial configurations (e.g., eyebrow position or mouth open or closed) without assigning specific emotional meanings to them.

Between 4 and 9 months of age, infants become more emotionally responsive to the expressions they observe (Striano & Vaish, 2006). Infants of this age range can match their

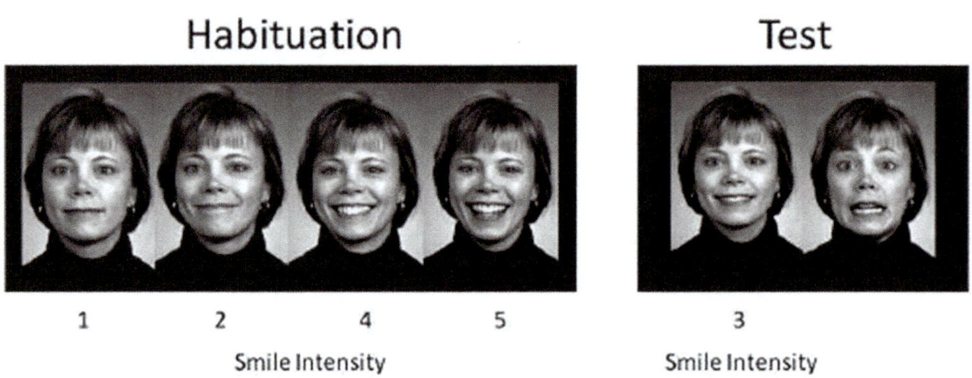

FIGURE 10.2 Stimuli used to test 5-month-old infants' categorization of the facial expression of smiling. Note that in the test display, the smile exemplar was not presented earlier in the habituation phase and that it represents a midpoint along the smile intensity continuum (1 is a slight smile, and 5 is a broad toothy grin). The far right expression is fear.

expressions to the emotional expressions of adults, and they may also acquire more enduring socioemotional dispositions when, for example, their caregivers are depressed (Bridgett et al., 2009). In fact, infants of depressed mothers might process facial expressions differently from infants of well mothers. Using a habituation test procedure, Bornstein and colleagues (2011) compared discrimination between a smiling and a neutral expression in infants of depressed and nondepressed mothers. Most infants of nondepressed mothers distinguished the two facial expressions, but most infants of depressed mothers did not. Infants of depressed and nondepressed mothers habituated to repeated presentations of the habituation stimulus in the same way (Box 6.1), suggesting that results were not due to some general difference in information processing. Thus, the experience of having a depressed mother could affect infants' perception and subsequent responsiveness to facial expressions.

Starting around 8 to 9 months of age, infants begin to appreciate that others' emotional messages pertain to specific objects or events. **Social referencing**, or the deliberate search for information to help clarify uncertain events, involves using others' emotional expressions to understand such ambiguous situations (Kim & Kwak, 2010; Figure 10.3). For example, infants may not approach a stranger unless a trusted adult (a parent or a newly acquainted experimenter) indicates that it is okay to do so by smiling or otherwise providing positive signals (Schmitow & Stenberg, 2013; Stenberg, 2017). Similarly, infants stop playing with unusual toys when their mothers show disgust as opposed to pleasure, and they continue to behave in this way even after their mothers stop posing distinct emotional expressions and are instead silent and neutral (Hornik et al., 1987). Infants

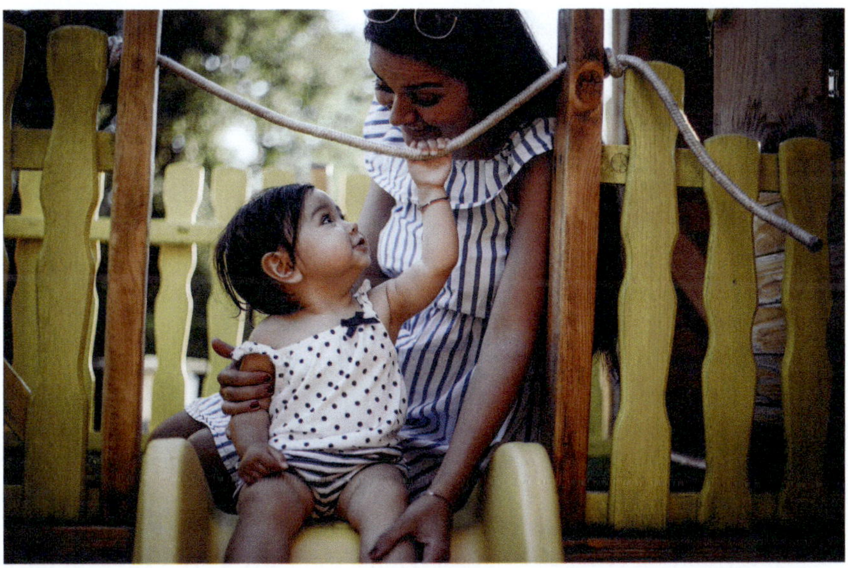

FIGURE 10.3 An example of social referencing, where infants monitor the emotional reactions of adults to help them interpret new situations. In this case, the mother's smile indicates that it is okay to go down the slide.

also reference emotional information presented by televised models (Mumme & Fernald, 2003), and 14-month-olds retain information gained in social referencing contexts for 24 hours (Hertenstein & Campos, 2004). These developments are hardly surprising. Emotional expressions are among the most important social signals, and thus we should expect that babies become attuned to them from early in life.

Section Summary

During the infant period, infants' emotional repertoire continues to broaden. Infants experience sadness, disgust, anger, interest, and joy early in the infant period, and fear emerges later. As infants age, situations that elicited one emotion (such as distress) may come to elicit another (such as fear). Emotional development is affected by the emotional expressions infants observe in others. In extreme cases, infants of depressed mothers have different experiences with emotional expressions, and this experience shapes their perception of emotions in others. Infants also reference others' emotions to interpret ambiguous situations.

TEMPERAMENT

Emotions are immediate responses to ongoing experiences and circumstances. In contrast, **temperament** reflects stable individual differences in behavioral functioning (Bornstein et al., 2015, 2019a; Rothbart, 2011). As children grow older, their temperament might lead them to prefer certain environments over others, especially settings that best suit their behavioral style. Highly active children might choose to become involved in sports, whereas low-activity children might select settings that foster sedentary activities, such as reading or conversation. Admittedly, this kind of **niche picking** (preferring certain environments over others, especially those settings that best suit a behavioral style) is harder for infants to accomplish, but similar preferences might be expressed by their selective interest in certain activities (e.g., vigorous play with one parent versus more low-key interactions with the other), which in turn have different developmental implications.

Of course, infants' primary caregivers play a large role in shaping the context in which temperament develops. For example, in their daily interactions with their babies, mothers can influence their infants' attentional styles and expressions of negativity (Bridgett et al., 2009, 2011). Such results have given researchers rich insights into the ways individual characteristics in temperament interact with environmental demands to shape and guide developmental outcomes.

Temperament is influential in the development of the individual but is not determinative. Rather, in the transactional view, children's long-term adjustment depends on interactions of their temperament and demands of their environment. Specifically, what may be most important is the **goodness of fit**, or match, between children and their developmental contexts (Johnson et al., 2025). Easy infants who have a low activity level, positive mood, and good adaptability likely fit well in a home or day-care setting that makes few demands and provides many opportunities for self-direction. But such an environment is likely a poorer fit for difficult infants who have a high activity level, unhappy mood, and low adaptability. In this light, temperamentally difficult infants will not inevitably experience later problems if parents understand, are tolerant of their infants' behavioral style, and provide activities in which their infants' characteristics can be channeled and valued. Conversely, even temperamentally easy children might experience problems if parents impose excessive demands or ignore reasonable needs. As a consequence, the sensitivity and adaptability of parents to their children's temperament are an important predictor of children's long-term adjustment.

Developmental scientists agree that temperament is defined by reciprocal influences between biology and environment (Rothbart, 2011). Moreover, contrary to simplistic views that good features of temperament lead to optimal developmental outcomes and bad features predict later behavioral problems, it appears that the outcomes of particular temperamental profiles depend on several factors. These factors include infants' biological endowments, the demands of environments in which the infants grow, the sensitivity and adaptability of their social partners, and the ways in which temperament itself guides children's choice of activities and interpretations of their experiences. Thus, temperament reflects stable individual differences in behavioral functioning, temperament can be described in terms of temporal and intensive features, and the match between the biology of temperament and the demands of the environment is key to the development of personality.

It is clear from this discussion (and from inspection of Table 5.1) that theorists conceptualize and study temperament in different ways, but it is unclear whether this diversity of approaches is desirable or not. On the one hand, different conceptualizations of temperament have led researchers to ask varied questions of different behavioral processes, often concerning individuals at markedly different periods of development. The diversity of empirical approaches has complicated the integration of findings from different research groups. On the other hand, multiple viewpoints are a common and desirable feature of scientific investigation in general. Indeed, the willingness of most theorists to revise their theories, and the current generation of new research findings that may contribute to such revisions, is promising in that a diversity of research efforts will yield useful findings that converge on common issues. If, in the end, the value of these theories is measured by their usefulness in explaining individuality of temperament, this heterogeneity of theory might converge on a common definition.

Stability of Temperament

Because contemporary theories of temperament in infancy include underlying biological (hereditary and constitutional) processes, it is tempting to expect temperament to be stable across the lifespan. After all, MZ twins show higher concordance in temperament dimensions than DZ twins (Gagne & Goldsmith, 2011). Generally, temperament is stable. For example, across the first year, infants, regardless of sex, birth order, term status, and SES, showed remarkable stability in temperament, as rated by their mothers (Bornstein et al., 2015). Moreover, infant temperament is equivalently stable in Chilean, United Kingdom, and American infants (Spinelli et al., 2022).

Stability of temperament is perhaps best illustrated in a 21-year longitudinal study by Kagan (2010; Kagan & Snidman, 2009). In this study, Kagan first classified 4-month-old infants as either high or low in reactivity and then examined them into adolescence. Reactivity was assessed by measuring infants' motor activity and responses to auditory, olfactory, and visual stimuli. Reactivity in temperament was fairly stable. Children classified as highly reactive in infancy were significantly more likely to react fearfully to novel stimuli at 14 and 21 months than were children classified as nonreactive. By 4 1/2 years, highly reactive children showed less spontaneity and sociability with adults than nonreactive children did, but highly reactive children were not as likely to appear fearful in response to novelty than they were at younger ages. By 7 years, highly reactive children were more likely to behave anxiously than were nonreactive children and were also more likely to have a higher diastolic blood pressure than were nonreactive children (diastolic blood pressure, the bottom number in a blood pressure reading, measures the period between heartbeats and is indicative of hypertension). By adolescence, inhibited children were more likely to have generalized social anxiety disorders (Chronis-Tuscano et al., 2009).

Kagan and colleagues speculated that inhibited children have a lower threshold of reactivity in limbic structures (such as the hypothalamus and amygdala) that mediate fear and defense, whereas uninhibited children have higher reactivity thresholds. Because of these neural differences, inhibited children show more fearful, wary, and shy behaviors, whereas uninhibited children are generally more outgoing and emotionally flexible. As predicted, fMRI examinations at 21 years of age revealed that individuals classified as inhibited as children showed more activity in the amygdala when they viewed novel, as opposed to familiar, faces than did individuals classified as uninhibited as children (Schwartz et al., 2003). The amygdala may not be the only region involved. Similarly, different levels of activity in the striate and caudate regions of the brain differentiate children who vary in reactivity and signs of social anxiety (Lahat et al., 2018).

These studies indicate that indexes of autonomic reactivity are related in a predictable manner to stable behavioral measures of reactivity and inhibition/self-regulation. According to Kagan (2007), however, these characteristics sometimes change when parents make concerted efforts to modify their children's attributes. For example, intervention programs have successfully taught parents to help their 3- to 5-year-old children who are at risk for social anxiety disorders to be less anxious (Lau et al., 2017). Thus, even though temperament is relatively stable, it is not immutable.

Section Summary

Although temperament is relatively stable across the lifespan, it can change during development on account of genetics and maturation, experiential influences, the contexts in which temperament is expressed, and the integration of facets of temperament into emerging personalities. Temperament patterns vary across cultures, with different patterns corresponding with different cultural orientations and genetic compositions.

EMOTIONS AND TEMPERAMENT

Emotional expressions and individuality of temperament share many features. Most theorists regard variability in emotionality as important, and babies' emotional expressions influence the caregiving environment in ways that are similar to the effects of activity level, sociability, and other dimensions of temperament. Current findings convincingly show that newborns and young infants express a variety of emotions that are predictably related to specific eliciting conditions. These findings support structural and functional portrayals of emotions and emotional development. With subsequent growth in a variety of developmental domains, the infants' emotional repertoire continues to broaden. Infants become emotionally responsive to a greater range of eliciting conditions, they are increasingly capable of coping with or regulating emotional experiences, and as a result, more complex emotions and emotional interrelations emerge. Emotional development not only involves these internal changes but also changes in the behavior of adult partners. Early emotional development is currently characterized by a variety of theories, but existing shortcomings of specific theories are balanced by contributions each makes to explaining emotional development – in terms of learning influences, the emotional climate of parent–infant interaction, cognitive development, or the biological heritage of the human species. Each theory helps explain small but important features of emotional development in infancy.

In focusing on emotional development and temperament, developmental scientists increasingly acknowledge that infants make significant contributions to their social interactions and that these interactions help shape development. Infants' emotional worlds are complex, as are their temperaments, both of which influence their social relationships. Moreover, emotions and temperament are impacted early in development by caregiving influences that accommodate, interpret, and channel infants' socioemotional characteristics. All this takes place in a cultural context, which also shapes the nature of infants' important early interactions.

CONCLUSIONS

Across infancy, emotions broaden. Infants express sadness, disgust, anger, interest, fear, and joy. Situations that initially elicit one emotion may come to elicit another. Emotional development in infancy is affected by the emotional expressions infants observe in others. Infants of depressed mothers have different experiences with emotional expressions from infants with typical mothers, and their experiences shape their perceptions of emotions in others. Temperament is relatively stable across the lifespan but can still change during development. Forces that operate to modify temperament include genetics and maturation, experiences, and the contexts in which temperament is expressed.

KEY TERMS

Emotional contagion
Goodness of fit
Niche picking
Social referencing
Temperament

SUGGESTED READINGS

Dukes, D., Samson, A. C., & Walle, E. A. (2022). *The Oxford handbook of emotional development*. Oxford University Press.

Tan, P., & Cole, P. M. (2019). Infant temperament and early self-regulation. In R. DelCarmen-Wiggins & A. S. Carter (Eds.), *The Oxford handbook of infant, toddler, and preschool mental health assessment* (pp. 175–223). Oxford University Press.

CHAPTER 11

Infants

Communication and Relationships

Language and communication begin to resemble understandable forms as infants develop from their first vegetative sounds and gestures to seemingly meaningless coos but very meaningful cries to the production and explosion of real words. Among infants, individual differences in all aspects of language comprehension and production are impressive. Language and communication, in turn, advance and intensify the development of interactions with parents and others. The heart of infant interactions is the development of meaningful relationships called attachments. The development of attachments occurs in identifiable stages and reflects the operation of a small number of behavioral systems. Infants develop attachments with particular attachment figures, and depending on the nature of their interactions, infant attachments fall into different types. Parents bring individual characteristics to their interactions with infants, just as infants bring a variety of idiosyncratic characteristics to their interactions with parents, and the eventual goodness of fit between them comes to define the nature of the parent–infant relationship.

COMMUNICATION: LANGUAGE DEVELOPMENT

Between 4 and 17 months, infants make tremendous gains in language. Although most 4-month-olds are beginning turn-taking in vocal "call-and-response," many 17-month-olds understand a lot of common language directed at them, and many can engage in rudimentary conversations. By the threshold of childhood, infants know the meanings of many words and likely have spoken their first real words. Here we chronicle language development during this compelling stage of acquisition, from first sounds to first words, and the extraordinary variability that typifies reaching these milestones.

Babbling

By the end of the newborn stage, babbling emerges as the result of a surprising amount of physiological coordination of movements of the mouth, tongue, and lips in combinations with the flow of air from the lungs to produce consonant-vowel combinations. It was once thought that babbling and true speech were distinct and discontinuous periods of vocal production (Jakobson, 1968). Such a conclusion seems intuitive; after all, babbling in newborns sounds random and makes no sense, whereas the sounds and plausible

DOI: 10.4324/9781003381709-13

words of infants carry meaning. However, continuity between babbles and first words is now recognized. Infants' babbles and first words are articulated by the same brain and oral anatomical mechanisms, and the two types of vocalizations share the same fundamental speech sounds. Moreover, babbling production continues to coexist with first words for several months, and infants frequently draw their early vocabulary from the repertoire of sounds established in the course of babbling (Lee et al., 2018). Fine-grained acoustic analyses have revealed that infants' first words incorporate frequently produced babbling sounds.

Early experiences influence the development and production of infant babbling. All infants use at least two sources of perceptual information when beginning to speak: the speech they hear and feedback from their own speech. Infants who do not hear speech at all or not very well, such as those who are hearing-impaired, babble as much as 5 to 19 months later than hearing infants (Oller, 2000). Deaf children almost never learn to articulate speech in the same manner as hearing children. The parameters of deaf children's speech production vary significantly in such dimensions as intonation, rhythm, and stress patterns, although, of course, their language production in sign may be perfectly fluent (Mora et al., 2012). Thus, auditory input is necessary for the timely development of normal spoken syllables and words. In addition, some components of babbling resemble the infant's local language and so must be positively influenced by local auditory input. Babbling infants come to match the consonant–vowel (CV) frequency and accent characteristic of the language around them (Majorano & D'Odorico, 2011). Moreover, vocalizations in infants can be shaped by contingent social reinforcement. Goldstein and Schwade (2008) studied the role of feedback from mothers for their 9-1/2-month-old infants' vocalizations. Half of the mothers in their study were instructed to provide responses to their infants' babbling with social feedback (smiling, moving closer to the infant, touching) contingent on infants' vocal production. The other half gave non-contingent responses; that is, they responded only whenever the experimenter told them to. Infants receiving contingent responses increased in their number of speech sounds, and they restructured their babbling to incorporate vocal patterns from their mothers' speech. Also, other, larger linguistic and cultural contexts shape the development of infant vocalization. The amount of language input has important implications for the detection of sounds and words as well as for language processing speed and vocabulary development.

First Words

Infants cry, babble, and even gesture to communicate effectively before they acquire and use words. But these methods of communication are severely limited. For example, it is impossible for infants to use gestures to share a memory, and all parents attest to their frustrations at the ambiguity of infants' cries and babbles. The next steps are for infants to learn that specific sounds have specific shared meanings and to communicate with them.

Insofar as infants are learning language from the language washing over them – by imitation or observation or reinforcement – a major obstacle confronting language-learning infants is the problem of **reference**, the link between sounds and their meaning. Consider this sentence: *Yourteddyislyingonthecouchsweetie.* To understand this simple statement, even after parsing the acoustic signal into separate meaningful sound units correctly, infants must determine which unit refers to them ("*Sweetie*"), which to objects ("*teddy*," "*couch*"), which to an action ("*is lying*"), and so forth. Connections between sounds and word meanings are essentially arbitrary, which makes the decoding task all the more difficult. The main questions about infant word development turn on how reference is defined, when it begins, and what its origins are.

What Is a Word?

Appreciate the challenge of even the most basic aspect of the problem, namely, defining what an infant's first word is. This challenge is problematic because what a word is for a newly talking infant is open to dispute. Is "*baba*" (for bottle) a real word, even if used consistently to refer to bottle and nothing else but bottle? Some developmental linguists argue, yes, it is. Others would say that the infant has to clearly articulate "*bottle*" to count as a word; for them, "*baba*" is a proto-word. Regardless of the disagreement over what a word is, linguists agree that producing a word reflects **nominal insight** – an understanding that things have names. First words can appear as early as the infant's first birthday.

Developmental linguists can be quite picky about awarding infants credit for saying a "word." By 9 months, many soon-to-be English-speaking infants use single sounds in regular or stereotyped ways: "*mama*" upon request, "*dat*" to show, "*bam*" for things falling. Therefore, infants might not have pronunciations and word meanings that align with those in their target language, but they have taken the important step of using specific sounds to mean specific things, even if this usage only occurs in specific and limited contexts. This is a least-conservative definition of using a word. For example, an infant might use "*bam*" to refer to falling, but only for an object falling from a high chair and not when they themselves fall down, or "*car*" to refer only to the family car and not to any other cars. For conservative linguists, such **context-restricted** "words" do not give evidence of true word use because these sounds are not applied to *classes* of people, objects, or events. More conservatively, infants might attain reference only when they use sounds that clearly name people, objects, or events. By the time they are 12 or 13 months of age, infants might use "*mama*" to mean *mother* in a variety of settings and situations and not exclusively when their mother is in a particular place or performing a specific activity. More conservatively still, crediting infants with reference might have to wait until around 16 to 18 months, when infants use single words to convey a full sentence's worth of meaning. This strictest attribution of word knowledge involves infants' understanding or using labels even when the referent is not present, for example, a child saying "*dog*" to ask where the family dog is. In both comprehension and production, this development gives evidence of a true shift from context-restricted to **context-flexible** usage, signifying a distinct, mature level of understanding of what words mean.

Nouns Versus Verbs

To what do infants' first words refer? One might expect that infants' first words would be those that they hear most often and that the part of speech (noun, verb, adjective, etc.) of first words would be proportional to the number of words infants hear in each part of speech. But this is not true – or at least the story is not that simple. The two most frequent

English words in speech to infants are "*you*" and "*the*," which are rarely, if ever, in the top 50 of infants' first-produced words. Thus, word frequency is not the sole key to early vocabularies. Most studies of English and other languages have found that a large number of early words are nouns, at least if the words are identified in terms of their adult part of speech (Bornstein, Cote, et al., 2004). As language development progresses, infants' vocabulary expands to include more verbs, adjectives, articles, and pronouns (MacWhinney, 2015).

A number of explanations for the noun advantage in infants' early vocabularies have been proposed (Bornstein, Cote, et al., 2004; Waxman et al., 2013). One or all of them may be true to some degree. The standard view is that the key factor is the ability of infants to learn the concept to which a word refers. Nouns often refer to concrete people or objects or events, and verbs often refer to relations between things. Because noun notions like *dog* are easier to see, hear, feel, etc. than verb notions like *give*, infants learn nouns more easily and quickly, and so they know more nouns. A second view is that understanding the meaning of verbs depends on understanding nouns. It is nouns that engage in actions (e.g., *dad gives a kiss*). A third view is that the noun advantage is language-specific. Some languages are noun-friendly in that they require nouns to be spoken to convey meaning. In contrast, other languages are verb-friendly, because speakers may drop a noun if the context is sufficient to support the meaning. So infants learning noun-friendly languages (such as English and French) learn more nouns than verbs compared to infants learning verb-friendly languages (such as Japanese and Korean). A fourth view is that input factors play a role. Adult speech consists of more nouns than verbs, and so infants first speak more nouns than verbs. A fifth argument is that nouns are much more likely to appear at the beginnings and ends of utterances. It is easier for infants to remember and recognize words that appear in these prominent positions in utterances, suggesting that this structural feature of language might influence rates of word learning as well. Additional support for this argument is that, when verbs appear at the end of utterances, such as those ending in *-ing* (*He is running.*), infants have less difficulty acquiring their meaning than verbs that appear in the middle of utterances. Although there is evidence for and against each of these arguments, on balance they together tilt word acquisition in favor of nouns.

Individual Differences in Vocabulary

Like many other domains of development, infants differ vastly in their comprehension and production of words. Various attempts have been made to account for widespread individual differences in infants' early vocabularies. Many explanations focus on variation in infants' experience, primarily in the speech infants hear from their parents. The types and amounts of speech parents use vary systematically with their socioeconomic status (SES, a principal component of which is education), ethnicity, multilingualism, and other factors (Hoff, 2015). For example, parents lower in SES tend to talk substantially less to their infants than parents higher in SES do. This difference in input is believed to affect infants' own vocabulary development and language processing efficiency, and its effects may span generations: Lower-SES parents speak less to their children who learn and know less language and, in turn, use less language with their own children (Fernald et al., 2013; Sohr-Preston et al., 2013). Additionally, parents' use of specific kinds of language also differs along class lines. Higher-SES mothers tend to elicit conversations with their infants, whereas lower-SES mothers tend to direct their infants' behavior. Furthermore, infants exposed to more than one language acquire vocabulary in each language at levels that match the ratio of exposure to one language versus another. So infants whose linguistic environment is predominantly Spanish with some English will speak more Spanish words than English words (Song et al., 2012). Similarly, teen parents and older siblings caring for younger siblings talk less to infants than adult parents do, and infants in these caregiving situations acquire vocabulary more slowly and experience other delays in language development (Hoff, 2015).

Generally speaking, input matters. Not only does input affect vocabulary development, input also affects language processing speed and other aspects of cognition (Friend et al., 2018; Teepe et al., 2017). Moreover, input can have longer-term consequences: The amount and types of language input (unusual words) at early stages of development predict language usage at later stages (Bornstein, Cote, et al., 2012; Pruden et al., 2011). Importantly, interpretation of the direction of influence is uncertain. Language acquisition by children illustrates transaction. It could be that maternal speech influences infant speech *or* that infants who use more language earlier promote language use by their mothers or both. In addition, systems infuse language development in infancy: Infants' ability to pay attention shapes how long language interactions with parents will last, and so their exposure to language (Teepe et al., 2017).

That input matters does not negate what individual differences in infant brain development, information processing, memory, and cognition generally, as well as their emotions and temperament, all bring to promote or inhibit infants' acquisition of language. In the end, infants' mental and social lives, in combination with their verbal experiences, fuse to make up the speaking and comprehending child.

Section Summary

Infants transit a set series of stages on their way to becoming more able conversationalists. The consonant-vowel pairings that emerge with babbling allow infants to practice the sounds they eventually use to form words. The earliest sounds that infants produce are not specific to their linguistic environment. Very soon, however, both sound perception and production become subject to the linguistic environments provided by parent and culture. Language exposure promotes the development of language. The appearance of first words is a significant milestone, likely representing a cognitive revolution in infants' understanding of what language is and what it is used for. How infants learn words is still under debate, but it is likely that they employ principles or constraints that aid them in doing so.

RELATIONSHIPS: DEVELOPMENT OF ATTACHMENTS

Attachments are critically important in infants' early relationships. Recall that attachments are specific, enduring, emotional connections between people. In proof of the systems perspective in developmental science, they have significance across many domains of development. Bowlby (1969) described four phases in the development of attachments, the first of which – the newborn phase of indiscriminate social responsiveness – was described earlier in the "Newborn" section of this book. The next two phases apply in infancy: discriminating sociability and attachments.

The second phase of attachment moves from the newborn's indiscriminate social responsiveness to the infant's **discriminating sociability**. Bowlby (1969) wrote that discriminating sociability began in the second or third month of life. Presumably because significant others (such as parents) have been associated with pleasurable experiences (e.g., feeding, cuddling, rocking, and playing) and with relief of distress, those familiar people become the people with whom infants prefer to interact. Initially, infants' preferences manifest themselves in fairly subtle ways. Certain people will be able to soothe them more easily and to elicit smiles and coos more readily and regularly. Parents are enormously rewarded by this change to discriminating sociability in their infants' behavior. Such preferences indicate that infants view their parents as special and that infants appreciate the effort parents put into caregiving.

During this second phase of social development, infants are also far more coordinated behaviorally than they were earlier. Infants' arousal levels are less variable, and they now spend larger proportions of their awake time in alert states. Distress is less frequent, and interactions with adults more often involve play (Roopnarine et al., 2005). In many Western cultures, face-to-face games make their appearance in this second phase of attachment, becoming prominent when infants are around the middle of the first year. In earlier face-to-face interactions, adults assumed primary responsibility for keeping adult–infant interactions going. However, infants are less and less simply passive partners in face-to-face games, like peekaboo. Two- to 3-month-olds respond with boredom, distress, or withdrawal when their mothers become unresponsive, shedding their previous indifference for a more typical interactive and responsive stance (DiCorcia et al., 2016). Infants now seem genuinely concerned when adults fail to follow basic rules of turn-taking in interactions, indicating that infants understand something of these rules, find synchronized and reciprocal interactions enjoyable, and expect their partners to follow the rules.

From repeated experiences in face-to-face play and distress–relief sequences, infants are learning at least three important lessons. The first is **reciprocity**. In social interactions, partners take turns acting and reacting to others. The second is **effectance**. Infants learn that their behavior can affect the behavior of others in a consistent and predictable fashion. The third is **trust**. Their caregiver can be counted on to respond when signaled. Incorporating these lessons is key to becoming social. As infants realize that their coos, cries, and smiles elicit predictable responses from others, they develop concepts of themselves as individuals who significantly affect others and develop a more coherent view of the social world. The degree to which significant others in infants' lives are predictable instills growing confidence regarding infants' reliance on those others – that is, the degree to which they trust or have faith in the reliability of specific people. In turn, trust builds the security of their attachment relationships.

Phase 3 heralds and consolidates infant attachments which endure to childhood. By the middle of their first year, infants give evidence that they understand and respect the rules of reciprocity in their interactions, and they have preferences for interacting with **attachment figures** (normally parents). Their confidence in others reinforced, infants at this age enjoy their newly acquired ability to creep around and begin to move close to those attachment figures instead of waiting for others to come in response to their coos or cries. In the second half of their first year, infants are increasingly likely to initiate interactions using directed social behaviors (by calling or pointing, for example), and they begin to balance physical proximity to parents and exploring their environment. At this phase, parents provide their infants with a **secure base** for venturing farther afield and exploring the world beyond the dyad.

Attachment figures have now come to occupy a unique and significant place in the lives of their infant. As they assume an increasingly active role in their relationships, infants also begin to protest (by crying) when separated from attachment figures. According to Bowlby, separation protests are signals aimed at making attachment figures return. These protests are a sign of **separation anxiety**, fear when the attachment figure is not present or is preparing to leave. Infants quickly learn that some adult activities, like picking up keys, putting on a coat, or packing a bag, predict leaving, and they are not shy about expressing displeasure when these activities begin. The emergence of separation anxiety is linked to infants' attaining a concept of **person permanence**, the notion that people have a permanent existence (Ainsworth, 1973).

Major changes in social relationships take place between the beginning of this third phase of attachment and again around the advent of the second year and the end of phase 3. Infants become increasingly sophisticated in their abilities to behave intentionally, communicate verbally, and respond appropriately in different contexts. As infants grow older, they initiate an increasing proportion of their social interactions. They also come to tolerate growing distances from attachment figures, and they become more adept at interacting with peers and unfamiliar adults.

Attachment Figures

The onset of phase 3 is marked by the formation of attachments. Two key questions arise about this time. The first is by what processes attachments form, and the second is to whom infants become attached. The first question is about processes, and ethologists have turned to the animal world to gain insights into those processes. Studying young ducklings, the Austrian zoologist and Nobelist Konrad Lorenz (1935/1970) described what seemed to be ducklings' innate predisposition to **imprint** on an object. Shortly after hatching, ducklings remain close to whatever salient moving object is present, usually the mother, during a sensitive period. Attachment formation is not as instantaneous and takes longer in humans than in ducklings. Moreover, it is unlikely that imprinting in ducklings and attachment in humans result from similar mechanisms (Roisman & Groh, 2011). At the same time, attachment and imprinting share some commonalities in terms of dependence on exposure and the lasting sense of offspring–parent relationships. Bowlby was influenced by Lorenz's work on imprinting when he proposed a comparable predisposition in human infants to form attachments (Oates et al., 2005).

With regard to the second question, according to Bowlby, the consistency of adults' presence and their availability during a sensitive period – the first six postnatal months – determine to whom infants will become attached. If there is no consistent caregiver over this period (as might occur in institutions such as orphanages), infants would not form attachments. Bowlby and his co-theorist, Mary Ainsworth, believed that most infants develop a hierarchy of attachment figures and that their primary caregivers – those persons who spend the most quality time with infants, usually a parent – become primary attachment figures before infants form any other relationships as strong. Once infants have this foundation, they may, and often do, form relationships with others, for example, grandparents, older siblings, and day-care providers (Ahnert, 2021).

Substantial evidence has now accumulated that infants develop attachments to both parents (Brown et al., 2022). In the normal course of development, 7-, 8-, 12-, and 13-month-olds tend not to show systematic preference for one parent over the other on several measures of attachment (such as staying near, approaching, touching, crying to, and asking to be held). Infants tend not to show protest or greeting behaviors in preferences for either parent. In brief, most infants form attachments to both parents and do so at about the same age. When infants are distressed, their displays of attachment behaviors increase, and they may appeal to whichever parent is present. When both parents are present, however, distressed infants tend to turn preferentially to their primary caregiver, most often the mother (Umemura et al., 2013).

Behavior Systems

Certain characteristics distinguish infant–parent attachments from nonattachment relationships. Being ethologically oriented, attachment theorists have been interested in biologically adaptive functions (i.e., survival value) of infants' attachment behavioral tendencies. Bowlby (1969) stressed the fact that attachment behaviors (like crying and approaching) promote proximity between infants and adults; staying close to protective caregivers is a good way to ensure survival of helpless infants. Bowlby termed this process the *attachment behavior system*. In addition to the attachment behavior system, attachment theorists have posited that three other systems mediate infants' social behaviors – a fear/wariness behavior system, an affiliative behavior system, and an exploratory behavior system. Each system controls behaviors that may be used to achieve an adaptive goal.

The **attachment behavior system** controls or coordinates infants' activities that are most related to attaining and maintaining proximity to or contact with attachment figures. Examples of behaviors in this system are gestures or signals (like crying) that indicate a desire to be held. These attachment behaviors are frequently directed to infants' attachment figures, and researchers have actually attempted to identify attachment figures by determining the people to whom infants direct those behaviors. The function of the attachment behavior system is to ensure that infants maintain access to persons on whom they can rely to meet their needs. Such behavioral propensities would have adaptive significance in maximizing the probability of infant survival.

The **fear/wariness behavior system** coordinates avoidant, wary, or fearful responses to strangers. These behaviors are unlike those controlled by the attachment behavior system, although both systems have adaptive value. For the same reason that it is important for infants to ensure access or proximity to protective adults, it is adaptive to avoid encounters with unknown and potentially dangerous people and situations. Apprehension over the appearance of strangers becomes marked in many infants around the beginning of the second half of the first year. This apprehension is thought to be an expression of the fear/wariness system.

Although it may be adaptive to be wary when first encountering strangers, it is not adaptive for infants to avoid all contact or interaction with nonattachment figures. Of course, many people other than parents have a profound impact on infant and child psychosocial development, as most interactions in later life involve people to whom children are not attached per se. Consequently, it is not surprising that the potency of the fear/wariness behavior system diminishes over time, as infants eventually enter, if only tentatively at first, into friendly interactions with nonattachment figures. These kinds of interactions typically involve social behaviors at a distance, such as smiling and vocalizing, and are mediated by the third behavior system, the **affiliative behavior system**. During an intermediate period, when both affiliation and fear/wariness are activated, coyness (which has both approach and avoidance overtones) may be prominent.

The existence of the affiliative behavior system speaks to the importance of infants' interactions with people to whom they are not attached. In the course of interactions with other people, infants have the opportunity to gain social competencies and to learn social skills through processes such as modeling and reinforcement. Affiliating with a variety of individuals sets the occasion for infants to learn how to adjust their style of interaction to match those of others. Infants likely benefit from these varied social interactions in a variety of ways.

Infants also engage in interaction with their physical environment to develop competence in and mastery over it (Wachs, 2015). Just as social encounters are mediated by the affiliative behavior system, the **exploratory behavior system** mediates contact with the material nonsocial environment. The exploration and manipulation of objects also enhance the development of perceptual and cognitive competencies.

Attachment theorists claim that the four behavior systems are interrelated and complementary to, not independent of, one another. However, the immediate goals of all four behavior systems usually cannot be attained simultaneously. Consequently, the more likely scenario is that the degree to which one system is activated arouses or inhibits the others. The specific effects that any one system has on arousing or inhibiting the others can be predicted by considering the adaptive functions of the four systems. A few examples suffice to demonstrate how these behavior systems operate and interrelate.

The appearance of an unfamiliar individual should, according to attachment theory, arouse infants' fear/wariness behavioral system. In most cases, infants' responses involve both an attempt to avoid interaction with the stranger (fear/wariness behavior system) and an attempt to move closer to the familiar attachment figure (attachment behavior system). The activation of either (or both) of these systems is incompatible with the affiliation and exploration behavior systems. Consequently, the affiliation and exploration behavior systems are typically inhibited when either the attachment or the fear/wariness behavior system is activated. The corollary is also true. When infants are not distressed and are in familiar (and thus not anxiety-provoking) surroundings, they might feel free to engage in interaction with less-familiar persons (as the affiliative behavior system is activated) and to explore the environment actively (as the exploratory behavior system is activated) without notable concern for remaining near their attachment figures. In these situations, apparently, the attachment behavior system is either not activated or is inhibited.

Types of Attachments

Taken together, the four behavior systems begin to offer predictions about how infants might respond in situations of uncertainty. Infants may feel comfortable exploring the objects around them if their attachment figure is present. The attachment figure in this case serves as a secure base. Infants may also show less fear/wariness and more affiliation (like smiling or greeting) to strangers if the attachment figure is present. If the attachment figure is not present, infants are more likely to engage the attachment behavior system to bring the attachment figure close (like crying). At the same time, infants may experience more fear/wariness and be less likely to affiliate or explore. A compelling question provoked by these complementary forces is whether these patterns are the same for all infants. The short answer is that they are not. Attachment quality (called type of security) varies, and as a result, individual infants show differences in expressing the different systems.

To assess different types of security of attachment, Ainsworth (1973) developed the **Strange Situation** procedure (Box 11.1), which allows investigators and clinicians to

Box 11.1 *How Do We Know This?* The Strange Situation

The Strange Situation procedure has become a popular technique to study attachment. It is used when infants are old enough to have formed attachments and are mobile yet are not so old that brief separations and encounters with strangers are no longer noteworthy. As a result, the Strange Situation procedure is appropriate for infants ranging in age from about 10 to 24 months. The procedure has seven episodes, which are outlined in Table 11.1. Briefly, the procedure is designed to expose infants to increasing amounts of stress to observe how they organize their attachment behaviors around their attachment figure when distressed. An unfamiliar environment, the presence of an unfamiliar adult, and two brief separations from the parent induce stress.

TABLE 11.1 Sequence of Episodes in the Strange Situation

Episode	*Sequence of Events*
1.	Parent and infant enter a novel play room.
2.	An unfamiliar adult joins the parent and infant.
3.	The parent leaves the room, and the infant and stranger are alone together.
4.	The parent returns and the stranger leaves.
5.	Parent leaves the infant alone in the room.
6.	The stranger returns to the room.
7.	The parent returns and the stranger leaves.

Note. Each episode usually lasts 3 minutes, but episodes 3, 5, and 6 can be curtailed if the infant becomes too distressed, and episodes 4 and 7 are sometimes extended.
Source: After Ainsworth and Wittig (1969).

observe how individual infants respond under increasing stress with and without the presence of an attachment figure. In brief, the Strange Situation takes place in an unfamiliar space (or room) where an unfamiliar adult appears (a stranger). Across the procedure, the attachment figure comes and goes. At the start of the procedure, infants should be able to use attachment figures (usually a parent) as a secure base from which to explore the novel environment. Considering the four behavior systems, a stranger's entrance to the room should lead infants to inhibit exploration and draw a little closer to the parent, at least temporarily. The parent's departure at this point should lead infants to attempt to bring the parent back by crying or searching as well as to reduced exploration and affiliation. Following the parent's return, infants should seek to re-engage with the parent, and if distressed infants may wish to be cuddled and comforted. The same responses should occur, with somewhat greater intensity, following another separation and reunion. In fact, this is precisely how about 65% of infants studied in the United States behave in the Strange Situation (Thompson & Virmani, 2010). Ainsworth and her colleagues deduced that infants who behave in this way have a **secure attachment**; their behavior conforms to theoretical predictions about how infants should behave in relation to their attachment figure.

By contrast, some infants seem unable to use their parent as a secure base from which to explore. Furthermore, although these infants are distressed by their parent's absence, they behave ambivalently on reunion, both seeking contact and interaction and angrily rejecting it when it is offered. These infants are conventionally described as having **insecure-resistant (ambivalent) attachments**. They typically account for about 10 to 15% of infants in U.S. samples (Thompson & Virmani, 2010).

A third group of infants appears unconcerned by the parents' absence. Instead of greeting their parent on reunion, they actively avoid interaction and ignore their parents' bids to interact. These infants are said to exhibit **insecure-avoidant attachments**, and they typically constitute about 20% of infants in U.S. samples (Thompson & Virmani, 2010).

A fourth group of infants displays behaviors that appear disoriented and/or disorganized, and they are described as having a **disorganized attachment** (Main & Solomon, 1991). These infants (5–10% of U.S. samples) may simultaneously display contradictory behavior patterns, freeze or make undirected movements, and appear confused or apprehensive about approaching the parent. This type of attachment is often found in cases of child maltreatment (Granqvist et al., 2017).

Section Summary

The earliest and most significant infant relationships are attachment relationships, which develop in phases. Initially, infants appear indifferent to specific people. Once they recognize significant others, infants interact preferentially with them, and attachments are gradually formed with those individuals who are consistently and reliably accessible to infants during the first months. Four behavior systems mediate infants' interactions with others: the attachment behavior system, the fear/wariness behavior system, the affiliative behavior system, and the exploratory behavior system. Most infants first form attachments to their two parents, but infants eventually form relationships with siblings, peers, and nonfamilial caregivers. Individual differences in infants' security of attachment relationships are often identified using the Strange Situation procedure, with infants developing secure, insecure-resistant, insecure-avoidant, or disorganized attachments.

PARENT–INFANT INTERACTIONS

Why some infants develop secure attachments whereas others do not has generated considerable debate. According to attachment theorists, infants count on attachment figures to protect them and to be accessible when needed. Almost from birth, infants learn about people from their interactions with them. Because adults differ in their style and sensitivity, differences should be evident in the extent to which infants come to trust and have confidence in others' reliability and, as a result, in their own effectance in acting on the environment or significant others successfully. As a consequence, infants do not trust all attachment figures equally, and differences in security of attachment appear to affect how willingly infants use different attachment figures as bases of security in situations like the Strange Situation.

Bowlby proposed that the consistency of adults' presence and their availability determined to whom infants became attached. Many developmental scientists have attempted to test this attachment hypothesis in independent longitudinal studies (Roisman & Groh, 2021). One outcome of this work is a refinement of what parents are doing, beyond being consistent and available, to support attachment. In this work, specific support has emerged for the notion that **sensitive parenting** is nurturant, attentive, nonrestrictive parental care. Synchronous infant–mother interactions are associated with secure infant behavior in the Strange Situation, and this support appears to describe U.S. samples of varying ethnicities as well as samples from cultures outside the United States (Mesman et al., 2016).

Insecure-avoidant attachments are associated with intrusive, overstimulating, rejecting parenting, and insecure-resistant attachments are linked to inconsistent, unresponsive parenting (Raby et al., 2021). Although the antecedents of disorganized attachments are less well-established, disorganized attachments are more common among abused and maltreated infants and among infants exposed to other pathological caregiving environments. Moreover, disorganized attachments may be consequences of parental behaviors that infants find frightening or disturbing (Roisman & Groh, 2011). Rather than considering insecure attachments as nonoptimal, however, a more constructive interpretation might view them as adaptive responses to nonoptimal caregiving (Weinfield et al., 2008). For example, if a parent is not consistently responsive to infants' needs, an adaptive strategy for infants may be to not rely on the parent.

Stability and Individual Differences in Attachment

Because attachment relationships emerge out of ongoing interactions with parents, they could be relatively stable. According to Waters (1978), 48 out of 50 infants (96%) obtained the same attachment classification on two testing occasions. Later, Main and Cassidy (1988) reported a high degree of stability between 12-month and 6-year assessments. Indeed, Pinquart and colleagues (2013) have suggested that attachment security is moderately stable into adulthood.

These impressive examples aside, short-term test-retest reliability for attachment classifications is not always high and shows considerable variation (Thompson & Virmani, 2010). In some cases, instability of attachment classifications is related to changes in infants' environments. For example, Sroufe and colleagues (2005) found that many infants in a low-SES sample changed from one classification to another between 12 and 18 months of age and that these changes were asymmetric. When the families experienced considerable social stress during the 6-month period, infants with secure attachments often changed to insecure, but when families experienced a low degree of stress, insecure attachments did not necessarily become secure. Attachment theory predicts that changes in infant attachment classification over time should be associated in some way with changes in parental sensitivity. For example, a change from secure to insecure should coincide with a decrease across the same time period in parental sensitivity.

At this point, a coherent explanation of stability or instability in attachment classifications remains open. It could be that stability and instability of attachments are explained by continuities and discontinuities in parental behavior, although such conclusions await studies of representative samples of parents and infants in several different contexts over time, such as at home, at day care, and on the playground, to provide an adequate test of this possibility. It could also be that changes in attachment security are partially independent of parenting and relate to normative family life transitions. For example, the birth of a second child predicts a decrease in attachment security among firstborn children, and that decrease is not necessarily linked to changes, from before to after birth, in mothers' sensitivity with their firstborns, mothers' psychiatric symptoms, or mothers' reports of marital harmony (Teti & Cole, 2011). Indeed, the change in firstborn attachment security might reflect changes in infants' perceptions of their relationships with their mothers in response to the introduction of the new family member, who may be perceived as a threat (Teti, 2002).

Attachment classifications intrigue developmental scientists because they appear to predict aspects of children's future behavior. Attachment theorists believe that, when infants encounter people for the first time, they tend to assume that those people will treat them in the same way that other people have treated them in the past. Thus, infants who have developed trust in their attachment figures will tend to regard the new people they encounter as trustworthy too. As infants get to know each individual, of course, they develop a set of expectations about that specific individual.

Factors That Affect the Quality of Caregiver Attachment

Attachment theorists have usually assumed that parental sensitivity reflects adults' enduring personality traits and that sensitive parenting is more likely to occur when parents are psychologically healthy (Belsky & Barends, 2002; Bornstein et al., 2011). Parents' adaptability may be important in the infants' first few months, when infant state and activities appear unpredictable and disorganized, and their cues less distinct and undifferentiated. For example, parent self-centeredness can lead to insensitivity when adults fail to put infants' needs ahead of their own. Other parental factors are depression, parenting cognitions, stress and social support, and parents' own attachment history. Moreover, infant characteristics play a role as well.

Parent Depression. One of the strongest predictors of parenting is depression. Many people – including mothers and fathers – experience depression. Sometimes depression reflects an enduring personality characteristic; other expressions of depression may be transient, as a response to poor economic or social circumstances. These feelings influence parental perceptions and behaviors toward infants. Depressed mothers fail to experience – or may convey to their infants – much happiness with life. Depressed mothers tend to be less responsive to infant signals and, therefore, more often engage in inadequately coordinated interactions (see Box 6.2).

Parenting Cognitions. One type of parenting cognition is parents' informal theories of child development (Holden & Smith, 2019). Most parents implicitly assume particular relations between their infant's age and the infant's behavior, and parents continually assess their infants' level of development when deciding how best and most productively to interact with them. Parents develop scripts about what should happen in development, and these scripts constantly update, as parents acquire new information about their infants through observation, feedback, experimentation, and so forth. In consequence, parental cognitions help shape parental behavior. For example, when parents see infants as active participants in their own development, parents are more likely to use teaching strategies in their interactions. However, when parents believe that they have little or no effect on their infants' intelligence or temperament, they might not assume a very active role in teaching infants. Thus, the ways in which parents choose to interact with their children reflect parents' own general cognitions.

A central parental cognition is parents' perception of their **efficacy**, or competency, as a parent (Schuengel & Oosterman, 2019). Parents who believe that they are efficacious see themselves as competent caregivers and interpret interactions between themselves and their infants as enjoyable for infants. Parents who feel incompetent may feel rewarded by even modest levels of success. Perceived efficacy likely affects parental sensitivity because parents who feel effective are motivated to engage their infants in further interactions, which in turn provides additional opportunities to read infants' signals, interpret those signals more accurately, and respond to those signals more appropriately. Mothers' feelings of efficacy in the parental role are a stronger predictor of parenting competence (i.e., sensitivity and warmth) in interactions with their infants as long as their knowledge of child development is also high (Hess et al., 2004). Mothers who have poor knowledge of child development appear to be naively confident about their parenting skills, but they show the least amount of sensitivity when interacting with their infants.

Parental Stress and Social Support. Stress and the availability or lack of social support can also influence parents' behaviors toward infants (Crnic & Coburn, 2019). Financial and social stress demand attention from parents and, as a result, can reduce their attentiveness, patience, and tolerance as well as undermine their general well-being and psychological health (Hoff & Laursen, 2019). It is not surprising, therefore, that child maltreatment is more common when parents are subjected to high levels of economic or social stress and/or are socially and emotionally isolated from potential support networks (Sturge-Apple et al., 2019). However, the availability of support from others can mitigate those negative effects. For example, support from fathers predicts parenting quality of mothers and can serve as a buffer against other environmental stressors (Bornstein et al., 2012b). Finally, reducing stress in infants leads to reduced stress in parents, and vice versa (see Box 11.2).

Box 11.2 *Application:* Reducing Stress in Infants

Parents (and educators and health-care workers) might think that infants naturally differ when it comes to reacting to stressful situations; some are highly reactive, whereas others are calm. In fact, there are ways to help all children react less to stress. One way parents can help reduce their infants' stress is to simply maintain physical contact with the infant. Skin-to-skin contact with young infants has tremendous effects on reducing stress (Pavlyshyn & Sarapuk, 2023). For example, through skin-to-skin contact, levels of cortisol, a hormone indicator of stress, were decreased in young infants, accompanied by improvement in infant sleeping and mood. Another way parents can reduce their infants' stress is with music. When preterm newborns were played music for 15 minutes three days in a row, the cortisol levels of the newborns were lower both immediately and 4 hours later (Schwilling et al., 2015). Also, pain scores in the newborns improved on all three days of music exposure. Lavender-scented baths appear to help as well! Field et al. (2008) tested the effects of a lavender bath on the parents while bathing their 6-month-old infants. Mothers who washed their infants in a lavender bath smiled and touched their infants more while also being more relaxed, as shown by mothers' decreased cortisol levels. For their part, infants looked at their mothers more during the bath and cried less when in lavender baths compared to a non-aroma bath. Additionally, infants had lower cortisol levels and spent more time in a deep sleep after the bath.

One skill that parents can practice to reduce infant stress is to be responsive to their infants. Responsiveness, which is described as being emotionally supportive as well as sensitive toward their infants by responding with appropriate reactions, is correlated with protection of telomeres, a part of a chromosome associated with health and longevity (Asok et al., 2013). Stress typically shortens telomeres, which can result in changes in DNA replication. The shortening of telomeres is a natural process of aging, but an accelerated rate of shortening can result in long-term risks, such as higher risk of death due to disease, as well as other general symptoms associated with aging (Shammas, 2011). Exposure to stress speeds the shortening of telomeres. Thus, emotionally supportive parenting can help reduce stress in the moment and better health in the longer term for both parent and infant.

All these methods reflect positive caregiving practices. Some come naturally, and others can be learned easily and practiced, so hopefully in the end everyone experiences less stress and its deleterious outcomes.

Parents' Own Attachment History. Parents were once infants who also had attachments to their own parents. Because researchers do not usually know what parents' early relationships were like, researchers try to infer them by asking parents (or any adult) to reflect on their early relationships. One way that has been developed to do this is the **Adult Attachment Inventory** (AAI; George et al., 1984). On the basis of the AAI, mothers are classified into different categories of attachment, and notably parental AAI classifications have been found to be predictive of corresponding infant–parent attachment classifications. For example, mothers classified with the AAI as autonomous (the analog of a secure attachment in infancy) are likely to have securely attached infants (Verhage et al., 2016). Relations have also been found between categories of insecure attachments in mothers and infants: Mothers classified as dismissing (analogous to insecure-avoidant infant–mother attachment) are likely to have insecure-avoidant infants. Mothers classified as preoccupied (analogous to an insecure-resistant attachment in infancy) are likely to have insecure-resistant attachments. Finally, mothers classified as unresolved (conceptually akin to insecure-disorganized attachment in infancy) are likely to have insecure-disorganized infants. In addition, autonomous mothers are more sensitive toward their infants than are non-autonomous mothers. However, these effects are less robust or sometimes show cross-overs between types of insecure attachment (Shah et al., 2010; Verhage et al., 2016).

The AAI has opened opportunities to chart transgenerational continuity of attachment relationships from parent to infant; however, much of this research is based on self-report measures of mothers of their AAI and of their children's attachment, and so this kind of research is open to criticism. First, the data for both constructs come from the same individuals (the mothers), and, second, many individuals who self-report may attempt to look good and bias their responses in a positive way. A more valid way to study the concordance of parenting representations with infant attachment classifications would be to know the attachment classification of parents and the type of parenting they experienced when they were infants and then independently observe their parenting and their infants' behavior in the Strange Situation. Of course, such data depend on a longitudinal design (Box 1.1). The Minnesota Longitudinal Study of Risk and Adaptation positioned itself to make such a comparison (Sroufe, 2021). Families were enrolled in this study before the birth of their first child, and many families were followed until the infants themselves became parents. Comparing the parenting the parents received as infants to the parenting they showed their own infants revealed that many parents parented the way their parents did. Such findings identify parenting as a mechanism for the transmission of attachment classification across generations.

Infant Characteristics

In the transaction perspective, parent characteristics alone are not determinative of parent–infant relationships. Infant temperament and other characteristics, such as responsiveness, readability, and predictability, are also influential. **Responsiveness** refers to the extent and quality of infants' reactivity to stimulation. **Readability** refers to the definitiveness of infants' behavioral signals. Easily read infants produce unambiguous cues that allow caregivers to recognize infants' states quickly, interpret infants' signals promptly, and thus respond contingently. **Predictability** refers to the degree to which the infants' behaviors can be anticipated reliably from infants' own preceding behaviors or from contextual events. Moreover, the same parental practice might rapidly soothe one infant but be ineffective with another infant, leading the parents of different infants to reach very different conclusions about their own competence as parents despite similarities in their behavioral styles. In essence, attachments are two-way affairs: Attachment figures contribute to parent–infant attachment just as infants contribute to parent–infant attachments.

What about infants might contribute to their attachment? Temperament, the aforementioned characteristics, as well as the quality and contingency of infant responses might present pathways through which infants could influence the ways parents perceive their own effectiveness as well as infants' own contributions to parent–infant attachment. Attachment researchers have tended to reject the notion that infant temperament has a direct effect on whether infants are classified as secure or insecure (Groh et al., 2017; Sroufe, 2021). However, indirect effects may be at play because infant temperament likely affects the quality of infant–parent interaction. Distractible infants, for example, might be less affected by their parents' behavior than attentive infants are. Thus, the extent to which parenting is sensitive to infants' needs would determine whether infants become securely or insecurely attached, but constitutionally based differences in infant irritability would determine whether infant insecurity will be manifest in a low-distress (i.e., avoidant) or high-distress (i.e., resistant) fashion. It seems likely that temperament and attachment security are interdependent dimensions, with temperament affecting irritability and emotionality, and so attachment security indirectly, but not security of attachment directly.

With maturation and experience, infants begin to interpret the behaviors of others. For example, by 9 months, infants are able to predict others' actions (Southgate et al., 2010). In one study, 12- to 13-month-old infants viewed animations of sensitive versus insensitive responding to a crying infant (Johnson et al., 2010). In actuality, the objects involved in the interactions were ovals of different colors and sizes (Figure 11.1). A small oval represented an infant, and a large oval represented an adult (a parent). The animation begins with the two ovals near each other. As the animation continues, the large oval moves away from the

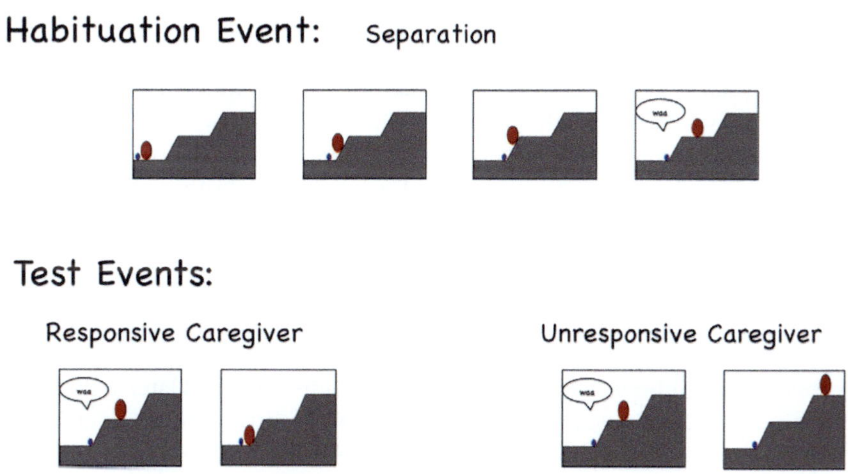

FIGURE 11.1 Habituation and test events have been used to assess infants' expectations regarding relationships. In the habituation event, the large oval (a "parent") moves away from the small oval (an "infant") and the infant cries. The two test events show a sensitive response (moving toward the infant, as in the responsive caregiver event) and an insensitive response (moving away from the infant, as in the unresponsive caregiver).

small oval, and the small oval cries. In the sensitive condition, the large oval moves closer in response to the crying. In the insensitive condition, the large oval moves away. Infants classified as securely attached looked significantly longer to the insensitive response (a violation of expectation; Box 6.2), suggesting that they found this reaction novel. Insecurely attached infants showed the opposite pattern: They looked significantly longer to the sensitive response. Thus, it appears that infants bring expectations about actions and appropriate responses to their interactions with others.

Moreover, infants appear to draw on inborn behavioral tendencies that provide contingent feedback to their parents, which in turn feed feelings of effectance in their parents. Infants' readiness to respond to social stimulation, mutual eye contact, and soothing when held indicate to parents that their practices are effective and enjoyable. Under ordinary conditions, specific infant behaviors appear to predictably elicit parental practices that allow infants to develop notions of effectance as well. Successful dyadic interactions thus help parents and infants alike to perceive themselves as effective and their relationships as positive.

The health and developmental maturity of infants also affect parents and the quality of infant–parent interaction, as has been illustrated in the research on preterm infants and their parents (Gattis, 2019). Studies of healthy preterm infants and mothers consistently show that these infants are more passive and reactive and that their mothers are more active and directive than are full-term infants of comparable postnatal age with their mothers. However, this finding does not necessarily mean that mothers of preterm infants are less sensitive; rather, the differences could arise in part because preterm infants are immature and call for more directiveness from their adult partners. Thus, such differences might actually attest to the genuine sensitivity of mothers of preterms. Support for this view can be found in the fact that the interaction styles of preterm infants and their mothers are similar to those involving younger full-term infants, that is infants who are of the same conceptional age but have spent a briefer period of time outside the womb. The maturity level of infants might influence their social interactions.

Again, pursuing the systems perspective, advances in motor development over the first two years likely enrich infants' opportunities for interaction, both with people and with objects. Self-produced locomotion affords opportunities to engage more with people and enjoy the attendant rewards (Thurman & Corbetta, 2017). Once infants can reach, they can engage with the objects that others give them, and they can explore the people around them by touching parts of their bodies (putting fingers in someone's mouth and grabbing hair, glasses, and jewelry are common at this time). Crawling versus walking also changes the way mothers and infants interact. Once they begin to crawl and later walk, infants take more initiative in interactions, such as maintaining proximity to familiar people or moving away from parents to approach strangers. They also begin to share. While exploring their world, they may turn to an adult, usually a parent, and show or give an object.

In the end, what may be most important is the goodness of fit between newborns, infants, and children with their developmental contexts (Lerner, 2018). Easy infants who may have a low activity level, positive mood, and good adaptability may likely fit well in a home or day-care setting that makes few demands and provides many opportunities for self-direction. But such an environment is likely a poorer fit for difficult infants, who may have a high activity level, unhappy mood, and low adaptability. In this light, temperamentally difficult infants will not inevitably experience later problems if parents understand, are tolerant of their infants' behavioral style, and provide activities in which their infants' characteristics can be channeled and valued. Conversely, even temperamentally easy infants might experience problems if parents impose excessive demands on them or ignore their reasonable needs. As a consequence, the sensitivity and adaptability of parents to their infants' temperament are important predictors of parent–child relationships and long-term child adjustment. From this perspective, the nature of children's temperament or other characteristics is less important than the fit between temperament or other characteristics and parents' character and caregiving.

Section Summary

A number of factors influence parent–infant interactions, and both parties contribute to the parent–infant relationship. Infant factors include temperament and developmental status (whether full-term or preterm), attentiveness, and/or mobility. Parents bring a number of factors to the interaction, including their mental health status, parenting cognitions, social supports, feelings of self-efficacy as parents, and their own experiences being parented.

CONCLUSIONS

Infants develop from mute and inept organisms to increasingly capable interactional and conversational partners. Infants first coo and babble, but soon their syllabic pairings (at first barely specific to the language they will develop) form comprehensible (language-specific) words. The language infants hear fosters their use of language. Language development feeds parent–infant relationships. Both parents and infants contribute to both the growth and the depth of those relationships. Infant temperament, developmental status as term or preterm at birth, attentiveness, and mobility are prominent characteristics that contribute to the formation of parent–infant relationships. For their part, parents bring a number of factors to relationship formation, including their mental health status, cognitions, social supports, feelings of self-efficacy, and own experiences being parented. The development of communication and parent–infant relationships is a good example of transactional perspective. Infants not only perceive and interpret their social and material environments in their unique ways and are uniquely influenced by their social and material environments but also alter their social and material environments as they interact with them.

KEY TERMS

Adult attachment inventory
Affiliative system
Attachment behavior system
Attachment figures
Context-flexible
Context-restricted
Discriminating sociability

Disorganized attachment
Effectance
Efficacy
Exploratory behavior system
Fear/wariness behavior system
Imprint
Insecure-avoidant attachments
Insecure-resistant (ambivalent) attachments
Nominal insight
Person permanence
Predictability
Readability
Reciprocity
Reference
Responsiveness
Secure attachment
Secure base
Sensitive parenting
Sensitive period
Separation anxiety
Strange Situation

SUGGESTED READINGS

Bowlby, J. (1969). *Attachment and loss, Vol. 1: Attachment*. Basic Books.

Golombok, S. (2020). *Parenting: What really counts*. Psychology Press.

Scaff, C., & Cristia, A. (2025). Language development. In M. H. Bornstein & M. E. Lamb (Eds.), *Developmental science: An advanced textbook* (pp. 362–406). Routledge.

Sroufe, L. A., Egeland, B., Carlson, E. A., & Collins, W. A. (2005). *The development of the person: The Minnesota study of risk and adaptation from birth to adulthood*. Guilford Press.

CHAPTER 12

Infants in Context

With their advancing perceptual, mental, emotional, and verbal skills, infants become more engaged with the people, objects, and events around them. Their first important relationships develop, and their social spheres expand. In the systems perspective, newborns, infants, and children develop in families, which themselves are embedded in larger contexts. Parents play especially important roles in all phases of infant development. Through interactions with their parents, infants are developing confidence in their own abilities, trust in others, and an awareness of the reciprocal nature of social interactions. Meanwhile, experiences with a variety of other adults and children foster the development of an even more sophisticated and flexible repertoire of social skills by providing exposure to individuals who have different behavioral styles and provide contrasting patterns of interaction. Where and how infants interact with adults and children vary across cultures, but for many infants in Western contexts, day care is one option. Through these interactions, infants come to learn things about themselves, including their gender and the social expectations for boys and girls. In this chapter, we discuss some salient contexts of infant development, focusing on gender of infant and parent, nonparental care and its social and cognitive outcomes, infant–peer interactions, as well as socioeconomic status, ethnicity and culture, and time.

GENDER OF INFANT AND PARENT

The genders of infant and parent alike loom as significant factors in infant development and infant–parent relationships. Of course, girls and boys are born with different genetic compositions (XX and XY, respectfully), and gender has traditionally been associated with variations in infant behavioral style, just as gender influences the ways in which others perceive and relate to infants.

Infant Gender

Parents provide the initial influences on the development of their infants' gender, and parents have strong tendencies to treat infants differently by their gender, including what clothes they should wear (Figure 12.1). It is notoriously difficult to tell the difference between a newborn or an infant girl or boy who is swaddled. Classic Baby X studies

DOI: 10.4324/9781003381709-14

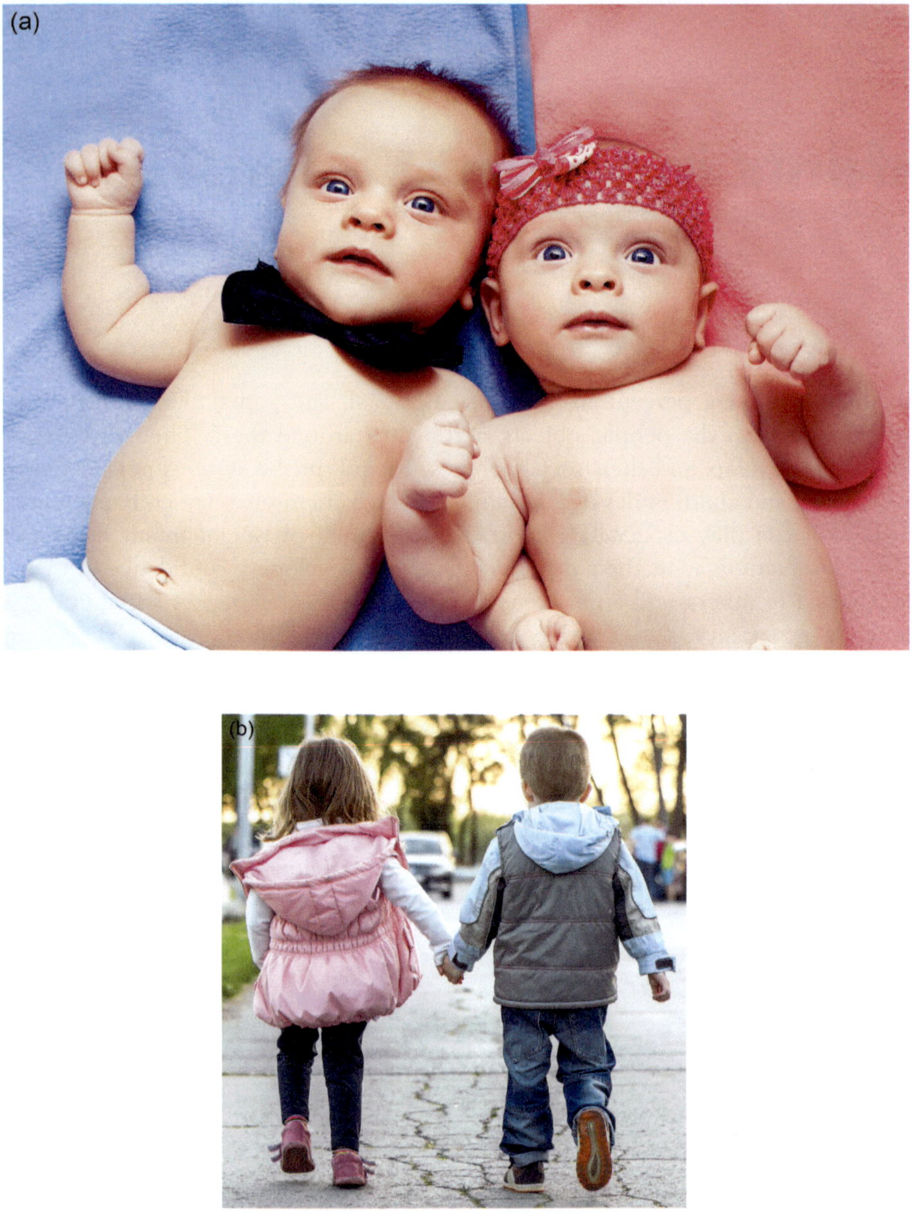

FIGURE 12.1 Well before infants are old enough to state clothing preferences, parents dress them in gendered clothes and colors (a), and these color preferences continue as children get older (b).

(where the gender of the infant is not known to study participants) have revealed that parents (and other adults) conceive of and behave toward infants differently depending on whether they *think* they are interacting with a girl or a boy (Seavey et al., 1975; Sidorowicz & Lunney, 1980). Infants dressed as boys are described as big and strong and are bounced and handled more physically than infants dressed as girls, who are described as pretty and sweet. Parents further emphasize gender differentiation in their infants by dressing them differently (pink for girls and blue for boys), and they purchase gender-stereotyped toys for them as well (dolls for girls and trucks for boys). Similarly, parents provide their male and female infants with different cognitive experiences in addition to teaching them what types of toys and activities are appropriate for girls and boys (Boe & Woods, 2018). Infant childcare providers also reinforce gender stereotypes by the types of activities they encourage, the toys they provide, and the comments they make, such as praising girls for their appearance and boys for their activity (Chick et al., 2002).

Gender expectancies spill over to other spheres of development. Before infants are able to label themselves as a boy or a girl (an ability that emerges around age 2), girls show preferences for dolls and boys show preferences for trucks (Jadva et al., 2010). Even girl and boy infants show differences in imitating actions. Benenson and colleagues (2011) showed infants aged 6 to 9 months videos of adults cradling and hitting a balloon. When given the chance to interact with a similar balloon, girls were more likely to cradle the balloon than boys, and boys were more likely to hit the balloon than girls.

The gender typing of infant–parent play is perennially fascinating because girls and boys gravitate in such distinctive directions, seemingly regardless of their parents' stated beliefs. Parents recognize that other people shape their infants' gendered behavior, but they are less likely to see themselves playing a role (Dinkel & Snyder, 2020). Evidence abounds, however, that parents play a determinative part of this drama. Infants who acquire gender labels before they near the end of the second year are also more gender-typed in their toy choices than late labelers (Zosuls et al., 2009). Moreover, parents' responses to their infants' gender-typed play at 1 1/2 years predict whether infants will be early or late in acquiring the ability to label gender. Parents of infants who label early give more attention (both positive and negative) when their infants play with either female- or male-gender-typed toys, regardless of infants' gender (Fagot et al., 2000).

In terms of temperament, female infants show more distress or fear to novelty than male infants, and male infants appear to be more active than female infants (Else-Quest et al., 2006). Given all the ways that people could differ, however, evidence about actual gender differences in infancy has become controversial, with increasing support for a gender similarities hypothesis (Hyde, 2014). That is, gender differences in infancy appear to be minimal. Developmental scientists who actually quantify gender differences must take into consideration the force of prevailing stereotypes about girls and boys as well as how differences in infants' early experiential histories are shaped by adult perceptions as opposed to actual infant preferences, capabilities, and behaviors. Mothers and fathers of 4-month-old infants tend to view their daughters in more negative terms as infants' crying increases, but no such negative perceptions emerge when sons cry more (Teichner et al., 1997). In fact, more crying by boys is associated with mothers' tendency to rate their sons as more powerful, whereas more crying by daughters is associated with mothers' tendency to rate their daughters as less powerful. Similarly, higher-pitched cries were attributed to girls, and lower-pitched cries to boys, even though acoustic analysis showed that there were no actual gender differences by cry pitch (Reby et al., 2016), and a study of motor development confirmed that mothers *under*estimate how well their 11-month-old girls would crawl down a sloped pathway, whereas mothers *over*estimate how well their 11-month-old boys would do (Mondschein et al., 2000) when subsequent tests of crawling ability on the sloped path revealed no gender differences in infant crawling.

Parent Gender

Despite the fact that father involvement in childcare generally increased in the 21st century, fathers typically see themselves (and are seen by their partners and others) as helpers rather than as primary caregivers of infants. Fathers typically spend less time than mothers do with their infants, and this is true of families in the United States, Australia, Belgium, and Great Britain, as well as families of varying ethnicity within the United States, such as European Americans, Latin Americans, and African Americans (Parke & Cookston, 2019; Roopnarine et al., 2005). All parties in traditional family configurations see income generation as the fathers' primary responsibility and contribution to their infant's life and well-being (although in contemporary modern North American and Western European societies, women are increasingly professional breadwinners in the family).

According to ethologists, women and men have different investment strategies in young offspring: Males are invested in reproducing, and females invested in childcare (Trivers, 1972). Among different species, responsibilities for infants are shouldered mainly by mothers, and maternal care is much more common than paternal care (Bjorklund, 2020). In mammals, males provide infant care in fewer than 5% of species (Moller, 2003). Contrary to popular conceptions, fathers are neither inept nor uninterested in interacting with their infants. Fathers are sensitive interaction partners; what differs is the nature of the interactions (Lucassen et al., 2011). That is, mothers and fathers tend to engage their infants in different types of interactions. For example, in face-to-face play with their 6-month-olds, mothers tend to be rhythmic and containing, whereas fathers tend to provide staccato bursts of both physical and social stimulation (Cerezo et al., 2017).

Section Summary

Parents tend to hold stereotyped beliefs about their infant girls and boys, beliefs that affect how they interact with their infants. Left on their own, however, infant girls and boys are not all that different in capability or action. Through their consistent cognitions and practices, however, parents begin to shape infants' gender-stereotyped patterns of identity and behavior.

NONPARENTAL CARE OF INFANTS

Infants today are cared for by many different people, on many different schedules, and in many different situations. Some situations are informal nonparental but still familial (grandparents), informal nonparental non-familial (neighbors), or formal nonparental non-familial (day-care centers). In 2021, parents of newborns and infants utilized a variety of options (Table 12.1). With age, the percentage of infants in nonparental care increases, as does the type of care, such as a decrease in relative care and an increase in center-based care.

TABLE 12.1 Percentage of Infants in Different Types of Nonparental Care Arrangements as a Function of Age

Type of Care	*1–12 Months*	*12–24 Months*
At least one placement per week	42%	55%
Relative care	58%	44%
Non-relative care	26%	25%
Center-based care	32%	47%

Source: National Center for Education Statistics (2021).

Across families, communities, countries, and time spans, an ongoing question is what the best way to care for infants is. Many parents – and rightfully so – want to provide the best option for their family and consider different options with an eye toward longer-term impacts, ease for family members, and cost. Policymakers and employers, who may subsidize day care, also want to know what is best and what the impacts are (see Box 7.1). For all these groups, day care is important.

Thus, it came as a surprise when some early reports indicated that the amount of nonmaternal care in the first 4 1/2 years of life predicted behavior problems (assertiveness, disobedience, and aggression) which persisted up to 15 years of age (Vandell et al., 2010); others have not replicated these findings (Love et al., 2003). For infants, beginning day care is difficult. Full-day placement in day care is emotionally and physiologically stressful for many, if not most, infants (Bernard et al., 2015). One way that stress is measured is by monitoring cortisol levels (Box 9.2). When under stress, levels remain high. Infants in day care show elevated cortisol levels compared to infants who are cared for at home (Drugli et al., 2018). Adjustment to day care may also be related to infants' attachment security, as securely attached infants fare better than those with insecure attachments, and to whether or not they have older siblings (Ahnert, 2021; Ahnert et al., 2022). To help infants adjust, many European day-care centers operate adaptation programs in which mothers are allowed to accompany their infants during the transitional period of enrollment. When mothers familiarize their infants to day care in a more leisurely manner and accompany their infants in the center, adjustment is easier, especially when infants are securely attached to their mothers (Rauh et al., 2000).

Many infants who attend day care show cognitive advantages over infants cared for at home (Narea et al., 2020), a pattern most strongly seen among infants from low-SES families who attend stimulating day-care centers (Burchinal et al., 2015). Infants from high-SES families do not seem to profit consistently from day care in this way, presumably because they enjoy stimulating environments at home. Indeed, positive family factors (such as greater family income and more sensitive parenting) are associated with more positive infant functioning and continue to affect infants positively even when they spend a lot of time in day-care settings (Belsky et al., 2007).

When researching the outcomes of day care, scholars often miss another important factor – day care's effects on parents and the family more generally. Availability of day care allows both parents to have meaningful work outside the home. Day care is essential for single parents to support their families; without it, they would need to rely on extended family support or government assistance. Moreover, from a biological systems perspective, there are indirect effects of the workplace on child development, including provision of material resources (Figure 1.6; Burchinal et al., 2023). The importance of day care was brought to light during and following the COVID-19 pandemic. Numerous formal childcare programs closed, and parents (especially mothers) of infants were forced to leave the workforce, balance infant care and work demands, and seek alternative childcare situations.

Section Summary

Nonparental care of infants comes in many different flavors and provides infants with opportunities to interact with same-age peers and adults who are not their parents. For some infants, nonparental care is associated with negative social behaviors, which may be due to stress. Transitioning to day care is also stressful for infants, but with time, stress responses return to normal levels. Cognitive benefits of day care are most notable in infants from low-SES families enrolled in higher-quality programs.

PEER INTERACTIONS IN INFANCY

For infants who do not have older siblings, interactions with other infants and children do not begin until they are enrolled in some alternative care setting. The development of peer relationships transits a series of stages (Bowker et al., 2025). In the first year, social interaction between infants is infrequent, and when it does occur, it is not sustained for very long. A short time later, peers seem to be interesting to infants. By 6 months, infants interact with peers and initiate exchanges and respond to one another's social overtures with combinations of looks, smiles, and vocalizations. Their sensitivity to social cues from peers leads infants to continue interacting when their partners are responsive, whereas they cease social bids when their partners are unresponsive. From 6 to 12 months and afterward, peer interaction increases, responsiveness to peer overtures and imitation becomes increasingly common, and interactions involving physical contact occur less frequently.

Infants do not engage in many prosocial behaviors, and their interactions on the surface appear to consist of a lot of conflict. To further understand infant–peer interactions, Williams and her colleagues (2007) observed peer interactions of infants between 12 and 17 months of age. All infants were observed in childcare settings and thus had plenty of opportunities to engage with same-aged peers. The researchers recorded three measures of social competence: peer sociability, active peer refusal, and passive peer avoidance. Peer sociability included smiling at peers, initiating play, imitating, and taking toys from peers. Active peer refusal included refusing peers' attempts to play, turning back to peers, and moving away from peers. Passive peer avoidance included watching rather than participating and acting as if they do not notice peers' attempts to initiate play. For infants, seemingly negative behaviors were not necessarily signs of poor social competence. For example, taking a toy away from another infant was taken to indicate a social interaction, rather than the hostile act it would be among older children. Hitting or biting, different types of aggressive acts, was interpreted as a way for infants to actively avoid interactions. Individual differences in infants' interest in engaging with others were found. Moreover, some infants simply prefer to play by themselves, a preference the authors attributed to differences in temperament.

The development of relationships with peers is influenced by infants' social, cognitive, and emotional attainments and by socialization practices within the family. Infants who experience warm, sensitive parenting and grow up in harmonious families tend to be well adjusted socially, unaggressive, and popular with peers (Ladd & Kochenderfer-Ladd, 2019). More generally, attachment theorists argue that infants who have secure relationships with their parents should be sociable and socially competent (Sroufe, 2017).

Section Summary

Infants interact with peers in addition to family members and other adults. These early interactions may be driven by curiosity. As infants' motor and cognitive skills develop, they engage in increasingly complex interactions with other infants. These interactions differ from the interactions of older children, likely due to infants' limited language skills. Parents and infant care providers play roles in facilitating positive peer relationships.

DISTAL SYSTEMS IN INFANT DEVELOPMENT

The bioecological systems model asserts that the individual grows and develops in a series of nested systems, some proximal to the individual and some distal from the individual (Figure 1.6). Examples of the more distal exosystem include the socioeconomic status, ethnicity, and culture in which the infant is embedded. Time constitutes the chronosystem.

Socioeconomic Status and Infancy

The social class in which infants are reared exercises profound effects over infant development. Differences in language used by middle-SES and lower-SES mothers with infants are illustrative. Middle-SES U.S. mothers talk to their infants in more sophisticated ways, with richer vocabulary than low-SES mothers, even though infants are not yet talking themselves (Hoff et al., 2019). Functionally, low-SES mothers focus more on directions and corrections instead of acknowledging their infants' actions or attempting to engage them in conversation. As far as discourse is concerned, low-SES infants are less likely than middle-SES infants to receive topic-continuing replies to their utterances (which results in more conversational turns and depth of conversation or opportunities for elaboration). Differences in lexical properties of language include middle-SES mothers talking more in total, talking more per unit of time, and sustaining longer bouts of verbal interactions than low-SES mothers. These amounts and types of language experience seen in infancy predict later language acquisition. In short, in a variety of ways, middle-SES mothers encourage their infants to converse and to expand their communicative abilities, which serve children well academically and professionally.

Of course, extreme economic disadvantage affects infant development in ways that go well beyond parental speech patterns, values, and expectations. When compared to infants growing up in middle-SES environments, infants living in poverty experience lower levels of emotional and verbal responsiveness, fewer opportunities for variety in daily stimulation, less appropriate play materials, and more chaotic, disorganized, and unstructured environments (Maughan et al., 2018). Moreover, worldwide, many families have inadequate housing and other basic necessities, such as clean water and adequate sanitation, resulting in increased exposure to toxins, poor nutrition, illness, and shorter life expectancies (Bradley & Rothenberg, 2022). These circumstances make parenting extremely difficult, and they have profound impacts on development (Bizzego et al., 2021; Fanning, 2021; Tella et al., 2018).

Ethnicity and Culture and Infancy

Culture exercises a pervasive influence over infant development. Using UNICEF's Multiple Indicator Cluster Surveys, Bornstein et al. (2015) explored relations among mother education, household resources, and infant growth in 117,881 families living in 39 low- and middle-resourced countries. Maternal education was associated with improved infant growth. Likewise, in a more modest five-country study (including two ethnic or regional groups in each of five countries, Argentina, Belgium, Israel, Italy, and the United States), Bornstein (2022) analyzed similarities and differences in base rates of 5-month-old infants' behaviors and their mothers' parenting practices. One of five infant behaviors – distress communication – proved common across cultures and groups within cultures, whereas all other infant behaviors (e.g., non-distress vocalization) varied in culture- and in group-specific ways. With respect to mothers' parenting practices, one kind of caregiving (nurturing) proved common across cultures and groups within cultures; nurturing might be conceived of as obligatory to the fundamental survival and well-being of infants. All other parenting practices (e.g., speaking to infants) varied in culture- or group-specific ways; they might be conceived of as discretionary and appear free to vary both between cultures and within countries, underscoring the significance of cultural influences on everyday maternal parenting practices. Furthermore, no one consistent country profile emerged: Neither infants nor mothers in any one country or group outstripped their peers in another country or group in all or even many domains of infant behavior or parenting. These kinds of findings confirm that, at the very heart of the social science constructs of ethnicity and culture, is the expectation that distinct peoples possess some distinct attitudes and act in some distinct ways.

One of the main differentiating characteristics of culture is language, and of course the language to which infants are exposed influences the language which infants will come to comprehend and produce. Clearly, infants born into different language communities rapidly grow up to speak different languages. Not unexpectedly, even some early babbling sounds are positively shaped by local auditory input. Boysson-Bardies and her colleagues (1984) first recorded pure samples of babbling among 6-, 8-, and 10-month-old French,

Arabic, and Chinese babies from Paris, Tunis or Algiers, and Hong Kong, respectively. The French, Arabic, and Cantonese languages differ from one another in voice quality, stress, and proportion of consonantal versus vocalic sounds. They then asked French monolingual adult judges – both experienced phoneticians and laypeople – to identify which babbling samples came from French babies. The phoneticians correctly identified the country of origin of 6-month-olds. Both the professional and lay groups correctly identified the country of origin of the 8- and 10-month-olds. Analysis of the speech samples revealed that the intonation in pitch and intensity contours specific to the different local languages strongly cued adults' perceptions. Because the language the infant hears is the only conceivable cause of such an effect, vocal production in infants as young as 6 months of age has already been influenced by components of the language they hear. The environment swiftly and surely channels early speech development toward the adult target language, and so very young infants must be extraordinarily sensitive to particular auditory experiences. Babbling production continues to coexist with infants' first words for several months, and infants frequently draw their early spoken vocabulary from the repertoire of sounds established in the course of babbling (Lee et al., 2018): Fine-grained acoustic analyses have revealed that infants' first words incorporate frequently produced babbling sounds. For example, Majorano and D'Odorico (2011) studied both babbling and word utterances in Italian infants between the ages of 10 months and 2 years. At around 11 months, babbling sounds mirrored the frequency and accent characteristics of Italian. Almost 49% of infants' first words contained sounds that first appeared in the infants' babbles.

Time and Infancy

The chronosystem likewise operates over development in infancy, and time (as pointed out earlier) runs on multiple schedules. For example, short-term test-retest reliability for attachment classifications is not always high and shows considerable variation (Thompson & Virmani, 2010). As mentioned in Chapter 11, the instability of attachment classifications is related to temporal changes in infants' environments. In a study of attachment stability in a low-SES sample, Sroufe and colleagues (2005) found that many infants changed from one classification to another between 12 and 18 months of age and that these changes were asymmetric. When the families experienced considerable social stress during the 6-month period, infants' secure attachments often changed to insecure; but when families experienced a low degree of stress, insecure attachments did not necessarily become secure. Attachment theory predicts that changes in infant attachment classification over time should be associated in some way with changes in parental sensitivity. For example, a change from secure to insecure should coincide with a decrease across the same time period in parental sensitivity.

Time also interacts with other systems. For example, Keller and Lamm (2005) observed that, as German society moved toward more individualism, mother–infant close caregiving practices changed from more body contact and less separation between mothers and infants to more physical separation and less body contact between mothers and infants. Long ago, Bronfenbrenner (1961) analyzed maternal infant feeding practices and observed that socioeconomic status differences varied over time in that middle-SES researchers consistently found ways to portray middle-SES values and practices as more desirable and appropriate than low-SES values and practices, even though the values and practices of both middle-SES and low-SES parents changed over time. When the same values and practices were held at different times by middle- and low-SES parents – say, the preference for bottle feeding or for breastfeeding – the preference was positively evaluated when held by middle-SES parents and negatively evaluated when adopted by low-SES parents. Such positive and negative evaluations clearly say more about the times (as well as the researchers and theorists) than about the parenting infants or health implications for infants.

Section Summary

In the bioecological systems model, infants exist in various nested distal systems, like family socioeconomic status, ethnicity and culture, and time. Each at least indirectly supports the expression of multiple domains of infant development.

CONCLUSIONS

As the bioecological systems model predicts, infants exist in various nested systems. Parents tend to hold stereotyped beliefs about their infant girls and boys, beliefs that affect how they interact with their infants. Left on their own, however, infant girls and boys are not all that different in terms of their capabilities and actions. In the context of the microsystem, parents' cognitions and practices shape infants' gender-stereotyped patterns of identity and behavior. Infants experience different kinds of nonparental care, which provides them with opportunities to interact with adults who are not their parents as well as with same-age peers. Nonparental care of different sorts is known to have positive and negative consequences for infants, given infants' own characteristics and the multiple parameters that compose the nature of such care. As infants develop, they engage in increasingly complex interactions with other infants. Infant development also unfolds in various nested distal systems of family socioeconomic status, ethnicity and culture, and all indirectly influence infant development. Last but not least, infants exist at specific times, and times change, so that infant development can be expected to change as well.

SUGGESTED READINGS

Bornstein, M. H. (2013). Parenting X gender X culture X time. In W. B. Wilcox & K. K. Kline (Eds.), *Gender and parenthood: Biological and social scientific perspectives* (pp. 91–119). Columbia University Press.

Bornstein, M. H., Putnick, D. L., Lansford, J. E., Deater-Deckard, K., & Bradley, R. (2016). Gender in low- and middle-income countries. *Monographs of the Society for Research in Child Development, 81*. https://www.ncbi.nlm.nih.gov/pmc/articles/PMC5860685/

Burchinal, M., Whitaker, A. A., & Jenkins, J. M. (2022). The promise and purpose of early care and education. *Child Development Perspectives, 16*, 134–140.

Seavey, C. A., Katz, P. A., & Zalk, S. R. (1975). Baby X. *Sex Roles, 1*, 103–109.

SECTION III

The Child

18 Months to 36 Months

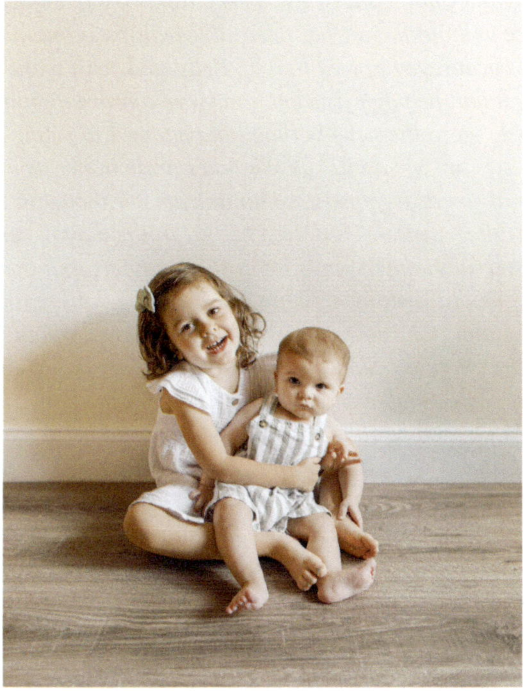

In only 9 prenatal months and 3 postnatal years, the initial union of the ovum and sperm turns into a fully formed walking, talking, perceiving, thinking, and relating human being. Continuing and systemic development before and just after birth and across the newborn and infant periods paves the way for the future development of the child. This section of *Newborn to Infant to Child* describes growth and action (Chapter 13), perception and cognition (Chapter 14), emotions and temperament (Chapter 15), communication and relationships (Chapter 16), and contexts of the child's development (Chapter 17).

Along with the many developments in the physical, perceptual, mental, verbal, and emotional domains, children's social world expands dramatically, and it is likely that first-born children will become a big brother or sister before they celebrate their third birthday. Some of the most dramatic changes in family dynamics occur when another baby is born into the family; the birth of a sibling alters the roles of each family member and

DOI: 10.4324/9781003381709-15

consequently affects the ways in which each family member interacts with all other family members. But first, meet mom Kelly and dad John, baby Liam, and big sister Charlotte.

Kelly and John have two children. Charlotte was 30 months old when her baby brother, Liam, arrived. Kelly and John already had a good routine for balancing work, childcare, and family life before Liam was born, but having a new baby in the family was still quite an adjustment. Luckily, Kelly's family lives nearby, so these new parents also have help from aunts, uncles, and grandparents, not to mention teenage babysitters in the neighborhood. Charlotte attends day care at John's work, which helps with the morning routine, and Kelly was able to take up to 12 weeks of unpaid leave and not lose her job after Liam's birth.

Charlotte is a big girl! She can now feed herself, and she has very strong opinions about what foods she likes to eat. Sometimes she becomes upset when something (often green) ends up on her plate that she really does not want to eat. Her parents try to encourage her to calm down and tolerate its presence without forcing her to eat it. Mealtimes continue to be messy as Charlotte is more and more encouraged to feed herself. Kelly and John want to promote Charlotte's independence, thinking it will help her develop hand–eye coordination in addition to a sense of agency. Charlotte likes to go to the neighborhood playground to swing and go down the slide. She often says "Watch me" or "Me do it!" as she takes pride in her new tricks. Her language is right on track, as she puts words together to communicate her thoughts, wants, and feelings, but she is not yet speaking full sentences. That does not get in the way of communication, however. Everyone around her generally understands what she is saying, and they engage her in conversation by asking questions, elaborating on what she is saying, and reading to her.

With the arrival of Liam, Charlotte seems overly concerned about where her parents are, not liking to be separate from them. She calls her brother "nicey baby," and she likes to give him kisses, but she also has some trouble sharing her parents' attention. She wants to know why Liam could not play or talk with her like her other friends, and her parents emphasizes that she needs to wait for little Liam to grow up.

Charlotte enjoys going "to school" (which is what her parents call her day-care center), especially to play with the other children. As her language matures, she is more able to use her words in interactions with other children. At school, she and her friends spend a lot of time pretending they are going to work and acting out different jobs and putting on costumes.

CHAPTER 13

Children

Growth and Action

Much of what is known about physical growth and motor action in childhood is based on research and observations of newborns and infants, as children's development in these domains moves fairly rapidly toward their mature state from those earlier stages. This chapter first connects growth and action in childhood as the two mutually reinforce each other, as growth affords opportunities for action and action supports further growth. A common child platform where the two converge and incorporate other developmental social, emotional, attentional, mastery, and cultural systems is play. Play develops dramatically and in stages across the early life period, starting from exploration and function and eventuating in symbolism and representation. Indeed, play is fostered during social interactions, especially with parents who are sensitively attuned to their children's emotional cues and developmental level. A second platform of children's cognitive accomplishment is children's acquisition of a theory of mind, their deepening acknowledgment, and their understanding of the thoughts and feelings of others.

GROWTH AND ACTION TOGETHER

During the childhood period, children make considerable gains in physical growth. The average U.S. 18-month-old weighs 23.75 lb (10.77 kg) and is 32.1 in (81.53 cm) tall. By 36 months, the average U.S. child will have increased in weight by a third, weighing 31.25 lb (14.17 kg) and standing over 3 ft tall (37.3 in, 94.74 cm; Centers for Disease Control, 2000). With these changes in body size comes increasing sophistication in control of body movements: Use of hands, arms, legs, and feet continue to mature, opening up many possibilities for action.

Physical growth and motor action go together in childhood. Children depend on continuing maturation of anatomy, musculature, and the like to execute gross motor actions (reaching) as well as fine motor actions (grasping). Table 13.1 shows the advances in actions that children undergo as a result of growth between 18 and 36 months. Notice that having increasing command and control over one's muscles allows more and more sophisticated activity, just as more and more practice in action improves musculature and coordination. Practice makes perfect.

The coordination of growth and action opens children up to more fully explore their world. Piaget (1952, 1954) brought the significance of action to center stage when he

DOI: 10.4324/9781003381709-16

TABLE 13.1 Motor Milestones for 18-, 24-, and 36-Month-Old Children

Age	*Action*
18 months	Walks without holding on to anyone or anything Scribbles Drinks from a cup without a lid and may spill sometimes Feeds himself with his fingers Tries to use a spoon Climbs on and off a couch or chair without help
24 months	Kicks a ball Runs Walks (not climbs) up a few stairs with or without help Eats with a spoon
30 months	Uses hands to twist things, like turning doorknobs or unscrewing lids Takes some clothes off by himself, like loose pants or an open jacket Jumps off the ground with both feet Turns book pages, one at a time, when you read to them
36 months	Strings items together, like large beads or macaroni Puts on some clothes by himself, like loose pants or a jacket Uses a fork

Source: Centers for Disease Control (2023).

proposed that simple sensorimotor behaviors constitute the foundations of knowledge. Piaget observed his own children in their own early life periods repeat their actions, first related to their bodies, then on simple objects, and eventually between objects. Psychologically, 9-month-old infants transited from simple manipulation and exploring object properties to relational and functional activities with objects as 18-month-old children.

Crawling and walking children draw on increasingly developed motor abilities to adapt their movements in response to changes in surfaces (Adolph & Hospodar, 2025). If the surface on which children are moving appears safe, locomotion proceeds without modification; if the surface appears to be unsafe in any way, children pause, look, and sway side-to-side or rock over their feet forward and backward to seek additional visual and vestibular information about the surface and their ability to maintain their balance when traversing it. Children use alternative forms of locomotion (e.g., backward rather than forward crawling) or refuse to move at all if surfaces appear to be too risky. They even modify their locomoting depending on the amount of friction surfaces provide. All these observations illustrate mutually reciprocal influences of growth and action from infancy into childhood.

Connections between growth and action are supplemented and enriched by parallel developments in related systems. For example, as children develop, they acquire more complex and sophisticated navigational skills based on advances in growth and action as augmented by improving perception and cognition. Among these important skills, wayfinding stands out as a quickly developing and significant navigational skill, denoting children's mounting ability to make use of environmental cues to reach their intended destinations (Farr et al., 2012). During the initial stages of crawling and walking, children heavily rely on landmarks to navigate their surroundings (Mangalindan & Schmuckler, 2017). Children are able to use landmark cues as early as 17 months to locate objects. The sophistication in how they use those cues develops through 30 months as children gain more and more experience (Learmonth et al., 2001; Mangalindan & Schmuckler, 2017).

Between 24 and 36 months, children acquire the ability to use distance and directional relations in more sophisticated ways (Fernandez-Baizan et al., 2021). Children who are more independent, with high scores in self-care activities and domestic and community interaction skills, tend to excel in orientation and cue utilization (van den Brink & Janzen, 2013). Twenty-four-month-old children are more successful in reorienting themselves after disorientation (such as being turned around with one's eyes closed; Learmonth et al., 2001).

Section Summary

Growth and action are intimately intertwined in childhood and in advancing development. Children use their eyes to explore surfaces, use their fingers and arms to explore objects, and use their bodies to approach far objects to explore them better. As a result of their actions, children grow in accuracy and specificity, and they learn more about their social and material worlds. Together, growth and action further promote children's learning about themselves and gaining mastery over their environment. Growth and action come together in especially telling ways in child play.

CHILD PLAY

Play coordinates multiple competencies in physical and motor as well as perceptual, cognitive, linguistic, and socioemotional domains of development, and play matures as these areas develop. Thus, peering through the lens of play opens a vista on the whole child engaging with the world and others in it. To set the stage for a more complete understanding of play and its centrality in children's lives, this discussion of play and its larger competencies and contexts stretches over infancy and into childhood to show how play develops and how it marshals social and contextual supports. Child play is far more than "something contented children do when adults are not bothering them to do other things; and play is something adults tell demanding children to do to get them out of the way" (Fein, 1991, p. 144).

This section therefore first describes the earliest developments of play, which begins as perception and action so central in infancy and moves gradually to symbolism and pretense so typical of childhood. The chapter then examines the ways in which play becomes embedded in social interaction. Play brings children into contact with many material and social features of the environment, and in a variety of ways play constitutes a significant type of self-initiated learning. Finally, other developments that either support the development of play or whose development is facilitated by advances in play are considered.

Development of Play

Play is fun, and it is social. Of course, it is. But for a moment, imagine what play looks like in its earliest stages. Play involves studying a doll, manipulating a busy-box, building with a set of blocks, or role-playing at a make-believe tea party. Play frequently imitates life, and it is common to observe children re-enacting specific events that they observe or which they participate in routinely (driving a toy car). Such play indicates that children explore and represent events mentally, reproducing them in play. In other words, play is also perceptual and cognitive, and it calls on motor skill development. The advent of **symbolic** or **pretend play**, play that is non-literal in quality, during the second year of life reflects an underlying developmental progression in the overall capacity for mental representation (Lillard, 2015; Smith & Roopnarine, 2019).

Piaget and Play

Piaget (1954, 1962) was among the first theorists to study play as a serious activity in human development. Piaget saw play as a platform for children to integrate and express their distinct and changing mental abilities, and he studied play for the light it promised to throw on cognitive development. After all, early play is exploration, and how exploration proceeds reveals much about the growth of the mind.

For Piaget, activities with a single object were the most primitive type of play. Young infants manipulate one object at a time, relying on their sensorimotor behaviors (for example, pushing, pulling, squishing, and so forth). Older infants move on to more advanced activities, manipulating the parts of objects or different objects together to examine relations among them (putting a spoon into a cup). For Piaget, the dynamic use of objects in play appeared to reflect developmental changes in children's cognitions. Many researchers since Piaget have studied play to learn what it tells us about cognitive development, what knowledge infants and children possess, how they acquire new knowledge, and factors that affect the acquisition and use of knowledge.

Studying his own children, Piaget articulated four major (and, as it turns out, enduring) principles about play:

1. Play follows an ordinal sequence in development.
2. Action is the basis of knowledge.
3. Representational (pretend) play, involving the use of one object to stand for another or pretending to engage in an action, has a late onset and slow development.
4. Pretend play shifts from play that involves only the self (pretending to sleep) through pretense involving self–object relations (pretending to drink from a cup) to pretense involving objects exclusively (having a doll pretend to drink).

Piaget's many successors have confirmed these principles, and along the way they have refined the ways that play is assessed (Smith & Roopnarine, 2019). Assessments vary depending on whether developmental scientists study infants' and children's naturalistic and unstructured free play, their modelling play, or parents' prompting play. Some scholars have also integrated play assessments into interventions, as for special-needs infants and children (Ravn et al., 2011).

The earliest forms of play involve the repetition of actions. Objects in the environment do not have an important role in play during the first 2 or 3 months of life. Instead, newborns play with their bodies. For example, 3-month-olds may coo repeatedly (as if playing with the sounds they can make) or kick their legs over and over while lying awake in their cribs. These actions are recognizable as Piaget's primary circular reactions – activities apparently repeated for their own sake. Even after infants develop more sophisticated manipulative skills around 4 to 6 months, they are primarily interested in the actions they can perform rather than in the objects being manipulated. Thus, young infants might look at a toy in their field of vision (Figure 13.1a). Even when two objects appear related to each other – two cups and a spoon – infants often still focus on actions rather than objects, such as banging the spoon in each cup rather than exploring the different cups (Figure 13.1b). Remove the spoon and the action is likely to continue, but this time with banging the cups.

At around 9 months of age, a major change in the complexity and quality of play occurs. Infants begin to engage in functional, relational, and functional-relational play. **Functional play** involves playing with an object in the way the object was intended to be played with (e.g., rolling a toy car on its wheels across the floor). In **relational play**, infants bring together two unrelated objects (e.g., a spoon and a block) with no indication of pretense (Figure 13.2a). **Functional-relational play** brings together two objects, but now in a meaningful and appropriate way. For example, infants may take a spoon and stir it inside a cup or place blocks inside a container (Figure 13.2b).

For the next several months, clear-cut pretense or symbolism is seldom evident. According to Piaget, pretense requires bringing to mind a physically absent object and hence involves representational skills, which he claimed were not attained until 18 months or so. Consistent with this notion, pretend play does not occur with any regularity until the second year of life, although some infants show this capacity as early as 13 months of age (Bornstein, 2007).

Symbolic (pretense) play can be clearly identified in the emergence of object substitution. When young children build a tower out of blocks, the tower seems to mean more to them than the characteristics of the blocks per se. Even when children are operating at the level of pretense, play initially centers on their own bodies and actions. In self-directed pretense play, children might pretend that they are going to sleep, drinking from a cup, or talking on a telephone (Figure 13.3). Later, children involve objects other than the self in their pretense. Children first pretend to sleep by lying down on a pillow and only later make a doll lie down and sleep. Even after this movement away from the self has taken place, significant developmental changes lie ahead. Play becomes more complex with age through the incorporation of combinations and sequences of pretend actions. Older children also make more elaborate plans for future play, as when they play "kitchen" and appear to prepare a whole meal.

The development of play from infancy through childhood can be broadly summarized (Lillard, 2015). In the first year, play is predominantly characterized by sensorimotor manipulation; infant play appears designed to extract information about objects, what objects do, what perceivable qualities they have, and what immediate effects they can produce. This form of play is commonly referred to as **nonsymbolic (exploratory) play** because play activities are tied to the tangible properties of objects rather than being

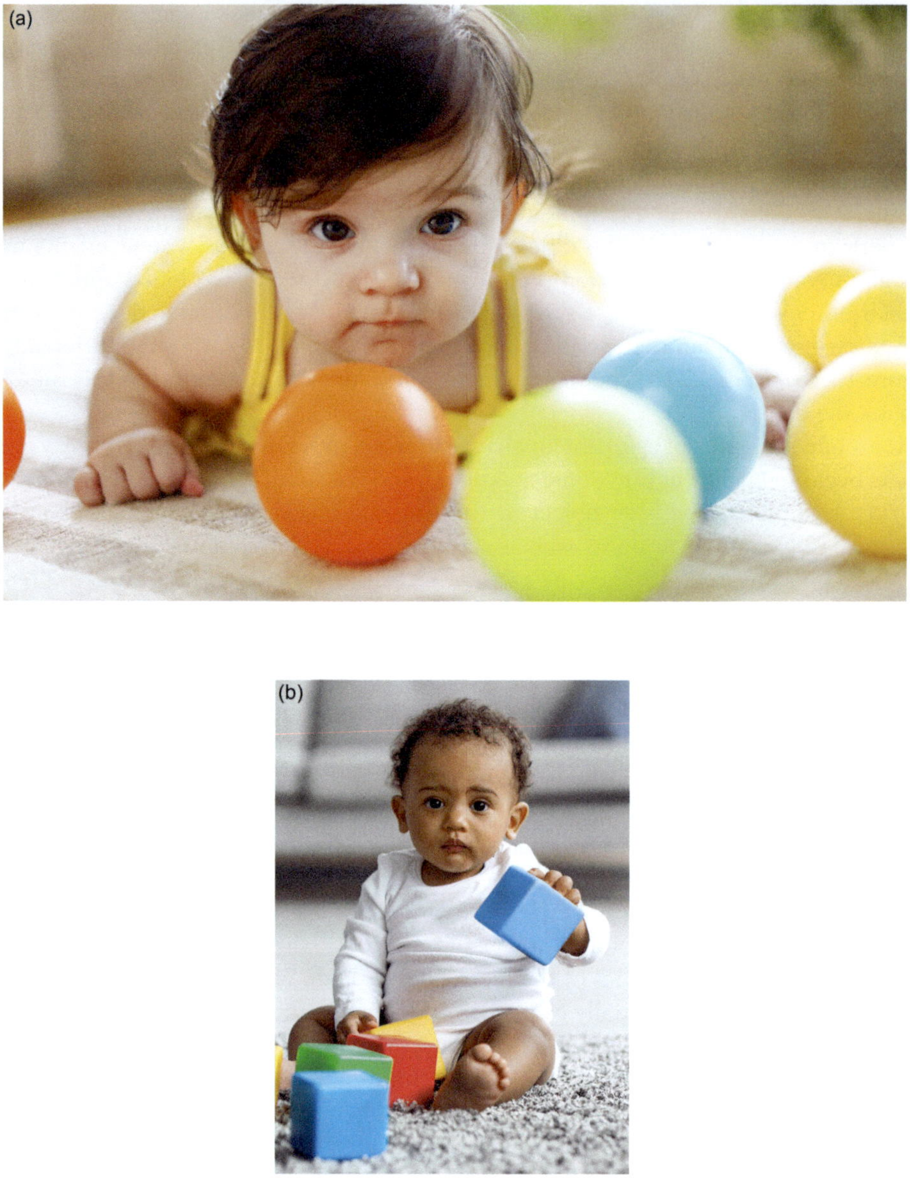

FIGURE 13.1 Infants in the earliest stage of play look at toys (a) but soon develop the motive and ability to interact with toys manually (b).

representational. In the second year, play actions take on more of a non-literal quality, commonly referred to as **symbolic (representational) play**. Play is also increasingly generative, as children enact activities performed by self, others, and objects in simple pretense scenarios, such as pretending to drink from empty teacups, talking on toy telephones, and the like.

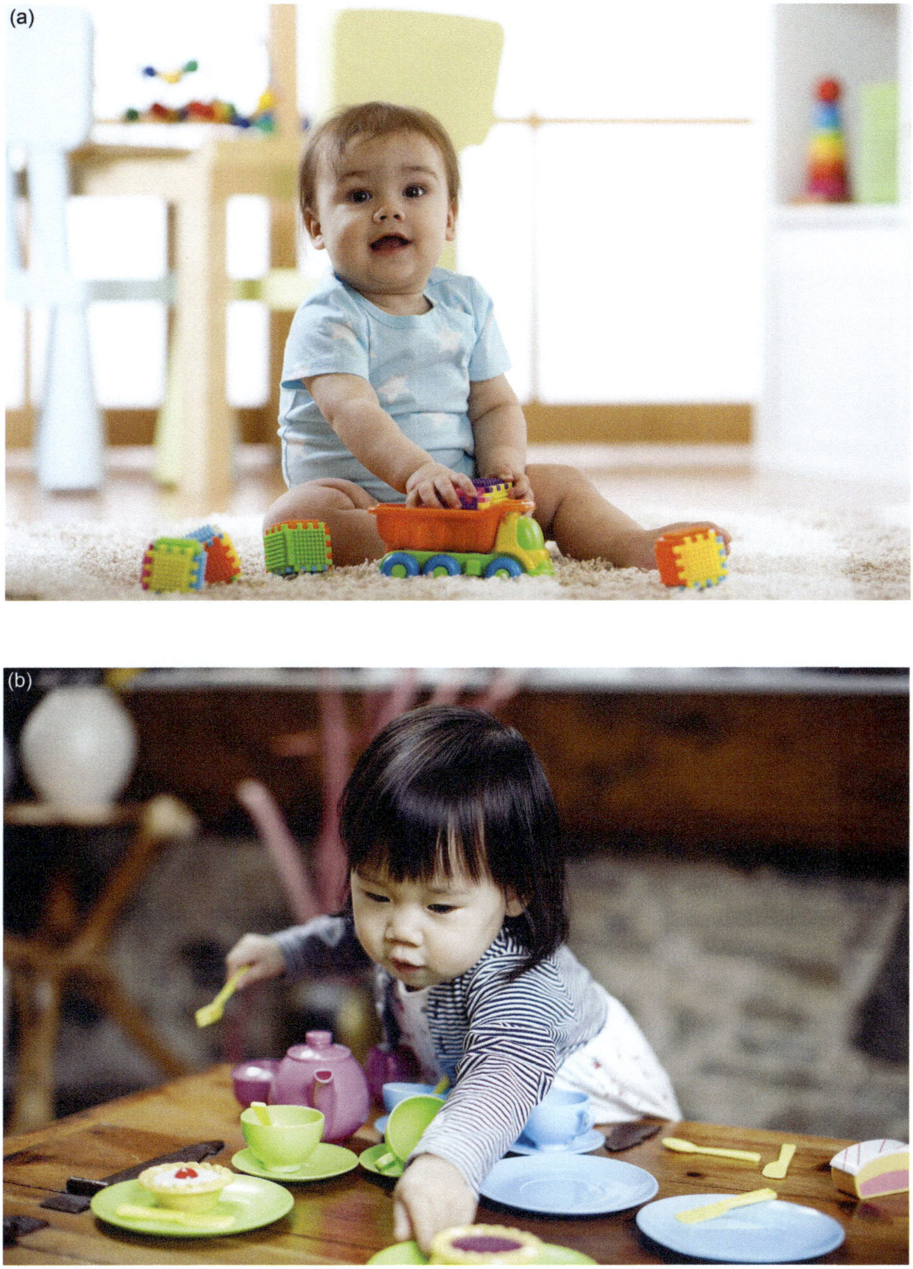

FIGURE 13.2 (a) Infants in the relational stage of play may bring two objects into juxtaposition, such as placing a block on a truck and then removing it (but not driving the truck). (b) Infants in the functional-relational stage of play may bring together objects in meaningful ways, such as placing eating utensils on every plate.

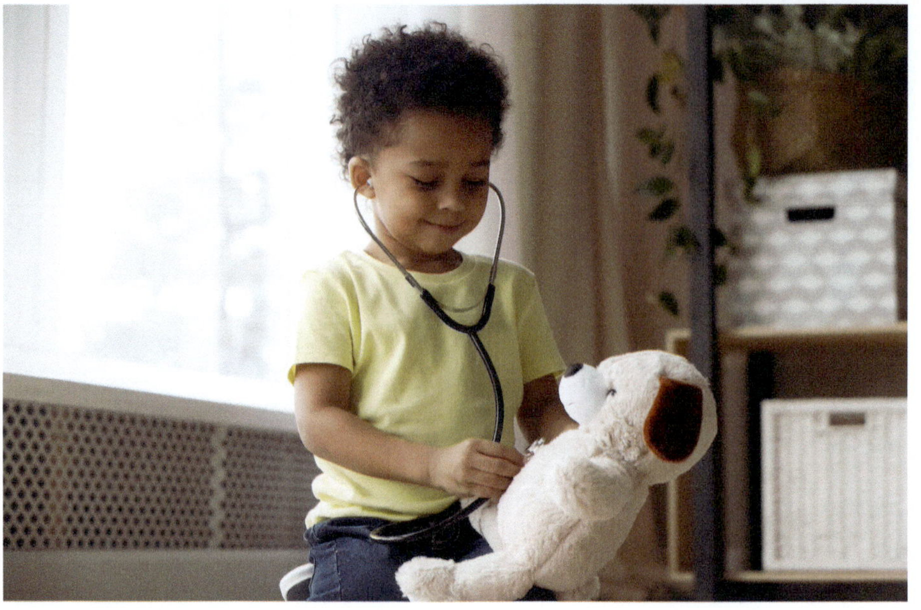

FIGURE 13.3 A child engaged in symbolic or representational play by pretending to be a doctor examining a patient.

This sequence portrays an idealized developmental progression: Most children progress this way, but (as stressed repeatedly in this book) children of a given age vary greatly among themselves, here with respect to their symbolic play. For example, Tamis-LeMonda et al. (2019) reported that 15% of 13-month-olds' total play was symbolic, but some individual 13-month-olds never exhibited symbolic play, whereas for others as much as 51% of their play was symbolic. At 20 months, 31% of children's total play was symbolic, but some individual 20-month-olds showed as little as 2% symbolic play, whereas for others 83% of play was symbolic. Furthermore, 13-month symbolic play levels predicted 20-month symbolic play levels – children who showed more representational play at 13 months also showed more representational play at 20 months – but stability in child play appeared to depend on the support of mothers.

Play in Systems Perspective

Play has broad implications for children's development and facilitates growth across five major developmental domains: emotional, mastery, cognitive, social, and cultural (Tamis-LeMonda et al., 2019). Emotionally, play calls on children to regulate their states of arousal, to express a range of emotions, and to resolve conflicts and traumas. For example, play partners (such as parents) who respond appropriately to children's needs for stimulation contribute to children's self-regulatory capacities. Play also expands the range of emotions which children express by enabling them to experience positive feelings of fun, excitement, and pleasure as well as negative feelings of anger, sadness, and frustration. The mastery function of play promotes **self-efficacy** in children, that is beliefs in their own abilities. The repetitive nature of play helps children perfect skills, which enhances their self-confidence. Play is associated with improved cognition, as expressed in greater attention span and persistence in problem-solving. In addition, during, and as a result of, play, children acquire information and skills, engage in creative and divergent thinking, and attain more sophisticated representational abilities (Onishi et al., 2007). Socially, play fosters children's understanding of others' feelings, intentions, and perspectives and thereby deepens their interpersonal interactions and relationships. Play also supports children's development of **reciprocity** (social exchanges, such as turn-taking) and **intersubjectivity** (shared meaning), which together forge a foundation for more mature forms of emotional and social understanding. Finally, play is a vehicle for the transmission of social roles and cultural values. In role-play, children practice behaviors they will need as functioning adults in their society, and role-play affords children opportunities to understand and acquire societal standards and beliefs. During play, children learn ways of thinking and behaving as appropriate to their culture (Clearfield & Nelson, 2006).

Section Summary

Both Piaget and contemporary researchers argue that play increasingly relies on representational abilities as infants age into children. Early play is nonsymbolic and exploratory, whereas later play is symbolic and representational. Infant-to-child play proceeds through a series of well-defined stages. Symbolic play can emerge as early as 13 months, and symbolic play in infancy predicts symbolic play in childhood. Individual differences exist both in children's progression through the stages of play and in the frequency of different types of play children engage in. Not insignificantly, play harnesses perceptual, mental, verbal, emotional, and social systems in development.

CONCLUSIONS

Growth and action mutually reinforce each other throughout the early life period. Growth opens gates to action, and the two come together and are well expressed in child play. Play changes dramatically from infancy to childhood, developing from exploration and functional manipulation of objects toward more sophisticated acts of representational pretense to self and the self with others in the material world. Play follows a species-typical development that, in turn, reflects broader cultural themes and values. Children engage in increasingly symbolic pretense that reflects the further development, refinement, and elaboration of their symbolic representational capacities. Additionally, play has systemic social, emotional, attentional, and mastery components and does not develop in isolation from culture but is shaped in development by cultural forces. Indeed, play is fostered during social interactions, especially with parents who are sensitively attuned to their children's emotional cues and developmental level.

KEY TERMS

Functional play
Functional-relational play
Intersubjectivity
Nonsymbolic (exploratory) play
Reciprocity
Relational play
Self-efficacy
Symbolic (pretend) play
Symbolic (representational) play

SUGGESTED READINGS

Lillard, A. S. (2015). The development of play. In L. S. Liben, U. Müller, & R. M. Lerner (Eds.), *Handbook of child psychology and developmental science: Cognitive processes* (Vol. 2, 7th ed., pp. 425–468). Wiley.

Veraksa, N., Colliver, Y., & Sukhikh, V. (2022). Piaget and Vygotsky's play theories: The profile of twenty-first-century evidence. In N. Veraksa & I. Pramling Samuelsson (Eds.), *Piaget and Vygotsky in XXI century. Early childhood research and education: An inter-theoretical focus* (Vol. 4, pp. 165–190). Springer.

CHAPTER 14

Children

Perception and Thought

In Piaget's theory of mental development, sensorimotor function dominated the newborn and infancy stages of the early life period. The advent of childhood changes that focus qualitatively as, for Piaget, this next stage in the mental life of the child represents a significant advance because of the onset of mental representation abilities. **Mental representation** refers to the ability to think about people, objects, and events even in their absence. As such, mental representation both constitutes a foundation of advanced cognition and reflects nothing short of a significant leap in the development of the mind. It turns out, however, that modern developmental scientists have recognized that Piaget likely underestimated infants' abilities, which have proved to be more advanced than Piaget originally supposed. Cognitive competencies, such as categorization, support this revisionist perspective on the development of cognition in childhood. Children are also learning by interacting with others in the form of imitation and observation, all facilitated by language. Of course, as childhood cognition proceeds, multiple developmental systems become more and more integrated, and so it becomes more and more challenging to disaggregate the contributions or constituents of any one system from the others. In short, it is beyond methodologically challenging to separate how children perceive the world from how they act on it, what they know about it, and how they talk about it.

MENTAL REPRESENTATION

In his systematic theory of mental development in childhood, Piaget asserted that children possess the emergent capacity to mentally represent people, objects, and events in the world at around 18 months of age, his sixth stage of mental development. According to Piaget, it is not until this stage that children command a fuller understanding of **object permanence**, knowledge that an object continues to exist even though the object is out of sight. With command of this mental ability, children can now imagine the whereabouts of an invisible object. They can also imagine invisible trajectories, so that when a ball rolls under a sofa, for example, children will move around the sofa and anticipate the re-emergence of the ball rather than attempt to follow its trajectory directly. These examples show successful representation of space and relations among objects. Children are also now able to imitate people even in their absence or imitate events they witnessed at some earlier point in time (**deferred imitation**). At this juncture and with this capacity as well,

DOI: 10.4324/9781003381709-17

children become capable of insightful problem-solving. Children's practical knowledge of the world is now so realistic that solutions to problems can be reached even prior to any direct experience with them. According to Piaget, however, attaining mental representation and insightful problem-solving is made possible only by many slow, struggling anticipatory accommodations. Thus, intrinsic tendencies of the organism, experience, and the emergence of new cognitive capacities play intertwined roles in the development of children's mental life.

Object Permanence

According to Piaget, understanding objects and their permanence develops across the first two years of life. Around 4 months of age, infants may retrieve an object that is partly covered. At 8 months or so, infants can retrieve an object that is fully covered, but if the location of the hidden object is switched, infants search at the first place they found the object (A) rather than at the correct location (B). They make the A-not-B error. Later, at 12 months, infants can find objects hidden in different locations, but they still have difficulty with invisible displacements, such as when objects are moved to a new location without them seeing the object (for example, when hidden in a hand; Figure 9.5). In these typical Piagetian tasks, infants show these behaviors very reliably: There is no question that infants respond as *if* they do not completely understand the permanence of objects. Out of sight *is* out of mind.

However, when infants are tested in tasks that do not require active search, they give evidence that they possess a better understanding of the continued existence of objects even when those objects are out of view. This more sophisticated understanding is shown in an experiment that tested infants' object permanence using looking, which is easier to control and develops earlier, than reaching, which is harder to control and develops later (Baillargeon et al., 1985). In a violation-of-expectation paradigm (Box 6.1), infants viewed a screen that rotated toward and away from them (Figure 14.1). Following habituation to the screen, a box was placed in the display area such that, as the screen rotated away from infants, the box was hidden from view. In one event, the screen stopped at the location of the now-hidden box. This event was a possible event because, if you believed the box continues to exist, the screen would have to stop. In a contrasting impossible event, the screen did not stop: It continued to rotate away from infants, apparently passing through the space occupied by the now-hidden box. This event is impossible because two objects cannot occupy the same space at the same time. Five-month-old infants looked significantly longer at the impossible than the possible event, suggesting that infants have an expectation that the box continued to exist even though it was out of sight.

Another example of early object knowledge, not predicted by Piaget's theory, is a study of newborns' perception of object solidity and trajectory (Spelke et al., 1992). Two-month-olds viewed an event in which a ball, starting at the left side of the display, rolled to the right side, moving behind a panel. After the ball stopped, the panel was raised and the ball was seen resting against a wall (Figure 14.2, left side). This was the habituation phase of the experiment. During a subsequent test phase of the experiment, newborns viewed two events. In both events, the wall was moved forward to a new location. In the consistent event (Figure 14.2, middle), the ball stopped at the wall in its new location, which is consistent with physics and thus expected (solid objects do not pass through

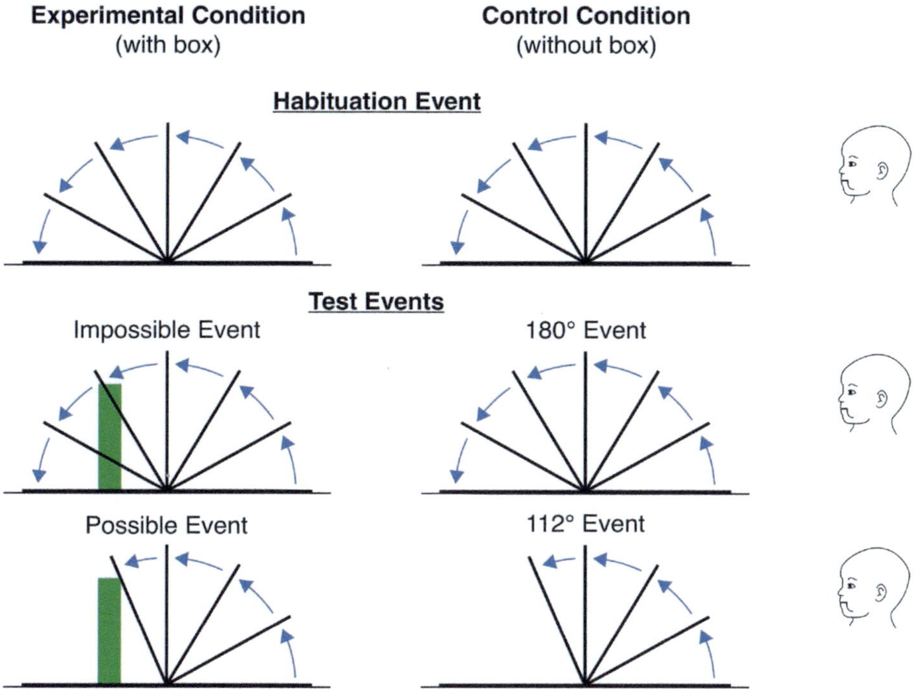

FIGURE 14.1 Impossible and possible events used to test infants' object permanence. Experimental conditions are on the left. In an impossible event, a screen moves from right to left through an arc and appears to pass through the box; in the possible event, the screen stops at the location of the box. The control condition is on the right. Here, the screen moves in similar manner to the experimental events but the box was not present.

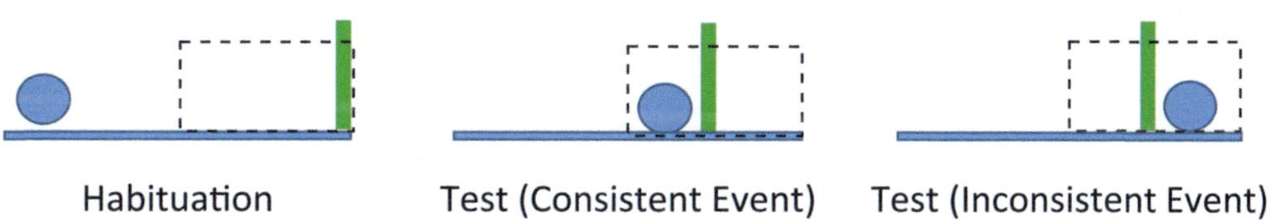

FIGURE 14.2 Schematic representation of events used to test 2-month-olds' understanding of continuity, trajectory, and solidity. In all three events, a ball rolled from left to right behind a screen (shown as a dotted rectangle). After the ball stopped, the screen was removed, revealing the location of the ball relative to the wall (green rectangle).

solid walls). In the inconsistent event (Figure 14.2, right side), the ball stopped at the old location, but to do so, it had to pass through the wall. If newborns understand that balls cannot pass through walls, then they should look longer at the inconsistent event (the one that violated physical principles) more than the consistent event. In fact, the newborns looked longer at inconsistent than consistent events. In Piaget's theory, 2-month-olds are only beginning to coordinate schemes in the primary circular reactions stage, so they have no expectations about how objects behave in relation to each other.

To explain these findings, some researchers have suggested that newborns and infants arrive in the world equipped with specific learning mechanisms that enable rapid acquisition of knowledge about object categories (animate objects, inanimate objects that move, and inanimate objects that do not move) as well as physical events (events in which objects collide with other objects, are hidden by other objects, or support other objects). For example, at 2 1/2 months of age, newborns' relatively simple understanding of collision lead them to expect any moving object to displace any stationary object on impact, and so they appear surprised when this does not happen. By about 6 months of age, infants seem to understand that a large moving object will, on impact, displace a stationary object farther than will a small moving object. By 8 months, infants begin to take the stationary object's shape into account in determining whether the stationary object will be displaced by the moving object.

This nativist attribution to newborns and infants is called **core knowledge** (Spelke, 2016) and, of course, is not without controversy. Some critics contend that these types of experiments are not well enough designed to eliminate alternative interpretations of newborns' and infants' responses (Cohen & Cashon, 2006; Jackson & Sirois, 2022). Another question is why different results arise based on tasks such as looking versus searching. Eight-month-olds successfully retrieve a hidden object, but they have trouble with changes in location (the A-not-B error). Yet 5-month-olds look longer at events where one object (a screen) moves through the space occupied by another object (a block; Figure 14.1). According to some researchers, newborns' and infants' search skills may be at issue, in that search errors reflect immaturity in inhibiting action or inability to integrate information in a search task (Baker et al., 2011). For example, infants successfully find an object in the dark before finding it hidden under a cloth, suggesting that they do not forget the object exists but instead may have difficulty integrating the actions involved in removing the cloth to then find the object (Shinskey & Munakata, 2003). This apparent disconnect between what infants and children may know versus what they actually do illustrates the important developmental distinction between competence and performance in attempting to plumb whether newborns, infants, and children represent the world mentally. In brief, newborns, infants, and children may possess the competence to understand something but may not possess the equipment necessary to perform that something. The plight of the early life period is thus: *I know the object exists, but I just cannot show or tell you that I know.*

Evaluation of Piaget's Theory

In many ways, Piaget's theory of cognitive development is unrivalled in elegance and scope, and there is empirical corroboration for many of his proposed developmental achievements as well as for the sequences in which they occur. His theory has served as the foundation for the study of the development of cognition. The topics Piaget identified, including conceptions of objects, number, time, space, and causality, have been principal subjects for research in cognitive development ever since Piaget identified them. However, no other theory in infancy has undergone such intense scrutiny, and the inevitable result of such attention has been the emergence of a body of work that takes issue with Piaget's assumptions, observations, formulations, and conclusions.

A basic tenet of Piagetian theory is that cognition is rooted in action, without which newborns, infants, and children would not be able to derive meaning from sensory and perceptual events. However, in grounding all knowledge in motor activity, Piaget mistakenly ignored the vital contributions of perceptual and sensory activity to representation and knowledge. An early (and tragic) natural experiment unearthed fault lines in Piaget's theoretical landscape. In Europe in the 1960s, some pregnant women were administered a drug called thalidomide to control nausea during the first trimester of pregnancy. During the first trimester, limbs are differentiating anatomically, and the drug thalidomide operated to inhibit limb differentiation. Mothers who ingested thalidomide at that time gave birth to limbless children (Décarie, 1969). However, these children developed a normal cognitive life despite the absence of normal sensorimotor experience throughout their early life. In addition, Piagetian theory does not give sufficient credit to the remarkable sensory and organizational capacities of newborns and infants, whose perceptions are multimodally integrated, rather than composed of disconnected bits of information coming from different senses.

Perhaps the greatest empirical challenges to Piaget's theory of sensorimotor development, however, come from those findings indicating that capacities for mental representation of the physical world appear much earlier in development than Piaget asserted. Lines of research that have contributed to this revolutionary conclusion include newborns' likely imitation of the facial expressions of others within minutes after birth, indicating that a rudimentary capacity to represent the external world might be present at birth, and research showing that newborns and infants possess the capacities for perceiving and representing the physical world.

Section Summary

According to Piaget, infant mental development across early life is based on active engagement with the world, often by using trial and error to solve problems. Piaget's stage 6 is a watershed moment, with children gaining representation skills, including object permanence. Tasks using looking time, rather than manual search, show earlier competencies that Piaget described, and children with physical limitations that result in reduced object exploration, as was the case with thalidomide exposure in utero, are cognitively on par with children who do not have limitations.

PROBLEM-SOLVING

The central developmental significance and implications of the competence–performance distinction are made plain in the study represented in Figure 14.2 and in related research. Recall that 2-month-olds who took part in that study looked longer at an inconsistent event, suggesting that even newborns find a ball that moves through a wall surprising. A similar task was used with older children (Berthier et al., 2000). In this follow-up research, children of two ages saw a ball move down a ramp, behind a panel with four doors. Visible above the panel was a wall, which would stop the ball, as the children saw during the familiarization phase of the experiment (Figure 14.3). Children were then asked to find the ball by opening one of the four doors. The 24-month-olds performed at chance; they seemed not to know which door to open to find the ball. Even 36-month-olds did not always select the correct door on the first try. This finding led Keen (2003, p. 79) to ask, "Why do infants look so smart and toddlers look so dumb?" In other words, do children forget or unlearn that objects do not move through walls between 2 and 24 months?

Arterberry and colleagues (2018, 2020) suggested that children in this age range might have trouble integrating perception and cognition with action. To solve the door task successfully, children need to perceive the location of the wall, reason that the ball cannot pass through the wall (when they themselves cannot see the ball hit the wall, as both are hidden behind the door), and then open the door to the correct side of the wall. This sequence may be a bit much for a 24-month-old to follow, hold in memory, and act on. This conclusion is reinforced by findings of a study in which 24-month-old children were tested on a variant of the door task. In this follow-up experiment, half of the children wore weighted wristbands, and the other half wore unweighted wristbands. The investigators reasoned that wearing weights would slow children's action planning so that they would have the time to consider all relevant information. Indeed, children who wore weighted wristbands performed better than children who wore unweighted wristbands. Curiously, however, the children who wore the weights did not do better immediately. For example,

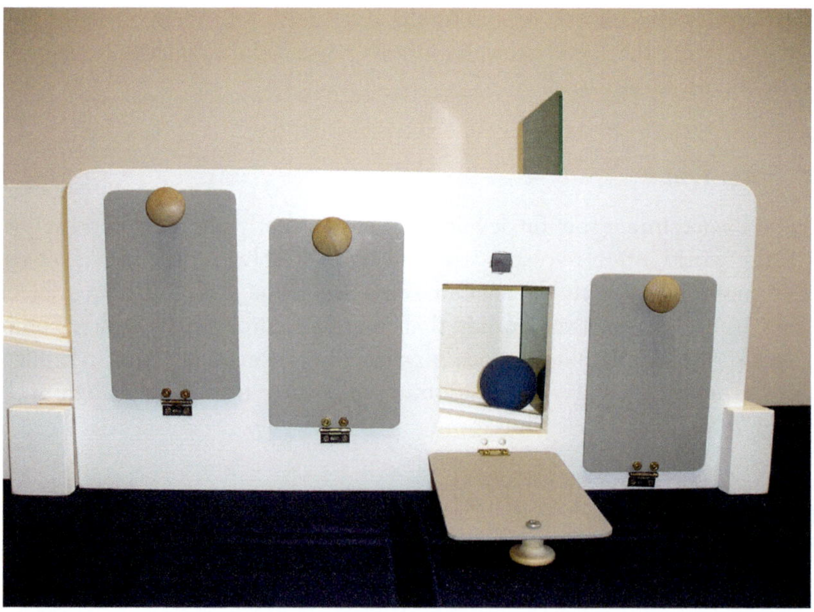

FIGURE 14.3 In this task, children saw a ball at the left roll down a ramp behind four closed doors. The ball stopped at the green vertical wall. Children were asked to find the ball by opening one of the four doors.

Source: Courtesy of M. E. Arterberry.

on their first search in the door task, they were just as likely as the children who wore unweighted wristbands to open the wrong door. When given the chance to search again, however, the children who wore the weights were more likely to meet with success.

Children 13- to 36-months-old are known to commit another common (and sometimes funny) cognition-action error. In making so-called **scale errors** (Figure 14.4), children surprisingly treat miniature toy versions of cars, chairs, and slides as though they were the appropriate real sizes for them. For example, they earnestly try to fit their whole body into a small-scale toy car (DeLoache, 2004; DeLoache et al., 2013). At least three types of such scale errors have been identified. *Body scale errors* occur when children interact inappropriately with objects in relation to their own body (like trying genuinely to fit into a toy car). Object and tool scale errors occur when children interact inappropriately with two or more objects, such as putting a doll to sleep in a bed that is too small for the doll or selecting a tool that is too small to achieve a goal (Casler et al., 2011; Ware et al., 2006). Body scale errors tend to emerge developmentally earliest, followed by object/tool scale errors (Jiang & Rosengren, 2018). Scale errors appear to peak when children are around 20 to 24 months of age (Ware et al., 2010). Different developmental scientists tend to favor different explanations for scale errors, but the common theme is that children appear to focus on object shape or function while ignoring size (Casler et al., 2011; Grzyb et al.,

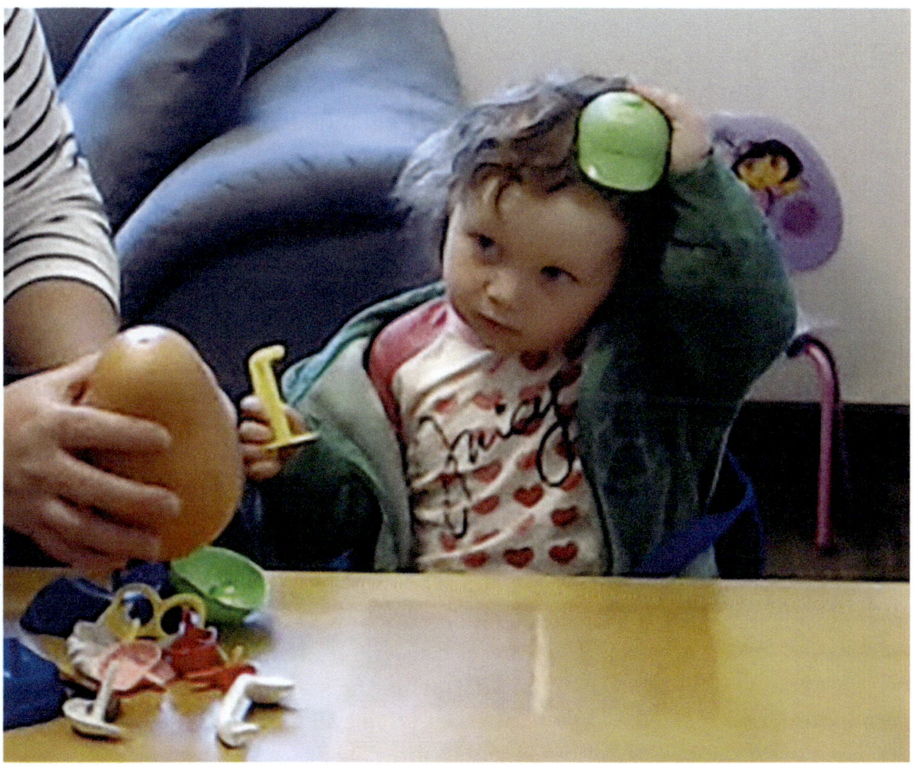

FIGURE 14.4 A child making a body scale error by trying to put a toy hat on her head.
Source: Courtesy of M. E. Arterberry.

2019; Hunley & Hahn, 2016). In a systems connection, these errors may be predicted by vocabulary development (Hagihara et al., 2024), but how word knowledge might account for scale errors is unclear.

Together, studies that explore the interplay among perception, cognition, and action and compare performance across ages on tasks that appear to rely on the same perceptual or cognitive knowledge betray the fact that a lot of cognition still develops across childhood, that is between 12 and 36 months of age. Moreover, scale errors and the like reinforce the caution that just because children may know something (competence) does not mean they put that knowledge to use (performance).

Section Summary

Despite impressive abilities documented in newborns and infants, children make errors in simple tasks. This situation is an example of the competence-performance distinction, and it is a reminder that newborns, infants, and children may understand something but are not always able to show it. It also is a reminder that there is still a lot of development that takes place in childhood.

REPRESENTATION

Mental representation abilities are diverse, and they grow considerably between 18 months and 36 months. The following discussion illustrates these two principles – diversity and development – in two domains of mental representation. One is **symbolic relations**, as exemplified in matching line drawings, scale models, or photographs to real objects, and the other is **categorization**, as exemplified in grouping conceptually similar yet discriminably different properties or objects into a set according to some rule.

Symbolic Relations

Infants sometimes show confusion regarding symbolic relations (DeLoache, 2011). For example, infants may confuse realistic pictures with their real objects or have difficulty equating pictures, particularly line drawings, with real-world objects. Later still, children have difficulty understanding equivalences between scale models and real spaces, like where a couch is located in a real room and where a toy couch is located in a dollhouse version of that same room (Troseth et al., 2007). In an example task, an experimenter hid a miniature toy under a couch in a scale model of a room while a child watched. The child was then brought into the actual room and asked to find the toy. Thirty-six-month-olds promptly searched for and retrieved the hidden toy, but 30-month-olds were flummoxed. The younger children did not find the toy because their memory of the hiding event was faulty; most could readily find the miniature toy in the scale model of the room. Instead, the 30-month-olds appeared unable to use the hiding event in the model to symbolize the hidden location of the real toy in the actual room.

These kinds of findings about early representation unveil the nature of children's minds, and they remind us how children use their minds. In the scale model task, children must understand that the model represents the room. A moment's reflection reveals that the appreciation of books and television calls on similar abilities. When and to what degree do children believe that what they see and hear represent actual reality? The answers to these questions have implications for when and how parents introduce children to media, including digital media, a topic we discuss in Chapter 17.

Categorization

Our world consists of infinite numbers of people, objects, and events, and without conscious thought, we group instances or members of each into categories: girls versus boys, animals versus vehicles, schools versus cinemas. Try to imagine how confusing and jumbled the world would be to children if they did not exercise some similar forms of unconscious or automatic categorization. According to Rakison and Oakes (2003, p. 4), "categories are collections of things in the world and concepts are the internal mental depiction of those collections." Categories vary along all sorts of dimensions and features (the category of "red things," "kitchen utensils," or "things that are human-made"), and a given instance or member can be grouped into different categories (e.g., a dog is both an animal and a living object). Thus, members of a category may be grouped together because they share a common attribute, element, or relation. Categorizing calls for grouping otherwise discriminable properties, objects, or events, like phonemes (/b/ and /b'/ as opposed to /p/) and colors (blue and blue' as opposed to green), and different types of dogs (Labradors as opposed to Corgis).

Categories also have some distinguishing overarching attributes. Categories have **breadth** (the variety of instances or members which are included in the category), **prototypes** (instances or members of the category which are best examples of the category), and **boundaries** (instances or members whose inclusion in the category is marginal or debatable). For example, for the category of birds, all birds have feathers and beaks, but birds vary in color, size, manner of locomotion, and preferred habitat (e.g., trees, ground, water). Thus, the category of birds includes variation, but at the same time, the category of birds has boundaries. Penguins do not fly, but they lay eggs like other birds. Reptiles also lay eggs and do not fly, but they are not birds. Penguins have other characteristics in common with birds that reptiles do not, and as a result, they are included in the category of bird. The best category prototypes possess many (or perhaps all) of the identifying features of a category, and the prototype is often what we think of when we think of a category. For many, robin, duck, and pigeon are prototypes of the bird category, whereas ostriches, penguins, and road runners are not.

Another key attribute of categories is that they are organized into hierarchies. Developmental scientists have distinguished superordinate from basic and from subordinate categories (Figure 14.5). **Superordinate categories** allow for greater inclusiveness even though individual members of the category may not share much perceptual similarity. Animals (versus vehicles) are a superordinate category. **Basic categories** are subsumed under superordinate categories, and their instances or members are discriminable but still share many perceptual features. Cats (versus horses) constitute a basic category that falls under the superordinate category of animals. **Subordinate categories** are subsumed under basic categories; their instances or members are still discriminable, and they share many perceptual features. Siamese and Persians make up a subordinate category of household cats.

As categorization is pervasive, a long-standing question has been at what level infants and children first categorize. Do they begin by seeing and understanding superordinate categories, or do they begin by seeing and understanding more constrained basic or by seeing

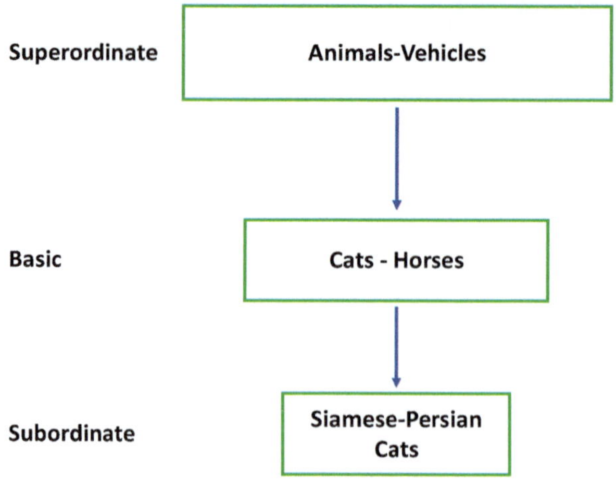

FIGURE 14.5 Hierarchical organization of categories into superordinate, basic, and subordinate levels.

Source: Created by M. E. Arterberry.

and understanding even more constrained subordinate categories? Charting the developmental order of acquisition of object categories has been difficult because no one method can be used across the span of the early life period. Habituation/novelty-responsiveness techniques (Box 6.1) have been used with infants, but children do not tolerate those techniques well. Object examining or sequential touching techniques have been used with children, but infants lack motor skills that are needed for them (Box 14.1). Unfortunately, different methods have revealed different developmental timetables for categorization, and even with infants of the same age (5 months; Mash & Bornstein, 2012). Generally, habituation/novelty-responsiveness tasks show earlier and more advanced categorization than object examining or sequential touching tasks. For example, 6- to 7-month-olds categorized different breeds of dogs in a looking-time task (Quinn et al., 2010), but 30-month-olds produced no parallel evidence of categorization in a sequential touching task (Bornstein & Arterberry, 2010). These different patterns of results led Westermann and Mareschal (2012) to suggest that different methods may be tapping into different cognitive systems underlying categorization.

To address the developmental question of the order of emergence of categorization level, it is necessary to test different-aged children at the different categorization levels using the same procedure. Bornstein and Arterberry (2010) used sequential touching with 12-, 18-, 24-, and 30-month-old infants and children, testing each age group with seven object sets representing superordinate, basic, and subordinate levels within the same domain (animals-vehicles or fruit-furniture). From 12 to 30 months of age, infants and children categorized at more inclusive levels (e.g., superordinate: animals versus vehicles) before less-inclusive levels (e.g., basic: types of animals or vehicles) and did not categorize the least inclusive level (e.g., subordinate: specific animals or vehicles). As a group, even 12-month-olds categorized at the superordinate level, and even the oldest children did not categorize at the subordinate level. Categorizing at the superordinate and basic levels might develop in parallel, rather than one before the other, but subordinate categorization is clearly the last to emerge. That subordinate categorization may lag behind categorization at the superordinate or basic level is also reflected in research conducted with infants

Box 14.1 *How Do We Know This?* Procedures for Testing Categorization

Three methods are typically used to study infants' and children's categorization. The first relies on attention or looking time, and it is a variant of the habituation–novelty responsiveness procedure (described in Box 6.1). In this categorization task, infants are first familiarized with several items from the same category (different animals) and are then presented with a novel item from the same category (yet another animal) and a novel item from a different category (a vehicle). Categorization is inferred if infants pay more attention after habituation to the novel out-of-category item (the vehicle) than to the novel in-category item (the new animal). Habituation procedures have been used to document infants' categorizing geometric forms, animals, vehicles, human gait patterns, phonemes, emotional expressions, and spatial relations (Park & Casasola, 2015; Quinn, 2011; Shin et al., 2018; Tsang et al., 2018).

Two other methods are appropriate for infants and children who have developed fine motor skills. One is **object examining** and is similar to habituation in that infants and children interact with one object at a time, and the amount of time they engage in active exploration of the object is measured (Oakes et al., 1991; Figure 14.6).

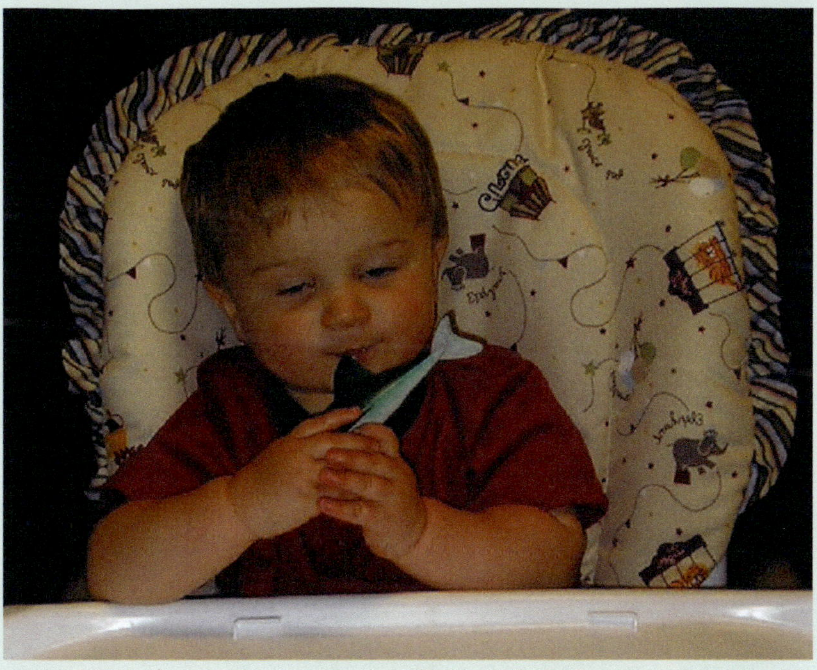

FIGURE 14.6 A 12-month-old infant exploring a replica dolphin in an object-examining task.

Source: Courtesy of M. E. Arterberry.

During a familiarization phase, infants and children explore instances or members of a single category (such as animals). During the test phase, infants receive trials with a new instance or member from the familiar category (another animal) and an instance or member from a new category (a vehicle). Ferguson and Casasola (2015) used this procedure to explore the role of stimulus features, specifically whether objects were plastic or wooden replicas, in 14- to 15-month-olds' categorization of animals and vehicles. Both infants in the United States and Malawi, Africa, categorized and generalized wooden replicas; however, Malawian infants did not generalize category membership to the plastic replicas, likely due to their unfamiliarity with plastic.

The other is **sequential touching**, typically displaying eight small three-dimensional models, four each belonging to two different categories, such as animals and vehicles (Mandler et al., 1987). The eight models are distributed randomly on a table in front of the child, and the experimenter encourages the child to play with them (Figure 14.7). Categorization is inferred if the child touches or manipulates objects within a category more frequently (i.e., at greater than chance levels) than objects between the two categories.

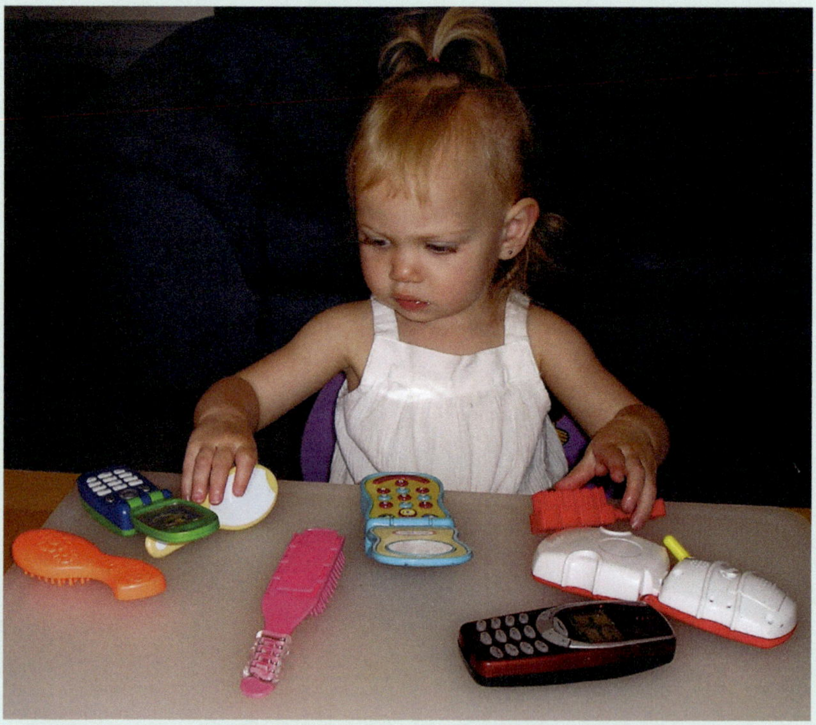

FIGURE 14.7 An 18-month-old explores eight objects, four from one category (mobile phones) and four from a different category (hairbrushes).

Source: Courtesy of M. E. Arterberry.

using looking-time tasks. Infants 3 to 4 months of age categorize at the superordinate or basic levels, whereas not even 6- to 7-month-olds categorize at the subordinate level (Arterberry & Bornstein, 2001; Quinn, 2004, 2011).

Section Summary

Categorization is a cognitive process that helps us organize the world. Categorization can be done at multiple levels, and we use prototypes to describe the best exemplars of categories. Young infants categorize, and with age infants and children are able to make finer distinctions within- and between-category members.

CONCLUSIONS

The study of perception and thought in children in the early life period focuses largely on the development of mental representation. Being able to represent people, objects, and events in the world as separate from manifest and immediate experience is liberating and opens up all sorts of possibilities to advanced cognition. On the basis of failures of object permanence, Piaget contended that children were incapable of mental representation until shortly before their second birthday. However, developmental scientists have devised numerous experimental strategies, such as symbolic relations and categorization, that have shown that infants and young children can represent the external world in their minds.

KEY TERMS

Basic categories
Boundaries
Breadth (as in category)
Categorization
Core knowledge
Deferred imitation
Mental representation
Object examining
Object permanence
Scale error
Sequential touching
Subordinate categories
Superordinate categories
Symbolic relations

SUGGESTED READINGS

Arterberry, M. E., & Bornstein, M. H. (2024). *Development in infancy* (6th ed.). Routledge. Chapter 8.

Corbetta, D., DiMercurio, A., Weiner, R. F., Connell, J. P., & Clark, M. (2018). How perception and action fosters exploration and selection in infant skill acquisition. In J. M. Plumert (Ed.), *Studying the perception-action system as a model system for understanding development* (Vol. 55, pp. 1–29). Elsevier.

CHAPTER 15

Children

Emotions and Temperament

As they develop from newborns and infants, children come to understand that they differ from other people – in other words, have a sense of self. Achieving that sense of self has implications for experiencing new emotions, such as shame, pride, and guilt, which reflect children's understanding of their own and others' expectations of them. With the advent of self-conscious and self-evaluative emotions, children's emotional world becomes considerably more complex. Children also show advances in social referencing, in that they now use the emotional displays of others to guide their behaviors. They make strides in regulating their own emotions, accomplishments due to biological maturation and children's social experiences. As we saw in Chapter 10, child temperament is relatively stable, but temperament also varies across cultures, as different patterns of child temperament correspond with different cultural orientations and population genetics.

DEVELOPING CONCEPTS OF SELF

A milestone in child development is understanding that the self is separate from others. Achieving such a sense of self usually occurs between 18 and 24 months of age. As in many other domains across the early life period, achieving an eventual mature sense of self is gradual and has identifiable roots in earlier achievements. When and how do newborns, infants, and children begin to differentiate themselves from the material and social world in which they are embedded? Glimmerings of a sense of self appear to be present much earlier than childhood, perhaps as early as birth (Rochat, 2019). That is, newborns' and infants' early actions with other people and objects suggest some understanding of their own selves.

One very early sign of an emerging sense of self comes from the fact that newborns and infants differentiate themselves from other objects. When newborns feel a touch to their cheek, they reflexively move their head toward it. This action is reflective of the rooting reflex, as typically such touch foretells the availability of nourishment. Even newborns differentiate between a touch from someone else and touching themselves (their own finger stroking their cheek; Rochat & Hespos, 1997): They only turn their head when someone else touches them. (This is like trying to tickle yourself; typically, it does not work so well as when someone else tickles you.) To differentiate self from other touches, newborns must have some level of understanding of their own bodies as differentiated from others.

DOI: 10.4324/9781003381709-18

A later example pertains to infants' reaching for objects. Infants adjust their body posture to reach for objects, and when objects are beyond reach, they lean forward (Yonas & Hartman, 1993). Moreover, when they attempt to grasp objects, infants modify their reach and hand shape in anticipation of the properties of the object (Yonas et al., 2005). These examples attest to the likelihood that newborns and infants must have some understanding of their bodies in relation to, but yet as separate from, other objects.

Even stronger evidence of infants having a sense of self was provided by Morgan and Rochat (1997), who demonstrated experimentally that 3- to 5-month-olds differentiate videos of their own moving legs from another infant's moving legs. Infants in this study perceived a difference between views of their leg movements that were congruent with their own actual movements from views that were incongruent with their own movements. Because infants distinguished videos of their own leg movements from those of another infant, infants had to know in some way that they were viewing themselves.

The traditional, definitive, and accepted measure of children's achieving a more mature **sense of self** is their self-recognition in a mirror or a photograph (Brownell et al., 2015). The mirror task, commonly referred to as the **rouge test**, involves surreptitiously placing a mark on the child's face, usually the nose or forehead, with a substance like rouge and then watching the child's reaction when looking at their reflection in a mirror. Children who have a sense of self, usually acquired between 18 and 24 months of age, typically touch the mark and/or avert their eyes from their reflection while showing embarrassment. Children who have yet to develop a sense of self do not show this reaction. Instead, they continue to look at the reflection or find something else to do. The onset of the sense of self is accompanied by the emergence of the so-called **secondary emotions**, such as shame, pride, and guilt, and it represents children's realization of how their self might be perceived by others. Before gaining this understanding, infants are unlikely to understand how others perceive them (Southgate, 2020).

Rochat (2019) claimed that behaviors like those just described require understanding of the self as differentiated from other people and objects. By 18 to 24 months, self-awareness seems to have consolidated, and in turn, it fosters a better understanding of others and their emotions. Later, recognition that other people are like the self develops from self-understanding and facilitates social cognition in children.

Section Summary

Children achieve a sense of self at around 18 to 24 months, but the road to developing that sense of self seems to begin as a newborn and continue into infancy. That children have a sense of self is measured by the rouge test, although earlier signs appear that newborns and infants command rudimentary abilities to differentiate themselves from others.

EMOTIONS

Self-Conscious and Self-Evaluative Emotions

Emotional growth between the ages of 15 and 24 months appears to be prompted by the development of self-awareness, at least as measured by the rouge test (Lewis, 2022). The emotions that children now display are called *secondary or self-conscious emotions*, and they include feelings such as embarrassment, empathy, and jealousy. These emotions depend on an ability to reflect on the self in relation to others. Later still, children develop the emotions of embarrassment, hubris, pride, and shame, called *self-evaluative emotions* (Lewis, 2022). These still later-developing emotions require an understanding of others' expectations and whether or not those expectations are met. Those expectations are also often culturally specific, reflecting standards, rules, and goals of the society.

Embarrassment is an example. Embarrassment is often the emotion shown in the rouge test, with children looking away from their reflection. Other signs of embarrassment are a smiling facial expression (or a sheepish grin), followed by alternating gaze aversion and looking, and/or touching parts of the body with the hands (Lewis, 2014; Figure 15.1a). Children also show embarrassment when they notice that someone is looking at them, when someone draws attention to them (such as a mother pointing and naming her child), and when they are asked to dance. Children show embarrassment as well when they are effusively praised by an adult.

Pride is another example of a self-evaluative emotion and also emerges around this time. Expressions of pride vary across cultures. Pride is based on achievement and results from a positive self-evaluation (Lewis, 2014). Signs of pride include an erect posture, smiling, looking at a parent, pointing to an outcome, applauding, and/or exclamations of positive self-evaluation, such as "Aah" and "I did it" (Lewis et al., 1992; Figure 15.1b). Success is defined by the standards, rules, and goals expressed by family or peers, which are often culturally prescribed. For example, elicitors of pride differ in U.S. and Chinese cultures (Liu et al., 2021). Via socialization, U.S. children and adults will readily feel pride when they accomplish something, whereas tranditional Chinese children and adults more often focus on what they could have done better (Mascolo et al., 2003). Many scholars attribute this difference to the dichotomy between individualist and collectivist cultures. In **collectivist cultures**, such as China, Argentina, Japan, and Korea, the social group tends to be valued over the individual, and interconnectedness of members of a community is emphasized. **Individualist cultures**, such as the United States, Belgium, Israel, and Italy, tend to value the individual over the social group and independence of the self more than interconnectedness. Thus, pride is an appropriate emotional expression in the United States and other individualist cultures, whereas expressions of pride are discouraged in China and other collectivist cultures which embrace modesty and unity with others.

Social Referencing

Still another noteworthy advance in children's emotional development is social referencing. *Social referencing* is children's use of other people's emotional reactions to help clarify uncertain or ambiguous events or situations. This ability is expanded to third-party displays of emotion by 18 months. For example, Repacholi and colleagues (2016) provided children with the opportunity to observe experimenters engaged in a novel action with an object. During the demonstration sequence, another experimenter in the room displayed either negative (e.g., "That's so annoying") or neutral (e.g., "That's so enticing") comments and emotional expressions. Later, when children were allowed to interact with the object,

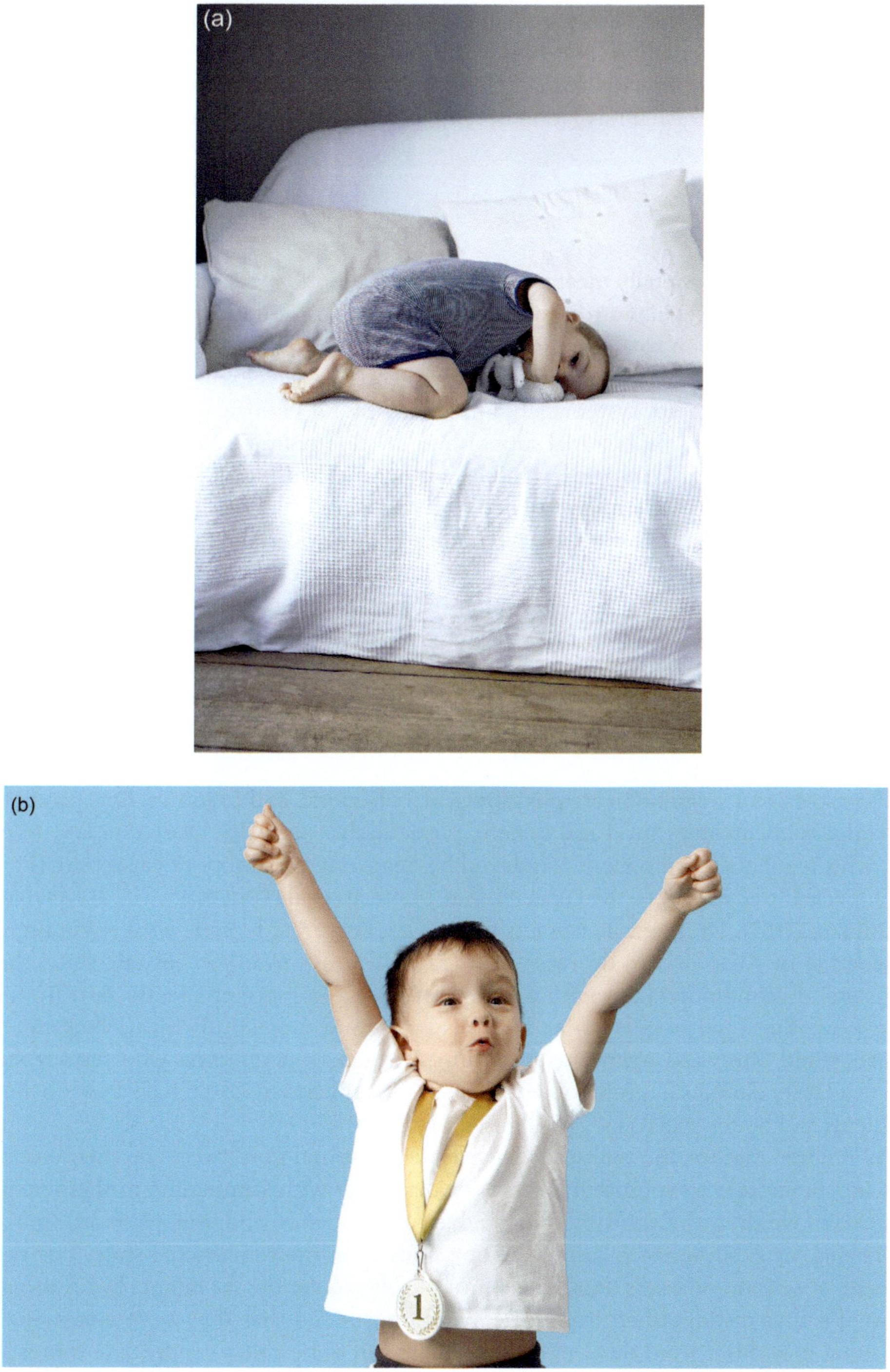

FIGURE 15.1 Two emotions that emerge around 18 to 36 months: (a) embarrassment and (b) pride.

those who saw and heard the negative interaction imitated less than those who saw and heard the neutral interaction. Not only can children guide their actions based on emotional communication directed toward them by trusted adults but also, by the middle of their second year, can use information obtained from communications between others to guide their own actions.

Emotion Regulation

Emotion regulation generally means managing one's emotions such that they match social situations. Emotion regulation is the regulation of one's emotion in a socially acceptable manner, in relation to a specific stimulus (Konishi et al., 2018). Emotion regulation develops gradually across the early life period, and the development and achievement of emotion regulation are systemically influenced by physiological, cognitive, and social development as well as by external supports to development (Bornstein, 2024; McRae & Shiota, 2017). Emotion regulation is important because without it social interactions and opportunities for learning are seriously compromised.

Newborns and infants have little voluntary control over their states of arousal and emotions. They rely on caregivers to soothe them when they are upset, to stimulate them when they are alert, and to help them transition from one state to another. Remarkably, by 3 or 4 years of age, children have mastered many of the physiological, cognitive, and social tools needed to self-regulate. Achieving such self-regulation at this point in development is important because children are also beginning to spend more time away from their caregivers, in settings such as day care, where they must be able to follow rules and control their impulses.

The tools of self-regulation are physiological, behavioral, and cognitive. One physiological component involves the vagal system, particularly control of heart rate and respiration. This regulatory component is indexed by heart rate variability or **vagal tone** (Porges, 2011). Vagal tone relates to the capacity to regulate arousal (Gao et al., 2022; Graziano & Derefinko, 2013). The vagus nerve acts to increase heart rate to cope with environmental stimulation or stress and to decrease heart rate to return to a homeostatic state, that is to a state of calm. Individuals with a high vagal tone can more efficiently shift from one state to another – self-regulate – and, in this way, more successfully meet environmental demands and afterward recover equilibrium. For example, children who display stable self-regulatory abilities in preschool are less emotionally negative and have fewer behavior problems and better social skills (Calkins et al., 2004).

As children mature, the tools they have at their disposal to self-regulate their emotions increase. Being able to voluntarily engage or disengage with stimulation in their environment gives children the ability to block adverse stimulation and seek pleasant, soothing, interesting, or exciting stimulation, thereby improving their emotional state. The development of self-awareness is another feature of self-regulation. As infants begin to gain a sense of self as distinguished from others and understand that they have intentions and goals that may differ from those of others, they begin to be able to appreciate things from another's perspective. Such appreciation is a significant milestone in regulation because children can now understand that others (namely, their parents) have intentions and goals for them with regard to appropriate behavior to which they are being asked to conform, for example, to not touch an electrical outlet or being encouraged to share a toy. This appreciation positions children to evaluate whether their behavior meets goals they or others set for them, which gives rise to emotions such as pride, guilt, embarrassment, and shame. These emotions help socialize familial and societal norms because they arise when children do or do not meet cultural norms and expectations.

Emotion understanding extends emotion regulation through social referencing. Children rely on trusted adults to help them assign appropriate emotions to ambiguous or uncertain actions or events. If a stranger enters their room, children might look to a trusted adult to determine whether the stranger can be trusted or should be feared, or whether a new toy or activity should be approached or avoided. Through their own demonstrations of emotions, children's caregivers help children know what emotions should be expressed in different circumstances.

At the same time, infants and young children are advancing cognitively in ways that are necessary to advance self-regulation. **Executive functions** control cognitive behavior, such as attention, and they can be enlisted to assist strategies for managing negative emotions (Hughes et al., 2023). In an expression of self-regulation, children can decide to engage in some alternative activity on their own, rather than waiting for adults to suggest an alternate activity. Relatedly, children can remember that there was a reward in the past when they waited, rather than waiting for a parent to remind them of a future reward.

Three executive functions appear to be critically involved in self-regulation and develop during this age period: **focused attention** (the ability to center on the task at hand or switch attention as necessary), **working memory** (the ability to remember and follow directions), and **inhibitory control** (the ability to resist inconsequential or irrelevant action in favor of consequential and relevant action). Other cognitive strategies children deploy to enforce or support self-regulation include switching perspectives, self-monitoring, error detection, and manipulating meaning of events (Thompson, 2015). Taking another's perspective, controlling the object of attention, creating alternative narratives, and intentionally using mental tricks such as distraction to modify thoughts and emotions are flexible, conscious, and effortful controls (Rothbart & Bates, 2006).

Children's developing language skills contribute to control because language enables and supports the formation and recall of mental representations. Children then use those representations to guide their behavior. They begin to understand that parents' directive "No, don't touch" requires them to moderate their behaviors accordingly. This compliance is followed by self-initiated inhibition. With age, children no longer need parents to say no. Children remember prohibited acts on their own and inhibit their own behavior. These achievements marshal several cognitive skills, including representational thinking and recall memory. At around age 2, children also come to understand the basic rules of behavior – how they are expected to behave. For example, they know when to say *Please* and *Thank you*, to hold an adult's hand when crossing a street, to sit at the table for dinner, and to help clean up their toys (although they may not always comply). Their knowledge often is conveyed by looks of defiance or looks of embarrassment or shame when they violate the rules. All these emotional expressions give further evidence of the emergence of self-awareness.

Ultimately, children need to assume control over their own emotional and mental states. However, parents play critical parts in this developmental drama. Initially, parents may soothe, stimulate, or distract. Early in life, parents spend a lot of time helping infants and children manage their emotions, such as picking up and trying to soothe a crying baby or helping a 2-year-old understand that it is time for bed rather than play. But as their children mature physically and cognitively, parents more often model, explain, and establish the norms of behavior to which they expect their children to adhere (as opposed to punish or reward).

Of course, not all parents are equally successful in helping their children regulate emotions. The links between parenting, emotional regulation, and child outcomes are many, including parents' own ability to regulate their own emotions (Zimmer-Gembeck et al., 2022). Some parents command better emotion regulation skills and have fewer difficulties in enacting more positive parenting practices with their children than others. These parents likely have children who themselves possess or command more emotion regulation skills; have fewer behavior problems or internalizing symptoms, such as anxiety, loneliness, or sadness; and enjoy more prosocial interactions with peers.

Section Summary

The emotional world of children is considerably more complex than that of newborns and infants. In childhood, new emotions emerge, including self-conscious and self-evaluative emotions. These emotions rely on children's understanding of expectations that others have for them, expectations which are often culturally prescribed. Children also show advances in social referencing in that they can use the emotional displays of others to guide their behavior in uncertain or ambiguous situations. Finally, children make strides in regulating their own emotions. Emotion regulation reflects both maturation or biological processes and the ways children experience their environments, including notably what parents do to help their children regulate their emotions.

TEMPERAMENT

Temperament generally reflects stable individual differences in behavioral functioning (Bornstein et al., 2015, 2019a; Rothbart, 2011). In this section, we highlight how temperament varies across cultures.

Temperament and Culture

When cultural groups are compared, culture and gene pool are naturally confounded, so it is difficult to determine whether observed differences in temperament are due to group differences in social customs and socialization practices or to variation in group genetics and heredity. This is why researchers have long focused on cultural differences in newborns or infants (Bornstein, 1989; Gartstein et al., 2015; Spinelli et al., 2022). Cross-cultural studies have shown that infant temperament varies considerably across cultures (Desmarais et al., 2021; Gartstein & Putnam, 2019; Putnam & Gartstein, 2017). Figure 15.2 shows rates of three temperament dimensions: **surgency** (the aspect of emotional reactivity in which a person tends toward high levels of positive affect), **negative affectivity** (fear, sadness, frustration, discomfort, and the ability to lower one's own arousal or distress), and **regulatory**

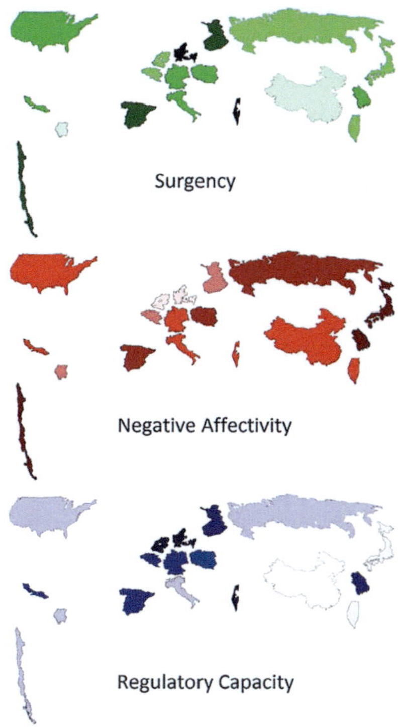

FIGURE 15.2 Relative rates of surgency, negative affectivity, and regulatory capacity across 18 countries. Darker shades indicate higher rates.

capacity (attentional abilities, behavioral control, and enjoyment of calm activities). To understand this cross-cultural variability, Desmarais and colleagues (2021) analyzed how these dimensions of temperament differed among 14 countries with different cultural orientations and with differences in salient features of their individualism/collectivism (Hofstede, 2011). Several cultural features were analyzed. One is **power distance**, which is the extent to which a culture accepts unequal power in society. A second is **masculinity/femininity**, which is the extent to which a culture is competitive and achievement-oriented (masculine) versus cooperative and nurturant (feminine). A third is **uncertainty avoidance**, which is the extent to which members of a culture are threatened by novel, surprising, or unknown situations. A fourth is **long-term/short-term orientation**, which is the focus on long-term goals, which is supported by persistence and thrift, versus short-term focus, allowing for satisfying immediate desires. A final dimension is **indulgence**, which is the extent to which members of the society can be unrestrained, thus not needing to defer gratification or adhere to strict codes of conduct. In their analyses, Desmarais et al. (2021) found that cultural orientation and gross national income accounted for a large amount of the variation in temperament. In addition, lower negative emotionality and higher orienting/regulation were found in higher-than-average resourced countries. Also, different cultural orientations predicted the different dimensions of temperament differently. For example, high levels of surgency were found in countries that were low in power distance, high in indulgence, and low in long-term orientation. In contrast, high negative emotionality was found in countries low in individualism and indulgence and high in power distance, masculinity, and uncertainty avoidance.

An interesting twist in the study of temperament across cultures is that peoples of different cultures could also differ in their genetic makeup, as for example their **allelic frequency**, or the incidence of a gene variant in a population. Putnam and Gartstein (2017) identified three gene variants that are related to mental health in adults and whose frequencies vary across regions of the world. 5-HTTLPR governs serotonin, and it has two common alleles, one short and one long. The short variant is most common in East Asian countries and less so in regions of Europe. A118G is an opioid receptor that regulates emotional states and is more common in East Asia than in Europe. The MAOA-uVNTR allele, which plays a role in neural plasticity, has a high and low variant, with the low variant more frequently found in East Asian countries than other regions of the world. Reports of children's temperament profiles followed geographic patterns and allelic frequency. For example, children inhabiting world regions with high A118G were reported to show high negative emotionality, and children inhabiting world regions with low expressions of MAOA-uVNTR and low frequency of short form of 5-HTTLPR showed high levels of surgency.

Overall, these findings illustrate how cultural and biological forces together shape children's temperament. People with similar genetic profiles live together and create cultural contexts that support (or not) certain temperamental proclivities. Children who are born in the same region of the world have similar genetic makeups, and their parents also likely socialize them in ways to match their shared cultural context, hopefully ensuring a goodness of fit.

From this discussion of cultural forces and genetic variation, it would be easy to conclude that one or the other is determinative, but neither is. In the transactional perspective (Figure 1.5), children's long-term adjustment depends on the interactions of their temperament and the demands of their environment. Specifically, goodness of fit between the two may be most important to children's optimal development and adaptation (Johnson et al., 2025). Children with one kind of temperament likely fit well in certain environments, whereas children with contrasting temperaments likely fit better in alternative environments. Neither biology nor environment alone is determinative of child temperament. An implication of the goodness-of-fit perspective is that mismatches between child biology and environment can steer the trajectory of personality away from optimal and adaptive.

Section Summary

Although temperament is relatively stable across the lifespan, it can change during development on account of genetics and maturation, experiential influences, the contexts in which it is expressed, and the integration of facets of temperament into emerging personalities. Temperament in children also varies across cultures, with different patterns corresponding with different cultural orientations and population genetics.

CONCLUSIONS

Children achieve a sense of self as they come to understand that they differ from other people. Achieving that sense of self helps generate a new set of emotions which reflect children's understanding of their own and others' expectations of them. The emotional world of children now includes self-conscious and self-evaluative emotions and so is increasingly complex. Children also use emotional displays of others as guides. At this point in their development, children gain greater control in regulating their emotions, reflective of both their biological maturation and experiences with emotional supports. Temperament is relatively stable across childhood, but patterns of child temperament vary systematically across cultures, reflective of both different cultural orientations and population genetics.

KEY TERMS

Allelic frequency
Collectivist cultures
Emotional regulation
Executive Functions
Focused attention
Individualist cultures
Inhibitory control
Masculinity/femininity
Negative affectivity
Power distance
Regulatory capacity
Rouge test
Secondary (self-conscious) emotions
Self-evaluative emotions
Sense of self
Surgency
Uncertainty avoidance
Vagal tone
Working memory

SUGGESTED READINGS

Lagattuta, K. H., & Thompson, R. A. (2007). The development of self-conscious emotions: Cognitive processes and social influences. In J. L. Tracy, R. W. Robins, & J. P. Tangney (Eds.), *The self-conscious emotions: Theory and research* (pp. 91–113). Guilford Press.

Leerkes, E. M., & Qu, J. (2019). Families with infants and young children. In B. H. Fiese, M. Celano, K. Deater-Deckard, E. N. Jouriles, & M. A. Whisman (Eds.), *APA handbook of contemporary family psychology: Foundations, methods, and contemporary issues across the lifespan* (Vol. 1, pp. 575–591). American Psychological Association.

Lengua, L. J., Gartstein, M. A., Zhou, Q., Colder, C. R., & Jacques, D. T. (2024). Temperament and child development in context. In M. H. Bornstein (Series Ed.), *Cambridge elements in child development*. Cambridge University Press.

Rothbart, M. K. (2011). *Becoming who we are: Temperament and personality in development*. Guilford Press.

CHAPTER 16

Children

Communication and Relationships

Children's advances in self-understanding and emotion regulation coincide with and support advances that they make in communication and their social relationships. The leaps in communication come in terms of expanding vocabulary comprehension and production, as well as the beginnings of grammar. At 18 months, children typically communicate using one word at a time; by 36 months, children use short sentences. Children growing up in multilingual homes or communities accomplish all the language acquisition tasks that children growing monolingual do, and they do so in both (or all) languages. Moreover, multilingual children may enjoy other cognitive advantages. The advances in relationships come as children move into a more mature phase of attachment, one that sets the stage for all later relationships. For many children, the social world expands with the appearance of a sibling and opportunities to engage with peers. Positive family relationships, such as marriage quality, predict the quality of children's ongoing relationships.

COMMUNICATION

From the appearance of their first words, children rapidly build their vocabularies – both words they understand (**comprehension** or **receptive language**) and the words that they speak (**production** or **expressive language**). Just as adults understand many more words than they say, children's comprehension far outpaces their production during language acquisition. At some point, children start to put their words together, and they do so following the rules of their language's grammar (**syntax**). Examples of early combinations of words spoken by children learning different languages are displayed in Table 16.1.

Syntax

Syntactic competence in children is a wonder. Children have the ability to detect syntactic rules and regularities even though they are hardly ever taught the rules of grammar. Moreover, those rules vary enormously across languages. In English, for example, subjects usually precede verbs, which usually precede objects. Thus, when you hear "The father kissed the daughter," you know who did what to whom. As English speakers, we are so accustomed to this subject-verb-object (SVO) word order regularity that it seems natural and perhaps even logical (Figure 16.1). But a great many languages do not work this way. For example, in Welsh the verb usually comes first (VSO). In Turkish and Japanese, many

DOI: 10.4324/9781003381709-19

TABLE 16.1 Children's Early Word Combinations Across Four Languages

Relations	*English*	*Russian*	*German*	*Samoan*
Agent–action	teddy fall	mama prua (mama walk)	Puppe kommt (doll comes)	pa'u pepe (fall doll)
Action–object	hit ball	day chasy (give watch)	tur aufmachen (door open)	tapale' oe (hit you)
Entity–location	there car	Tosya tam (Tosya there)	buch da (book there)	Keith lea (Keith there)
Possessor–possession	mama dress	pup moya (navel my)	mein ball (my ball)	lol a'u (candy my)
Entity–attribute	big truck	papa bol'shoy (papa big)	milch heiss (milk hot)	fa'ali'i pepe (headstrong baby)
Rejection–action	no wash	vody net (water no)	nicht blasen (not blow)	le 'ai (not eat)

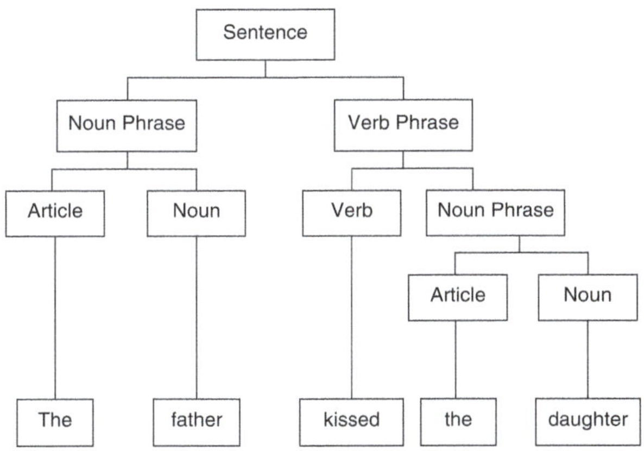

FIGURE 16.1 The basic structure of an English sentence, "The father kissed the daughter," and its grammatical decomposition.

Source: Created by M. E. Arterberry.

sentences place the verb last, but subjects and objects do not have a fixed order (SOV or OSV). To tell who is who, these languages attach an ending (suffix) to objects, and word order is used instead for focus, such as for emphasizing what is new and important in the conversation. Given that grammatical rules vary across languages and some rules are more challenging than others, they must be learned. For example, the English passive is learned late, and some Parisian adults need to look up some irregular French verb forms. Generally speaking, however, the rate at which children learn and the fact that children make far fewer errors than one might imagine suggest that children come to the task of language learning prepared to acquire grammar.

Across languages, words vary in communicating about tense, gender, animacy (living/nonliving), social status, aspect (whether an action is ongoing or completed), number, and many other properties. As we shall see, parents cannot be counted on to explicitly explain the rules: No mother tells her 19-month-old, "Listen carefully: In our language, *ed* at the end of a verb means something that already happened, except in some verbs like *run*." Children sort these things out for themselves, and they are surprisingly quick and good at it.

The Nature–Nurture Debate and the Acquisition of Grammar

Most developmental scientists (in this case, developmental psycholinguists) agree that there must be innate constraints on children's hypotheses when learning how combinations of words align with meanings. An innate constraint would be some channeling or limitation on the multitude of possibilities inborn or readily available to the child. Do such constraints exist, and what might they be? This easy question has brought philosophers and researchers to one of the great debates in the modern psychology of language. A nurturist view was advanced by Skinner (1957), namely, that children learn grammatical rules. On this account, grammar is characterized as an associative chain of words linked by transitions of different probabilities, and children learn **transitional probabilities** among words. Acquiring grammar is therefore simply a matter of learning that, in English, "The dog ate" is allowable ("dog" can follow "the," and "ate" can follow "dog"), but that "dog the ate" is not. Word-specific orders are learned by imitation and reinforcement. From this view, adults produce grammatical statements for children to imitate, and they systematically reward children's grammatically correct statements.

By contrast, Chomsky (1965) argued that Skinner's nurturist account of children developing syntax was oversimplified. Some of Chomsky's main criticisms were these: First, grammar involves more than transitional probabilities among units of language that otherwise have no intrinsic order. The grammatically correct use and meaning of an initial word in a sentence just as often depends on the end of the sentence (that is, on an overall sentence plan) as it does on the next word, as is implied by transitional probabilities. For example, the sentence "Colorless green ideas sleep furiously" is perfectly grammatical, although the actual transitional probabilities between the words are low (if existent at all). Thus, transitional probabilities from one word to the next do not provide a reasonable account of grammar and therefore cannot serve as the guiding principle for language learning. Second, Skinner's notion of reinforcement required parents to selectively reward children for producing correct grammatical utterances. Yet parents do not do this reliably enough to account for language acquisition. In fact, parents are much more likely to correct children's factual errors in a statement than the grammar of the statement. If their child says, "Me eat banana," parents are more prone to saying, "No, that was an apple" than "No, say 'I am eating a banana.'" Thus, parents do not directly teach grammar the way, say, your French, German, Spanish, or Mandarin teachers taught you grammar when you were in school.

One of the boldest of Chomsky's claims was that structure dependence and a number of other aspects of syntax are innate and are built into every infant in what he called **universal grammar** (UG). UG is said to account for the fact that, although language environments differ enormously, children's syntactic outputs are strikingly similar. Whereas variation in the vocabularies of language-learning children can be traced to environmental factors, such as amount of parent speech, variation in grammar hardly seems to exist among children learning a given language. Chomsky compared language learning to the growth of an organ such as the liver. As long as certain very basic preconditions are met, both develop in all children. The claim is not that language itself is innate; that would imply that an English child reared in a Cantonese family would speak English instead of Cantonese. Rather, the claim is that children are innately biased to interpret and produce language in certain ways.

A crucial feature of UG is that its innately specified knowledge is particular to grammar. In other words, UG applies to no other domain. For example, the notion that languages either require subjects of sentences or do not is not a kind of innate knowledge that could be shared with other cognitive processes, such as visual perception or memory. For scholars who do not share the Chomskyan perspective, this innate specification of linguistic structure is a key sticking point (Mehler et al., 2008). These researchers might claim that there are innate biases that concern children's ways of interpreting the world, including the interpretation of speech, but those biases are not special to language.

An alternative perspective to UG is **emergentism**, based on adaptive systems theory (MacWhinney, 2010, 2019). Emergentism is used to explain a wide variety of biological and physical phenomena, such as the various forces that result in mountains emerging from the earth's crust, to explain language development. Emergentism emphasizes the interconnectedness of the brain, the child, and the social context for facilitating language development. Adherents of the emergentist perspective emphasize the richness of the language that children hear, which allows them to extract rules and regularities. Moreover, they view language as a cognitive process, and it is supported by cognitive factors, such as information processing.

Regardless of how children learn language, motivation to communicate may guide many of the language acquisition processes discussed thus far. This motivation is strong: Even deaf children find ways to communicate if not exposed to a manual sign language (Goldin-Meadow, 2006). Moreover, this motivation illustrates an indirect strong social component of language development and the central importance of language in children's interactions with others.

Multilingualism

It was once the case that children might hear and learn only a single language, the language of their family or culture. This is no longer the case. Although exact statistics are not available, it is likely today that many more (perhaps most) children know and speak more than one language than know and speak only one language. That is, most children around the world live in multilingual environments and learn more than one language from birth. **Multilingualism** is increasingly the norm around much of the globe (De Houwer, 2021).

Some multilingual environments provide balanced input from two or more languages, such that children hear and eventually speak those languages with about equal proficiency. To take the simplest case of bilingualism (two languages), it could be that both parents speak both languages, one parent speaks one language and the other parent speaks a second language, or public national and personal (family or tribal) languages differ. In the latter case, parents may speak a language in the home that differs from the dominant language of the culture, and parents may not even be fluent in the dominant language. This situation characterizes the language context of many immigrant families, and in this context, it is often hard to maintain the minority language once children go to school and interact with peers. Social interaction is important for learning language, and children quickly learn which language is dominant in the wider community (De Houwer, 2021).

In contexts where children hear equal amounts of input from two languages, there is only a small amount of between-language confusion, and children reach language milestones in each language at around the same time as children learning only one language (Thordardottir, 2011). In comparison to monolinguals, bilingual children may have smaller vocabularies in each language; however, their total vocabulary across the two languages (when counting unique words) is equal in size to the vocabularies of their monolingual peers (Poulin-Dubois, 2023).

In learning any one language, children face and need to overcome a series of stiff phonological, lexical, and syntactic challenges. Consider the challenges faced by children hearing two (or more) different sound systems, words, regularities between words, and overarching meanings and intents of verbal exchanges with the same or with different people. The accomplishments of bilingual children are all the more impressive for doing so: Bilingual children need to determine the statistical regularities of each language, such that they can find boundaries for syllables, words, and phrases. They are learning different vocabularies and that the same object can have two names (like "dog" in English and "chien" in French). At the same time, they are learning different rules for word order, tense markings for verbs, etc. Finally, they are learning the social rules for each language. Moreover, they are doing this both to comprehend the two languages and to produce the two languages. The overall result is multidimensional representation of the two languages that need to compare and contrast with each other. As these representations develop, children sometimes engage in code-switching, using words from different languages to express themselves (Smolak et al., 2020). Code-switching does not necessarily indicate confusion between languages; often, it emerges from knowing the word in one language but not the other or finding that the word in one language better expresses some meaning than a word in another language. Thus, code-switching exemplifies a flexibility of multilingual learning at worst or creativity at best.

That flexibility is reinforced by claims for some cognitive advantages bilingual children enjoy outside of communication, such as in the speed of processing of information, inhibition, and imitation (Poulin-Dubois, 2023). Controversially, some developmental psycholinguists have contended that some cognitive advantages of bilingualism may even start before children produce language (Arredondo et al., 2022; Poulin-Dubois, 2023). Whether or not there are advantageous cognitive or socioemotional spillover effects from learning more than one language to other developmental domains, the value of children's being able to understand and speak more than one language should not be underestimated. Language is for communicating with others, and in a world that is increasingly multicultural and multilingual, children are doubly prepared. See Box 16.1 for how to support children learning multiple languages.

Section Summary

It is not exactly understood how children learn syntax. Children are exposed to a language that has a set of rules for putting words together, but they are not directly taught those

Box 16.1 *Application:* Raising a Multilingual Child

Parents who speak more than one language have a unique opportunity to foster multilingualism in their children. The first decision that multilingual families face is whether or not they want their children to speak multiple languages. Some parents may worry that learning multiple languages inhibits overall language development (it does not; Hoff et al., 2012). The second decision is when and how to do it. The ideal time to introduce children to a second (or third) language is before the end of their first year. Waiting to introduce a new language to children until they begin preschool (or even later) may make the language learning task harder.

Parents who speak multiple languages can continue to do so with their newborns, infants, and children using their multiple languages in the way they did before their child was born. Some parents, however, may not be fluent in multiple languages. Immigrant parents may not speak the language of their culture of destination, but they see the benefits of their child being multilingual. One important benefit is that children who speak the family language(s) and the language(s) of their new community can serve as so-called language brokers (López, 2020). That is, they can help their parents negotiate the culture of destination more advantageously. To achieve this goal, parents may rely on others in formal schooling contexts to expose their children to the language that they themselves do not speak (Mushi, 2002).

Best practices for fostering multilingual development include some of the same best practices for developing a single language, including using simplified speech, encouraging and engaging in turn-taking, and joint attention. In addition, language activities that involve active use of the language, such as talking to a person as opposed to listening to media, promote language acquisition. Engaging in social interactions in all the languages a child is learning encourages language development.

rules. Instead, every child must figure the rules out. Processes underlying the acquisition of grammar are likely innate and learned. Children may be neurologically prepared to extract its grammar, but exposure to a specific language helps shape specific grammatical rules. Children in multilingual contexts learn more than one language at the same time, and they do so remarkably well. Children growing up in multilingual environments need to accomplish all the language acquisition tasks that children growing up in monolingual environments do, but for two (or perhaps more) languages. Flexibility required for learning and using two (or more) languages builds a flexible brain that may enjoy other cognitive advantages.

SOCIAL RELATIONSHIPS

As mentioned earlier, children's advances in many areas of development support their social relationships. These relationships are guided by the final phase of attachment. Moreover, children's lives become socially more complex, including opportunities to develop relationships with siblings and peers. We begin this section by describing the fourth phase of attachment. Attachment not only affects relationships with other people; its quality may also impact health and other developmental outcomes.

Goal-Corrected Partnerships in Attachment

In phase 3 of attachment, infants develop specific attachments. During this time, infants and children explore their social and physical environment, relying (or not) on certain attachment figures. Moreover, they are deepening their relationships with others, including peers and siblings, based on their understandings of people, how they act, and what they can expect from them.

According to Bowlby (1969), the next major social transition occurs at the beginning of the third year of life, when children become able to take their caregivers' needs into account when interacting with them. For example, children now recognize for the first time (and begrudgingly) that parents must sometimes give priority to other activities and children's own needs or wants must wait. Key to this stage of attachment is mental representation of the parent–child relationship, referred to by some as a cognitive map of the parent–child–environment interaction or an **internal working model** (Cassidy, 2021). This model has actually been developing across the first few years of life. At this point, it is a representation or set of expectations for how social partners interact, and those expectations are theorized to guide future social interactions.

Attachment Across Cultures

Bowlby hypothesized that attachment is universal. Universality predicts that all newborns come into the world with proclivities or skills to form attachments. A simplistic test of this hypothesis is to explore whether attachment develops in different cultures despite their wide variation in patterns of caregiving. Figure 16.2 shows distributions of children in several countries who participated in the Strange Situation and were placed into three attachment categories. Note that most children were securely attached. There is variation, however, among countries in the percentages of children classified as insecure-avoidant and insecure-resistant (van IJzendoorn & Sagi-Schwartz, 2008).

This pattern of findings could mean that parents in the different cultures are similar in their child-rearing sensitivity, promoting mostly securely attached children, and promoting smaller and likely differentiating percentages of two insecurely typed children. Alternatively, the findings may point to the importance of factors other than the sensitivity of parental caregiving in explaining attachment classification. For example, Japanese and Israeli children typically show high degrees of stress in the Strange Situation, which may have led to increases in the proportions of children in those societies being classified as insecure-resistant. Japanese children might appear distressed either because they have much less experience with separations from their mothers than children in other cultures, such as the United States, or because their mothers are much more stressed by the Strange Situation and their children are responding to their stress. In either case, the situation would not be psychologically similar for Japanese and U.S. children. Likewise, for children growing up on traditional Israeli kibbutzim (where children were reared communally by professional day-care personnel while their parents worked outside the home),

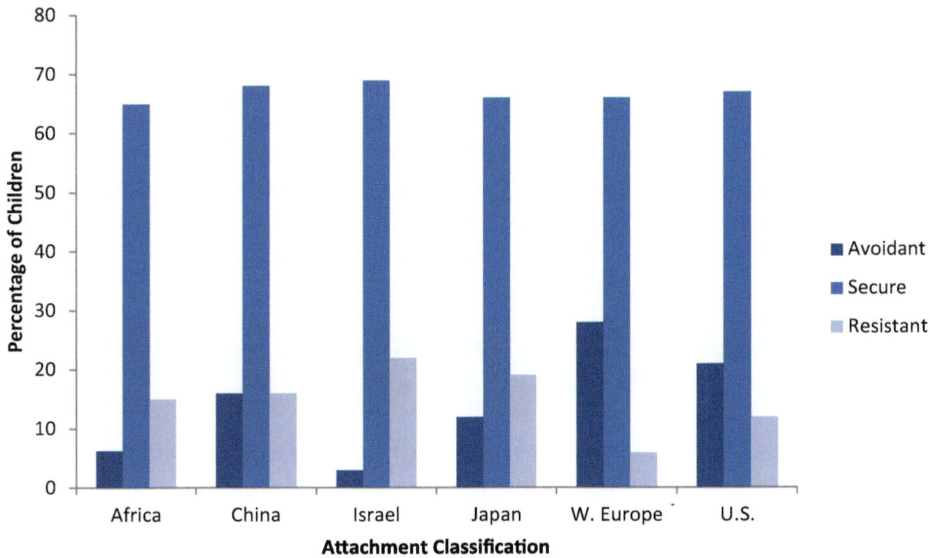

FIGURE 16.2 Percentages of children classified as avoidant, secure, and resistant from 39 samples across six locations. Africa includes samples from Kenya, Mali, the Central African Republic, and Black South Africans in Johannesburg.

Source: Created by M. E. Arterberry using data from Van IJzendoorn & Sagi-Schwartz (2008).

encounters with total strangers were unusual and thus elicited distress. Again, even though the Strange Situation procedure was structurally the same for Japanese, Israeli, and American children, the psychological experiences or meaning of the procedure for children from each culture may have been very different. Generally, cross-cultural researchers adamantly caution about applying a procedure and theory developed in one cultural context, such as the United States or Europe, to other cultural contexts (Amir & Bornstein, 2025).

Outcomes of Attachment

Relations between children's behavior in the Strange Situation and their styles of interaction with others are increasingly well documented (Roisman & Groh, 2021). Children with secure attachments to their mothers tend to become children who are more cooperative when interacting with a friendly stranger than are children with insecure attachments. Similarly, children's early attachment relates to social encounters with their siblings and playmates. Securely attached children tend to engage more frequently in prosocial and mature forms of interaction with their siblings and peers, sharing more and showing a greater capacity to initiate and maintain positive interactions than insecurely attached children.

Attachment classifications also relate to achievement motivation in children (Sroufe et al., 2005). Secure attachments at 18 months are associated with superior problem-solving abilities in a variety of stressful and challenging contexts in the same children between the ages of 3 and 5 years. Specifically, children who were securely attached to their mothers tend to persist longer and more enthusiastically in cognitively challenging situations than children who were insecurely attached. Secure infants also seem to be more resilient when stressed or challenged and appear more socially competent and independent when they later enter early education programs. Insecure attachment, and in particular the disorganized/disoriented classification, predicts elevated rates of antisocial behavior, depression, and anxiety in later childhood (Groh et al., 2012). Poor attachment histories are also associated with dropping out of school prematurely (Sroufe et al., 2005), and attachment classification may have long-term implications for health (Box 16.2).

Box 16.2 *Application:* Secure Attachments Decrease Adverse Health Outcomes

Children's early relationships with their parents have long-term implications for their relationships with other people, including peers, romantic partners, and even their own children (Aviles & Zeifman, 2021; Hedenbro & Rydelius, 2014). Secure relationships early in life lead to healthy social functioning later in life. But does this early relationship also spill over to physical health?

Childhood obesity is a national and global epidemic (Klingelhöfer et al., 2021; Ng et al., 2024), and children's security of attachment could be a contributing factor. Anderson and Whitaker (2011) investigated a possible connection between attachment security and childhood obesity. They observed mothers and their children playing at 24 months and later measured the children's growth at 4 1/2 years. The dyads' interactions were rated for children's level of engagement and negativity and the mothers' emotional responsiveness to determine children's attachment security. Children who showed signs of insecure attachments at 2 years were increasingly likely to be obese at 4 1/2 years: Obesity was found in 23.1% of insecurely attached children compared to 16.6% of securely attached children. Secure attachments help children regulate their emotions, which is particularly helpful when managing stress, and managing stress well could have longer-term consequences for nutrition.

Another potential mechanism linking attachment security and obesity may be inflammation. Short-term inflammation allows the body to respond to threats or injury, and it facilitates healing. Chronic inflammation is often the result of persistent stress. Bernard and colleagues (2019a) measured inflammation levels in 6-year-old children referred to child protective services and in control children who never received such services. The researchers measured attachment security in addition to inflammation. Later at age 8 years, they measured children's body mass index (BMI). Children classified as insecure or disorganized in the child protective services group showed elevated levels of inflammation, which predicted high BMI. In contrast, children in the child protective services group with secure attachments showed the same level of inflammation as children in the control group but were more likely to have lower BMI.

Thus, attachment security may have implications for long-term health. Is it the case that attachment insecurity is causing obesity? Unlikely. Instead, ongoing stress in one's relationships may lead to physical changes such as chronic inflammation that lead to obesity. The good news is that interventions that help parents be more sensitive in their caregiving show reductions in children's BMI from 2 to 4 years of age (Bernard et al., 2019b).

Sibling Interactions

Interaction with other children is an important component of child development. In rhesus monkeys, Harlow (1960) found that peer interactions were critical to many aspects of normal development (Figure 16.3). Through interacting with their peers, young monkeys learn how to play, how to fight, how to relate to members of the opposite sex, and how to communicate with other monkeys. When deprived of these interactions with peers, monkeys become socially incompetent adults even when they experienced good-quality care from their mothers. These findings led developmental scientists to pay attention to children's relationships with siblings and peers. Sibling relationships bridge between within-family relationships and relationships beyond the home.

The ways siblings interact with one another vary across contexts. In many non-Western, lower-resourced countries, older siblings assume a major responsibility for childcare, and they spend relatively little time simply playing with younger siblings (Kramer & Hamilton, 2019; Figure 16.4a). Instead, most of their interactions, like those of Western parents, involve protection or caregiving. In Western industrialized societies, by contrast, siblings seldom assume any responsibility for such kinds of caregiving, and sibling relationships revolve around entertainment (Figure 16.4b). Siblings tend to share common interests and have more similar behavioral repertoires than do parent–child dyads. At the same time, sibling pairs resemble parent–child pairs to the extent that sibling partners differ in experience and levels of both cognitive and social ability.

In the family systems perspective, parent–child and parent–parent relationships influence sibling relationships. Children who have secure attachments – close, trusting, and well-meshed relationships – with their mothers protest less and are less aggressive when

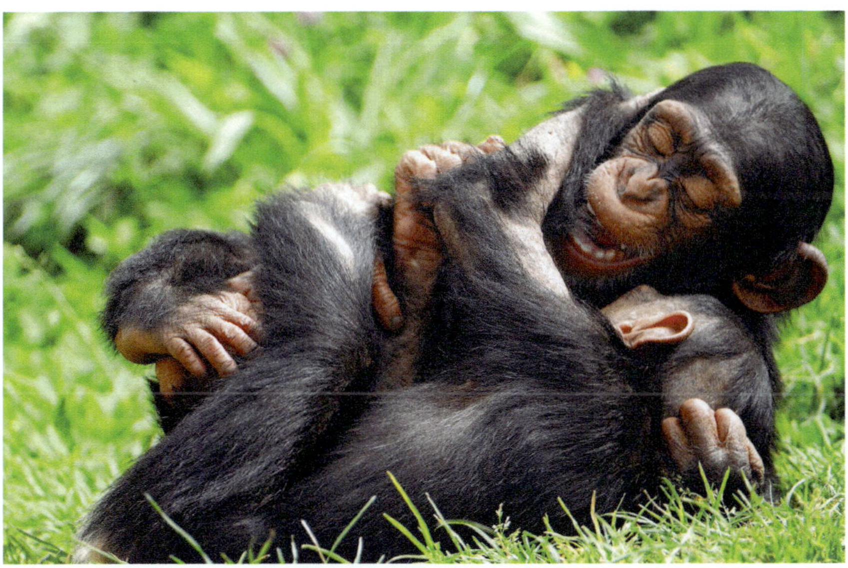

FIGURE 16.3 Primate peers playing. Such interactions are important in the social development of young primates, and peer play is important to human children as well.

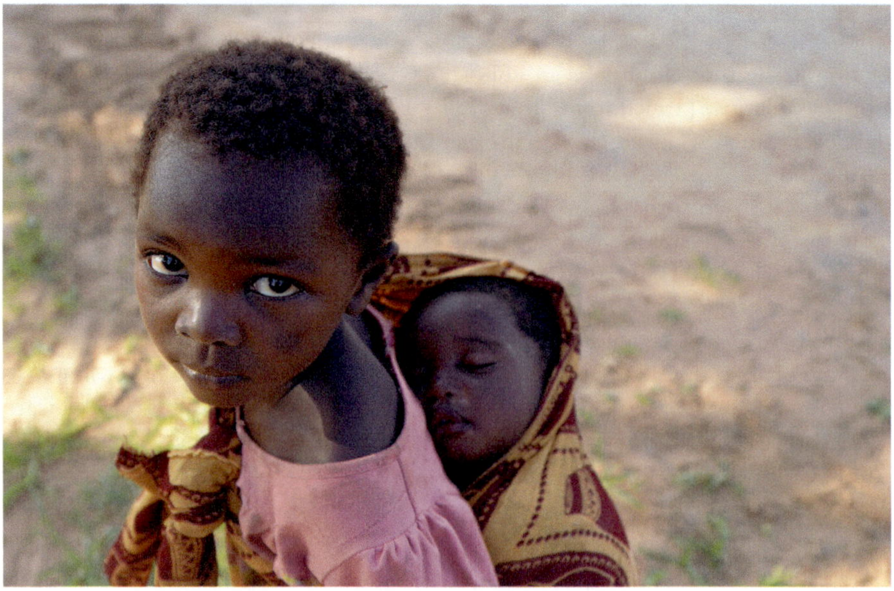

FIGURE 16.4 In some cultures, older siblings take a leading role in caring for their younger siblings. Here, an older sister cares for her younger brother by carrying him on her back, as many mothers do in her community. In other cultures, older siblings serve as playmates.

their mothers play only with their siblings. For their part, 4-year-olds who are securely attached to their mothers are more likely to respond to the distress of their infant siblings with nurturant behaviors than less securely attached older siblings are (Volling et al., 2017). Siblings are also more positive toward each other when they have nurturant relationships with their fathers. In addition, the quality of the marriage affects sibling relationship quality (Yu & Gamble, 2008). For example, Mexican American, European American, and Taiwanese mothers who reported higher levels of marital satisfaction also reported positive sibling relationships among their children. Moreover, that study showed a mutual influence of parenting styles and sibling relationships, such that it was not merely mothers' parenting that influenced siblings, but high-quality sibling relationships impacted the approaches mothers took toward parenting.

Siblings have ongoing access to their sisters and brothers. Older siblings can be sensitive to their younger siblings' needs, and they can respond to those needs by extending care and support (Kramer & Hamilton, 2019). They also serve as teachers, with older siblings teaching their younger siblings (Howe, 2015). In fact, siblings have been "expected to provide some caregiving in much of our history and in most cultures" (East, 2010, p. 56), and unlike in resource-rich countries, where sibling caregiving may be auxiliary to parental caregiving, according to Zukow-Goldring (2002, p. 257), "the majority of the world's parents assume their children will become competent caregivers and depend on their assistance in socializing younger sisters and brothers."

Section Summary

The fourth phase of attachment is goal-corrected partnership, where children have developed an internal working model of how familial relationships work. Children apply this model of how relationships work in the family to other relationships outside the family, such as to peers and nonfamilial adults. Some attachment classifications vary across cultures, and this variation could be due to differences in parenting practices, but it might also be due to the fact that the Strange Situation is not appropriate for measuring attachment across all cultures. Longitudinal studies show attachment stability across years and that attachment classification predicts other behavior, such as problem-solving. Children develop relationships with siblings, and some aspects of those relationships are similar to, and some different from, those with parents and other adults. Positive family relationships, such as marriage quality, predict the quality of sibling relationships.

CONCLUSIONS

Once children achieve an understanding of self and how to regulate their emotions, they advance in their communication capacities as well as the character and quality of their social relationships. In communication, understanding and speaking language are improving in terms of sheer vocabulary and in terms of the grammaticality (and so the comprehensibility) of their utterances. Children acquire language through exposure supplemented with lessons. More and more children around the world are multilingual. They pass all of the same language milestones as monolingual children, and they may enjoy additional cognitive and socioemotional benefits. At the same time, children have developed internal working models of how familial relationships work and will soon, if not already, apply them to relationships with peers and nonfamilial adults. Children with secure attachments have better health, mental, and social outcomes.

KEY TERMS

Emergentism
Expressive language (production)
Internal working model
Multilingualism
Receptive language (comprehension)
Syntax
Transitional probabilities
Universal grammar

SUGGESTED READINGS

Bohr, Y. (2010). Transnational infancy: A new context for attachment and the need for better models. *Child Development Perspectives, 4*, 189–196.

MacWhinney, B. (2015). Language development. In L. S. Liben, U. Muller, & R. M. Lerner (Eds.), *Handbook of child psychology and developmental science: Cognitive processes* (Vol. 2, 7th ed., pp. 296–338). Wiley.

Sroufe, L. A., Egeland, B., Carlson, E. A., & Collins, W. A. (2005). *The development of the person: The Minnesota study of risk and adaptation from birth to adulthood*. Guilford Press.

CHAPTER 17

Children in Context

Parents, siblings, and peers support children's development in some similar and some different ways. Children depend on each for their learning, as human interaction lies at the heart of advances in children's mental and socioemotional life. Today, screen time competes with human interaction for children's attention. Play is an example social context for learning, and some noteworthy developmental principles contribute to understanding children's learning and how what children learn carries over to their future mental, emotional, and social development.

SOCIAL AND CULTURAL INTERACTIONS SHAPE CHILD PLAY

Many people think, like early researchers, that play is a solitary activity in childhood. In your mind's eye you might see a young child playing alone in their room. In contrast, Vygotsky (1978) proposed that social interaction is a driving force in play and actually fosters the development of symbolic functioning (pretense). Indeed, Vygotsky motivated a conceptual shift in the study of play, regarding it not as a solitary activity reflecting underlying cognitive schema that infants and children already possessed but recasting play as a formative activity shaped by children's interactions with parents and others.

The achievement of symbolic play is now firmly seen as a reflection of children's individual growth through their interpersonal interactions and sociocultural setting (Lillard, 2015; Smith & Roopnarine, 2019). Play is enacted by children, but adults influence its development in many ways, by outfitting children's play environment, by engaging children actively, and by responding to children's play overtures. Many questions fall out of this interactive way of thinking, two of which are: (1) How does adult compared to sibling or peer interaction affect child play? And (2) how does play in this early life period affect later mental and social development?

Parent–Child Interaction and Child Play

The ways that adults influence child play have focused mostly on children's play interactions with their mothers (Bornstein & Tamis-LeMonda, 2007; Tamis-LeMonda et al., 2019). The play of 20-month-olds with their mothers is more sophisticated, complex, and varied than is children's solo play at the same age. Importantly, what mothers do

DOI: 10.4324/9781003381709-20

with their children during play appears to affect the quality of child play. For example, mothers of 20-month-olds who initiate symbolic play more frequently have children who engage in symbolic play more frequently, whether initiated by mothers or by the children themselves. Mothers and children also appear to be attuned to each other during play, with the play level of one partner closely matching the play level of the other. In addition, individual differences in symbolic play in mothers and children appear to be stable at least over the short term.

What mothers know about play and how it develops predicts the degree to which mothers facilitate the sophistication of their children's play (Tamis-LeMonda et al., 2019). Generally speaking, mothers of 21-month-olds recognize that exploratory play (mouthing and nonfunctional manipulation) is less sophisticated than functional play, and that functional play is less sophisticated than symbolic, pretend play. However, mothers differ a lot in their knowledge about child play; some mothers have more accurate knowledge of play than do others. These differences in accuracy, in turn, predict the degree to which mothers successfully support or scaffold their children's play. That is, mothers who know more about play tend to prompt their children to play at more sophisticated levels than do mothers with less accurate knowledge. Thus, the more parents know about play and how it develops, the more they may foster their children's play in daily interactions with them.

In addition to their sheer knowledge about play, mothers' ability to time and attune their own emotional displays relative to their children's emotional states during face-to-face exchanges in the first year of life predicts children's symbolic play at 24 months of age, suggesting that children's experiences with successful interpersonal emotional signaling and responsiveness in their first year lay a foundation for later symbolic development (Feldman & Greenbaum, 1997). When mothers respond to their 12- to 47-month-olds' object play in an options-promoting manner (encouraging, affirming, and/or expanding on the child's activities), their children engage in higher levels of symbolic play than do children whose mothers respond in an options-limiting manner (disapproving of or obstructing the child's play; Noll & Harding, 2003).

Moreover, mothers with different personality characteristics apparently contribute in different ways to the growth of symbolic play in their children. Mothers who score high on the personality characteristics of openness (the tendency to have a broad perspective on life and to approach life in intelligent, creative, philosophical, and inquisitive ways) and extraversion (the quantity and intensity of their interpersonal interaction, activity level, need for stimulation, capacity for joy, control, and assertiveness) demonstrate more symbolic play when playing with their children (Bornstein et al., 2011). Fathers, too, facilitate play in ways uniquely different from mothers (Cabrera et al., 2017). For example, fathers engage in more exploratory play and solitary play, and fathers who spend more time with their children (as primary caregivers) help create a more positive emotional tone during play sessions than fathers who are not engaged in primary care activities (Lewis et al., 2008). Clearly, both characteristics of parenting as well as parents' specific play practices help shape their children's play competence and development.

Siblings/Peers and Child Play

Siblings share common interests and have more similar behavioral repertoires than do adult–child dyads. At the same time, sibling dyads resemble adult–child dyads to the extent that younger and older siblings differ in experience and levels of both cognitive and social abilities. These incongruities often lead to differences in the ways younger and older siblings relate to each other and distinguish them from peer dyads. For example, consistent asymmetries emerge between the roles assumed by 3- to 6-year-olds and their 20-month-old siblings (Abramovitch et al., 1979). Older siblings tend to direct play interactions: They engage in more dominant, assertive, and directing activities than their younger siblings. Younger siblings, meanwhile, are very interested in what their older siblings are doing. They follow them around and attempt to imitate and/or explore the toys just abandoned by their older siblings. This strategy maximizes younger siblings' learning about their environment from their older sibling. Older siblings spend at least some time teaching object-related and social play and interaction skills to their younger siblings, and the amount of teaching increases with the age of the older child. These observations, along with the fact that younger siblings monitor and imitate their older siblings, corroborate the assertion that older siblings can influence the cognitive and social skills of younger children through combinations of teaching and modelling (Kramer & Hamilton, 2019). Unlike caregivers or older siblings, however, peers are playmates who share a similar developmental level and may relate to each other without a pre-established hierarchy. More than with adults, children's play with siblings and peers sustains attention, pleasure, and excitement.

A meaningful distinction between sibling and peer play are the contrasting circumstances in which the two commonly take place, circumstances involving both caregiver and place. Likely sibling–child interactions take place in the home under the watchful eye of a parent; peer–child interactions likely take place out of the home, perhaps in a formal childcare center, and under the supervision of a day-care provider. Consequently, criteria used for evaluating the quality of sibling–child and peer–child relationships differ. Moreover, childcare providers are entrusted to play significant roles in facilitating children's peer relationships (Williams et al., 2010). Providers accomplish this charge in several ways, including encouraging children to join a peer group, giving directives (*Wave hello*), and talking about other children's presence, objects, clothing, feelings, and intentions. In addition, helpful caregivers respond to actions initiated by children but not fully completed; for example, if a child is standing near a peer group looking on, a caregiver may assist the child with joining the group.

Sibling and peer play are important to child development, but in today's world, screen time competes with both. Putnick and colleagues (2023) evaluated whether screen time displaces reading and peer play time, which are subsequently associated with development in children aged 12, 18, 24, 30, and 36 months. Screen use in early childhood did not displace reported time spent reading but did displace peer play time. More peer play time was associated with a lower likelihood of developmental delay, and having more screen time increased the likelihood of developmental delay indirectly through reduced peer play time. Developmental delays were similar for fine and gross motor function, communication, and personal-social domains. Thus, different social partners contribute in unique and often complementary ways to children's cognitive and socioemotional advances in play.

Overall, different play partners have unique characteristics and styles that support different play functions at different periods in development. Adult caregivers, siblings, and peers all support multiple functions of child play, but with different emphases and in different ways (Lamm et al., 2015; Smith & Roopnarine, 2019). Adult caregivers are most important during the early years, and mothers are more effective than siblings and peers at all ages in helping children regulate their emotions by adjusting levels of stimulation and containing emotions in play. The cognitive skills that parents emphasize also differ from those common in sibling and peer play: Parents convey information about the real world and encourage conventional object use and convergent thinking, whereas siblings and peers tend to focus on play itself, and play with peers and siblings is often intense and emotionally charged. Siblings and peers are less likely than parents to transmit specific social roles or values through role-play, both because they lack competence in coordinating social pretense and because of their lack of deep knowledge of social and cultural values. By 2 to 3 years of age, however, peers' and siblings' contributions to play begin to outweigh those of adults. Thus, children play and develop in the microsystem of parent–, sibling–, and peer–child interactions. However, macrosystem forces also work in shaping partner, and so child, play.

Child Play and Culture

Who plays with children and how they play vary dramatically across ethnicities and cultures. Play also communicates information about cultural norms and about the roles of children in their society (Lamm et al., 2015). Around the globe, lower- compared to higher-SES parents typically provide infants and children fewer opportunities for variety in daily stimulation, have less appropriate play materials on hand, and engage in less total stimulation (Bornstein et al., 2022a, 2022c). Research on developmental milestones, individual variation, and parental correlates of play has almost exclusively involved Western families, although this trend is changing (Majdandžlć, 2017). For example, in Mayan and tribal Indian cultures, play is considered as predominantly a child's solo activity, whereas in middle-SES U.S. families parents have important roles as play partners (Bornstein & Tamis-LeMonda, 2007). Cultures also differ in how they value play. Some cultures believe that play provides important development-promoting experiences; others see play primarily to amuse (Bornstein, 2007). It is likely that cultural beliefs about play affect the nature and frequency of children's play, in addition to the way parents, siblings, and peers play with children.

In a larger cross-cultural framework, Bornstein and colleagues focused on mother–child play in the United States, Argentina, France, Italy, Japan, and Korea (Bornstein, 2007). Japan represents a provocative comparison with the United States in this respect because these two countries maintain reasonably similar levels of modernity and living standards and both are child-centered, but at the same time the two differ in terms of history, culture, beliefs, and child-rearing goals. Also, the activities which mothers in each country emphasize in interactions with their children differ. In general, U.S. mothers promote autonomy and organize social interactions with their children to foster physical and verbal assertiveness in children as well as interest in the external environment. By contrast, Japanese mothers organize social interactions so as to consolidate and strengthen mutual dependence within the mother–child dyad (Bornstein & Putnick, 2012). In other words, child-rearing practices in Japan emphasize closeness and interdependency between dyad members, whereas U.S. practices encourage interest in the environment and interpersonal independence supplemented by information-oriented verbal interactions.

Generally speaking, Japanese children and mothers engage in more symbolic play, and U.S. American children and mothers engage in more exploratory play. The difference in Japanese mothers' symbolic play is reflected in increased levels of other-directed pretense in their play with children (e.g., *Feed the dolly*). Thus, in line with their cultural preferences, Japanese mothers tend to organize pretend play with their children in ways that encourage their children to incorporate partners into their play. By contrast, U.S. mothers are more likely to encourage their children in self-exploration at functional play levels (e.g., *Push the bus*). Among Japanese mother–child dyads, the play setting and play toys facilitate social interaction and emotional conversation. By contrast, for U.S. mothers and children, play and the toys used during play are more frequently topics or objects of communication.

Section Summary

Parents, siblings, and peers support children's play in similar and different ways. Mothers engage children in pretense and help regulate emotions, and mothers' play that promotes options rather than limiting them results in higher levels of symbolic play. Siblings and peers share some key characteristics, but not others, which distinguish sibling– and peer–child play from parent–child play. Cultures differ in the extents to which parents serve as playmates and in the ways that parents engage their children in play.

DIGITAL MEDIA

Numerous forms of media target children, and numerous TV channels are devoted to children's programming. Infant-targeted media typically combine visual and auditory stimuli (e.g., 3D objects floating in space along with music), and some have words (spoken, written, and sometimes signed with American Sign Language) paired with objects. Child-targeted media are more sophisticated, replete with beautiful scenery, compelling characters, and elaborate storylines. With most parents owning a smartphone, tablet, or big-screen TV, infants and children likely experience some type of digital media every day. Children's experiences with screen media raise a number of cognitive and social questions. One germane to representation is whether infants and children understand and remember the information presented via digital media videos. As anyone around them will attest, videos are attention-getting and attention-maintaining. For example, 12- to 18-month-olds attend to 65% of a *Baby Mozart* video (Barr et al., 2008). Parents believe that their children learn from videos and other electronic media (Rideout & Hamel, 2006). But do infants and children actually learn and remember?

DeLoache and colleagues (2010) addressed this question experimentally. They asked a group of parents to show their 12- to 18-month-olds a popular video several times a week for 4 weeks. The video had a variety of scenes of a house and a yard, and a voice on the video labeled common objects. Half of the parents were asked to also interact naturally with their children while watching the video, and the other half were asked to allow their children to watch the video without interacting with them. Two more groups of parents and children who did not watch the video also participated in this study. One group of parents was asked to try to teach their children a list of 25 words (the same words presented in the video), and the last group was a control condition in which only the children's vocabulary was assessed. After the 4 weeks, all children were tested for their memory of the words. Children learned the most words when their parents tried to teach them the words; children in the two video conditions (with and without interaction) learned few words, and they did not differ from the control group. Thus, 12- to 18-month-olds did not learn vocabulary from digital media, even though some of their parents believed they did.

One barrier to learning words from a video may be making the connection between the object on the screen and real objects. Children have trouble equating scale models and full-sized spaces, and in other contexts children lag in their ability to connect line drawings to real objects (DeLoache, 2004). Moreover, learning new words in a media context involves communication, which more naturally takes place in interaction with others. Children who learn new tasks in an imitation context also learn better with an in-person human compared to an on-screen human or a robot (Sommer et al., 2021). Consistent with other research on this **video deficit** (Strouse & Samson, 2021), it appears that direct interaction with people and objects is the best context for promoting children's learning about and remembering features of the world around them. (See Box 17.1 for more on digital media and developmental outcomes.) Of course, it may be the case that children can learn some things, like social relationships, from watching media.

Box 17.1 *Application:* Digital Media

The American Academy of Pediatrics (2016) recommends no screen time (except for video chat) for children under 2 years and recommends that children between the ages of 2 and 5 years should watch no more than 1 hour of high-quality children's programming per day. The World Health Organization (2019) gives similar recommendations. Nevertheless, in many of today's families, children under the age of 3 years engage with digital media, either alone or with parents or siblings. Is this a problem? Maybe.

Use of digital media, defined as electronic media available on television, computers, tablets, and smartphones, is increasingly a part of children's environments and their daily lives. One concern is that infants and children do not learn via digital media. Moreover, infants and children sitting watching digital media are missing out on alternative active learning opportunities which involve engaging with people (Cycyk & De Anda, 2021; Dynia et al., 2021; Ramírez et al., 2021). Other concerns are that the amount of screen time correlates with the development of ADHD and disrupts sleep (Hill et al., 2020; Staples et al., 2021). A final concern is that screen time contributes to emotional dysregulation, such as more negative emotionality, poorer attention, and difficulty soothing, although cultural context also appears to play a role because these outcomes differ across 14 countries (Desmarais et al., 2021).

Parents use digital media. There is no getting away from it, and parents of infants and children resort to using digital media for all sorts of reasons. Sometimes digital media are used as a babysitter when parents need a break for personal reasons, as to prepare a meal. Sometimes digital media are used as a pacifier, as a distraught child can be distracted and effectively calmed by an appealing video. Sometimes digital media provide parents the opportunity to share a new experience with their little one. Instead of advising parents not to expose their infants and children to digital media (likely a hopeless and simply guilt-inducing policy), recommendations that focus on helping parents how to best use digital media with their infants and children may be more helpful and effective. Parents may not know the best ways to introduce new technologies to promote learning and/or positive interactions with their infants and children (Archer et al., 2021; Carr & Dempster, 2021). For example, parents can be coached to provide infants and children with scaffolded experiences that help make connections between virtual and real objects and their labels (Strouse & Ganea, 2021). Heller (2021) advocates for a harm reduction approach that would help families balance the benefits and risks of digital media use with infants and children. The result would be less-restrictive guidelines, such as no screen time, and instead suggestions to promote positive outcomes, such as selection of content, co-viewing strategies, and alternative activities.

Section Summary

Although the culture generally frowns on children's exposure to digital media, in today's world, exposure to digital media is inescapable. Digital media are not a substitute for human interaction, which all children need and crave. Digital media can be a force for ill, as when children are plunked down in front of a TV, tablet, computer, or smartphone to be used mindlessly as a babysitter. But digital media can also be a force of good in child development if used creatively, appropriated properly, and monitored judiciously.

LEARNING IN SOCIAL CONTEXTS

Whereas Piaget emphasized interaction with objects as a basis of cognitive development, Vygotsky emphasized the importance of interaction with people for cognitive development. This belief fits squarely with the transactional perspective. The transactional perspective states that child and parent alike bring distinctive characteristics to every interaction and are believed to change as a result of interacting (Figure 1.5). Vygotsky contended that the more advanced or expert partner (the mother) raises the level of performance of the less-advanced or expert partner (the child) through their social interaction. The difference between children's spontaneous performance on a task without guidance and their performance observed with guidance has come to represent a central concept in sociocultural theory known as the **zone of proximal development** (ZPD). Vygotsky's (1978, p. 86) idea of the ZPD centers on "problem-solving under adult guidance" even in early life.

Before children are old enough to enter formal social-learning situations like school, or even informal ones like play groups, the vast majority of their experiences stem directly from interactions within the family. Adult caregiving figures are responsible for determining most, if not all, of the children's early experiences. What, then, are prominent caregiving strategies that relate to children's cognitive development? In the home, parents take principal responsibility for structuring teaching exchanges with children: They engage them in turn-taking exchanges in early games as well as diverse learning situations. Wood et al. (1976) identified the informal teaching roles adults adopt in interactions with children under the rubric of **scaffolding**. As engineers do in constructing a building, parents sometimes use temporary aids to help their children advance in their mental understanding of the world. Later, the scaffold may be replaced or taken away entirely. Some scaffolding strategies may be more effective than others, depending on the nature and age of the children, and parents likely vary in the scaffolds they favor. Parental responsiveness is an important kind of scaffold (Valcan et al., 2018). Sensitive parents tailor their scaffolding to match their children's developmental progress, providing more scaffolding at the start of a new experience and less scaffolding as children's competency increases. Moreover, scaffolded actions and/or responses do not have to be verbalized (Pearson et al., 2011), and the environmental provisions that parents make available to their children in the forms of toys and books constitute all types of support (Bradley, 2010). Child gender plays a role here as well, as parents promote different kinds of activities for their girls and boys. Girls generally are encouraged to engage in small motor activities (such as exploring an object with their fingers), and boys generally are encouraged to engage in large motor activities (such as jumping or bouncing a ball; Dinkel & Snyder, 2020). Finally, parents vary in their scaffolding abilities, creativity, and implementation, as well as the appropriateness of their scaffolding strategies at any given time to their child, the task, and so forth, so individual variation among parents, children, and successes is expectable (Shannon et al., 2005).

Formal studies of maternal teaching in the early life period from the perspective of Vygotsky's ZPD reinforce the lesson that learning and socialization are interactive processes which require joint problem-solving (Rogoff, 2014). Cross-cultural investigations of role relations of children with their families in cultural communities as far-flung as Turkey, Guatemala, India, and the United States document how children from around the world experience different settings and different types of caregivers with widely differing outcomes in growing up. In all these interactions, however, children participate actively in culturally organized activities and, in this way, gain a deeper understanding of the world they live in. Children have been likened to apprentices: They must learn to think, act, and interact with all the central characters in their culture in order to grow up and adapt successfully.

In this connection, the concept of **intent participation** is relevant (Rogoff, 2003). Intent participation occurs when keen observation is motivated by the expectation that at a later time the observer will be responsible for the action in question. Intent participation might involve more experienced participants facilitating a learner's participation and participating along with the learner, or it could involve direct verbal instruction. Intent participation is a special form of learning by observation and contributes to ongoing activities that have cultural roots. It places a heavy role on observation compared to verbal instruction, which is a more prominent feature of formal schooling.

Parents bring more to interactions with their children than simple instruction. They promote their children's mental development through the structures they create and the meanings they place on those structures. At the same time, children bring an active mental life to their everyday interactions with adults, and they carry more away from their interactions than simply the specific contents of individual lessons.

Section Summary

Children learn in social contexts, and developmental scientists have arrived at some noteworthy principles of children's learning. For example, at any given time on any given task children may operate at a given level (zone of actual development), but with the aid of more expert partners, children can be guided (scaffolded) to more advanced levels of performance (zone of approximal development). What children learn effectively can then carry over to other and future problem-solving situations.

CONCLUSIONS

All the people who inhabit the child's world – parents, siblings, peers, and others – support children's development. They do so in some similar as well as many different ways. Generally speaking, children thrive on human interaction, and children learn in social contexts. Today, screen time competes with people for children's attention. Digital media cannot substitute for human interaction, but creative, proper, and judicious digital media can play a positive role in children's development. Developmental science has articulated some noteworthy principles of children's learning, and what children learn effectively can then carry over to other and future life situations.

KEY TERMS

Intent participation
Scaffolding
Video deficit
Zone of proximal development

SUGGESTED READINGS

Barr, R., Kirkorian, H., Coyne, S. & Radesky, J. (2024). *Early Childhood and Digital Media*. In M. H. Bornstein (Series Editor), *Cambridge Elements in Child Development*. Cambridge University Press Springer. https://doi.org/10.1017/9781108885751

Gauvain, M. (2022). *Cognitive development in infancy and childhood. Cambridge Elements in child development series* (M. H. Bornstein, Series Ed.). Cambridge University Press. https://doi.org/10.1017/9781108955676

Harris, P. L. (2022). *Children's Imagination*. In M. H. Bornstein (Series Editor), *Cambridge Elements in Child Development*. Cambridge University Press.doi:10.1017/9781009128216

Afterword

As we conclude *Newborn to Infant to Child*, we hope you have a new appreciation for how remarkable the early life period is. There is tremendous growth and development from conception through the first 1,000 days! Newborns, who cannot communicate very well and who sleep most of the time, quickly change into infants, who are becoming more responsive social partners, who then quickly change into children, who appear to never stop talking or moving. This fast transition challenges parents and developmental scientists alike, but in different ways. Parents need to adjust their parenting and other aspects of their life as their little ones grow. From the scientists' perspective, the objects of our attention – newborns, infants, and children – are changing by the month, by the week, or sometimes even by the day. We hope that you have gained an appreciation for the sophistication of the science behind the study of development in this early life period, including all the secrets that newborns, infants, and children have given up and the creative methods used to uncover newborns', infants', and children's competencies as well as the inferential nature of research and the many factors that limit interpretations of findings.

In this book, we have illustrated several themes that pervade the study and understanding of this formative period in development. We introduced and explored the nature and meaning of sensitive periods when discussing prenatal development and speech perception; we emphasized the deep and intricate coordination between nature and nurture when discussing visual perception and language development; we illustrated stages of development when discussing cognitive theory and attachment theory; we invoked the developmental constructs of stability and continuity in information processing, temperament, and mother–child interaction; and throughout we underscored the wholistic nature and the multiple systems of the newborn-infant-child as well as the many ways newborns, infants, and children are cared for but also shape parents' care of them. Moreover, we considered the wider social and material contexts of development – parents, siblings, day-care workers, peers, and social class, culture, and time. We also addressed a number of theoretical perspectives, including those associated with Piaget, attachment, bioecological systems, and transaction. At this point, we encourage you to re-read Chapter 1. This might strike you as an odd suggestion, but we hope that reading the first chapter from the vantage point of having an overview of the early life period will deepen your understanding of important themes and theories in *Newborn to Infant to Child*.

We hope you also now have a firm appreciation of how basic developmental science has informed society of how and when to intervene to promote optimal development of the next generation. We hope that learning about newborns, infants, and children has enhanced your interest in developmental science and that you will continue to study this fascinating topic, apply what you have learned, and benefit from this work when a new human being enters your own life. Our science has manifest implications for typically developing newborns, infants, and children as well as for those at risk for atypical development. Based on understandings gained from *Newborn to Infant to Child,* how would you approach your own newborn, infant, or child? What types of societal policies or interventions would you promote to support the development of newborns, infants, and children? What do you consider best practices for intervention to optimize human development beginning with the early life period?

Glossary of Key Terms

A-not-B error: A search task across several trials in which the location of an object is changed. When the object is hidden at location A, infants find it successfully. When the object is moved to a new location B, babies search at A.

accommodation: The modification of an existing scheme to apply to new information.

accretion-deletion of texture: When moving through the environment, closer surfaces are perceived to block more distant ones.

action potential: The electrochemical exchange along the axon fiber.

acuity: Ability to see fine detail.

adaptation: Processes wherein schemes are altered by experience with two complementary processes: assimilation and accommodation.

adult attachment inventory: A measure for researchers to infer adults' early relationships with their parents.

affiliative system: Social behaviors at a distance, like smiling and vocalizing, that communicate a desire to interact.

age of viability: The age at which the fetus can survive outside the womb.

allelic frequency: The incidence of a gene variant in a population.

alveolars: Sounds such as /n/ and /l/ that are produced by placing the tongue at the ridge just behind the teeth.

amniocentesis: A procedure in which amniotic fluid is drawn through the abdominal wall of the mother and examined to evaluate the chromosomal structure of a fetus.

amodal: Information that does not belong to a specific perceptual modality.

anoxia: Oxygen deprivation.

Apgar: A test administered to newborns to document normal functioning and to determine the need for intervention on each of five dimensions: appearance, pulse, grimace, activity, and respiration.

approach reflexes: Reactions concerned with intake, including breathing, rooting, sucking, and swallowing.

arborization: In reference to dendrites, the growth of spines connecting to neighboring cells.

assimilation: Processing information according to an existing scheme.

attachment behavior system: Controls or coordinates infants' and children's activities related to attaining and maintaining proximity to or contact with attachment figures.

attachment behaviors: Behaviors that ensure comfort and security by encouraging adults to approach, thus bringing infants and children close to protective caregivers.

attachment figures: People to whom infants and children have formed especially close and dependent relationships.

attachments: Infants' and children's specific, enduring, emotional bonds, the first of which are often with parents.

attunement: When certain experiences speed up the development of a structure or function or the final outcome is higher than it would be without that experience.
auditory localization: The utilization of sound arriving at different times to each ear to locate the origin of the sound.
auditory location: The ability to locate an object in space based on its sound.
auditory threshold: How loud a sound has to be for a person to hear it.
autism spectrum disorder: A neurological and developmental disorder that affects how people interact with others, communicate, learn, and behave. Symptoms generally appear in the first two years of life.
autonomic nervous system (ANS): An involuntary control system that operates at the level below consciousness and is responsible for heart rate, respiration, digestion, and other basic processes necessary for survival.
average temperament: Newborns, infants, and children who do not fit one of the other main temperamental profiles (easy, difficult, or slow to warm up).
avoidance reflexes: Reactions, such as sneezing and coughing, which keep foreign substances or stimulation away from the baby.
axon: The part of the neuron that transmits activity away from the cell body toward other neurons.
babbling: Pre-speech vocalizations.
Babinski reflex: The toes fan out when the bottom of the newborn's foot is stroked.
babywearing: Involves using a cloth material or commercial baby carrier to strap the newborn to the parent's body, often against the front torso.
basal ganglia: Located at the base of the forebrain, they play a role in the control of motor behavior.
basic categories: Categories that are subsumed under superordinate categories. Their instances or members are discriminable but still share many perceptual features. Cats (versus horses) constitute a basic category that falls under the superordinate category of animals.
binocular convergence: The convergence angle of the two eyes, when focusing on an object at some distance.when focusing on an object at some distance.
binocular cues: Depth cue based on the fact that our two eyes receive slightly different images of the visual world. The convergence angle of the two eyes and the disparity between the two images they yield provide some information about depth.
binocular disparity: A cue for depth perception that is based on the fact that we have two eyes and our two eyes receive slightly different images of the visual world.
bioecological systems framework: The nested set of systems of proximal to distal influences over development.
blastocyst: When the developing organism reaches 70–100 cells after conception.
boundaries: Regions or instances where category inclusion is marginal.
breadth (category): The variety of instances or members which are included in the category.
breech: When a newborn is born feet- or buttocks-first.
brightness: Luminance.
bronchopulmonary dysplasia: Chronic lung disease identified by the thickening and inflammation of the walls of the lung and a reduced airway, resulting in a significant decrease in the amount of oxygen the newborn can inhale.
canalization: The persistence of a developmental outcome despite less-than-optimal environmental circumstances.
canonical babbling: A stage in pre-speech vocalization in which consonant-vowel babbling emerges.
cataracts: A clouding of the lens, leading to the ability to perceive overall presence of light but not fine-patterned stimuli.

categorical perception: The propensity to treat as similar otherwise discriminable stimuli such as sounds.
categorization: The grouping of separate items into a set according to some property or rule.
cell body: Component of the neuron containing the nucleus.
central nervous system (CNS): The brain and the spinal cord, which play fundamental roles in thinking and acting.
cephalocauldally: Development proceeding from head to tail.
cerebral cortex: Outer covering of the brain that makes up 40% of the brain's mass, divided into four lobes: occipital, parietal, temporal, and frontal cortexes.
Cesarean section: A surgical procedure involving cutting into the uterus to remove the newborn.
chorionic villus sampling (CVS): A procedure for early fetal chromosomal evaluation.
chromosome: Contains genes that are composed of chemical codes of DNA that guide development of structure and function.
chronosystem: Refers to the time domain in development.
circadian clock: An internally driven biochemical, physiological, and behavioral process that adjusts to environmental cues, such as day–night light cycles.
classical conditioning: A type of learned association that involves pairing a neutral stimulus (CS) with a stimulus (UCS) that elicits a response.
co-sleep: Parent and newborn, infant, or child sleep in the same bed.
cochlea: The part of the inner ear responsible for perceiving sound.
collectivist cultures: The group tends to be valued over the individual, emphasizing interconnectedness of members of the community.
comorbid: Occurring simultaneously.
conditioned response: After repeated pairings of the unconditioned and conditioned stimulus, the conditioned stimulus takes on the properties of the unconditioned stimulus to elicit the same response – now called the conditioned response.
conditioned stimulus: A stimulus that is initially neutral that does not elicit an unconditioned response.
congenital: Structures or functions that are present at the time of birth but are not hereditary.
context-flexible (as in words): Words whose meanings are understood in the absence of environmental cues.
context-restricted (as in words): Words whose meanings are understood only in reference to specific entities.
continuity: Consistency in average group scores on some aspect of development over time.
cooing: A stage of pre-speech vocalization that involves consonants and vowels produced at the back of the mouth. (e.g., /gu/, /ku/).
core knowledge: Idea that newborns arrive with specific learning mechanisms that enable rapid acquisition of knowledge about event categories and object categories.
cortex: Outermost layer of tissue in the brain.
cortical association areas: Areas of the brain involved in higher-level processes, such as awareness, attention, memory, and the integration of information.
cross-sectional design: Comparison of groups of participants of different ages to determine whether and how structure and function vary depending on the age of the participants being tested or testing different newborns, infants, or children of different ages at the same time.
day care: A general term to describe nonparental care to newborns, infants, and children. Types include referring to relative care, home-based care, and care in centers.
deferred imitation: Imitation at some delay after observing an action.
dendrites: Part of the neuron that conducts information to the cell body.
dentals: Sounds created by placing the tongue against the teeth (e.g., /t/ and /d/).
didactic caregiving: How parents facilitate newborns', infants', and children's understanding of the world around them, including directing attention to objects and events, interpreting external events, and providing opportunities to learn.

difficult temperament: Newborns, infants, and children who are negative in mood, irregular in body functions, and slow to adapt.
directionality: A general principle of physical growth; examples include cephalocaudal and proximodistal.
discriminating sociability: During phase 2 of attachment, infants show preferences for engaging with specific people.
dishabituation: Change in looking time from the end of habituation to the test.
disorganized attachment: A type of attachment characterized by contradictory behavior patterns wherein infants and children make incomplete movements toward objects or their parents and appear confused or apprehensive about approaching their parents.
dizygotic or dizygotic twins (DZ): Twins born from different eggs fertilized by different sperm.
dose–effect relation: The function between amount of exposure to a substance and the resulting effect.
Dubowitz test: Estimates gestational age by scoring newborns on neurological items and external characteristics.
easy temperament: Newborns, infants, and children who are positive in mood, regular in body functions, and adaptable.
ectoderm: Predifferentiation of the skin, sense organs, and central nervous system structures of the brain and spinal cord.
effectance: Behaviors affect others in a consistent and predictable fashion.
effectors: Nerve fibers that end in structures that allow for action, such as muscles.
efficacy: Competence, such as in being a parent.
embryo: The prenatal organism from approximately 2 weeks to 8 weeks.
emergentism: A framework for understanding language development that emphasizes the interconnectedness of the brain, the infant, and the social context.
emotion elicitors: Internal and external events that trigger biological changes that are the basis for emotion.
emotion receptors: Structures in the brain that make it easier to register and encode emotion-relevant events.
emotion states: Psychophysiological activity reflective of the activation of emotional receptors.
emotional contagion: When one spontaneously resonates with another's salient emotional expressions, most often observed in response to another's distress.
emotional experiences: The interpretation and evaluation of perceived feeling affect states and expressions.
emotional expressions: Facial, gestural, and other behaviors that cue an internal feeling of affect.
emotional regulation: The ability to manage one's emotions.
emotions: Immediate responses to ongoing experiences and circumstances.
empiricist: Philosophers and scientists who believe all knowledge comes through the senses and mental development reflects learned associations.
encoding: Processes for the transformation of incoming information into memory.
endoderm: Predifferentiation of the digestive, respiratory, and internal organs.
endogenous: Naturally occurring forces internal to humans and other animals, such as how the circadian rhythm responds to light–dark cycles.
endometrium: Nutrient-rich lining of the uterus.
epigenesis: The hypothesis that new phenomena not present in the original fertilized egg can emerge over the course of development through the interaction of pre-existing elements with environmental influences.
epigenetics: Modern study of how experience and environment affect when and how genes express themselves.
ethology: The scientific study of animal behavior, often involving cross-species comparisons.

executive functions: Higher-level cognitive skills that control cognition and behavior.
exosystem: Elements of newborns', infants', and children's environment, such as the parents' workplace, the wider neighborhood, and the health-care system.
expansion: See *vocal play (expansion)*.
experience-dependent processes: Synaptic connections that are a product of experience with particular individual events.
experience-expectant processes: Synaptic connections that are a product of species evolutionary history.
exploratory behavior system: Mediates contact with the physical material environment.
expressive language (production): Language that is spoken or written.
external validity: Constructs investigated in one situation relate in a theoretically meaningful way to constructs assessed in another situation and perhaps at another age.
extrapyramidal system: Controls posture and coordination.
face validity: The obvious and commonsensical association with what is supposed to be measured.
facilitation: When certain experiences speed up the development of a structure or function but the final outcome is not higher than it would be without that experience.
familiar size: A depth cue using the known size of objects, such as people.
fear/wariness behavior system: Coordinates avoidant, wary, or fearful responses to strangers.
fetal alcohol spectrum disorder (FASD): A broad category of birth defects attributable to maternal alcohol use.
fetal alcohol syndrome (FAS): A birth defect with patterns of malformation, growth deficiency, central nervous system dysfunction, and mental retardation.
fetus: The prenatal organism from approximately 8 to 38 weeks.
figural coherence: The perceptual grouping of elements having an invariant set of spatial relations, as exemplified in the point-light display of a person walking.
focused attention: The ability to center on the task at hand or switch attention as necessary.
frontal lobe: A region of the cortex that governs higher-order cognition and voluntary activity.
functional perspective: The purposes and roles of emotion in ongoing transactions between individuals and their environments.
functional play: Play with an object in the way the object was intended to be played with.
functional-relational play: Play that brings together two objects in a meaningful and appropriate way.
functions: Mental processes and behaviors, such as seeing and walking.
gametes: Reproductive cells: sperm from males and ova from females.
gaze following: Looking to a new location based on the gaze (and sometimes head movement) of another person.
genotype: The genetic makeup of the individual.
gesture: Nonverbal supports to communication and language (e.g., pointing).
goodness-of-fit: The match between newborns, infants, and children and their developmental contexts.
gyri: Bumps or ridges on the cerebral cortex.
habituate: The decline in attention to a stimulus, suggesting recognition.
hierarchical integration: When simple separate skills become organized into more complex ones.
hue: What is typically thought of as color based on the wavelength of light.
ideology: Worldview of a cultural group.
imitation: The form of learning wherein an observed act is reproduced.
imprint: The predisposition in ducklings and other waterfowl to remain close after hatching to a salient moving object, usually the mother.
in vitro fertilization: A procedure where the egg and sperm are united outside of the mother's body and then introduced into the uterus.

independence of systems: Components that are differentially developed at a given time and develop along different trajectories.
indiscriminate social responsiveness: During phase 1 of attachment, infants do not show preferences for engaging with specific people.
individual differences: How organisms differ from each other, resulting from their unique combination of biology and experience.
individualist cultures: Tend to value independence of the self more than interconnectedness among members of the community.
induction: When a particular experience or set of experiences completely determines whether some aspect of development (a structure or function) emerges.
inhibitory control: The ability to resist inconsequential or irrelevant action in favor of consequential and relevant action.
innate: Present at birth or biologically programmed to develop at a particular time.
insecure-avoidant attachments: A type of attachment in which infants and children appear unconcerned by their parents' absence and actively avoid interaction when reuniting with their parents.
insecure-resistant (ambivalent) attachments: A type of attachment in which infants and children are unable to use their parents as a secure base to explore; although they are distressed by their parents' departure, they behave ambivalently on reunion or seek contact but angrily reject the parent.
intensive features: Descriptors of how strongly temperament behaviors are expressed (amplitude) and how sensitive they are to stimulation (threshold).
intent participation: Engagement when keen observation is motivated by the expectation that at a later time the observer will be responsible for the action in question.
internal validity: The ability to make causal statements about whether one variable causes another to change.
internal working model: A schema of how relationships work based on early interactions with caregivers.
interposition: A depth cue when contours of one object partially block another object from view; the first object is perceived to be closer than the second.
intersensory redundancy hypothesis: The importance of multimodal events in capturing infants' and children's attention, which then facilitates information processing, learning, and memory of multimodal events over unimodal ones.
intersubjectivity: Shared meaning among two or more people.
intonated babble: A stage of pre-speech vocalization that involves producing long strings of syllables having varied stress and tonal patterns.
intraventricular hemorrhage (IVH): Bleeding in the brain areas surrounding the ventricles.
introducing: A way for mothers to regulate their newborns', infants', and children's focus of attention, characterized by orienting the focus of attention.
invisible displacements: When an object that is hidden is concealed during the hiding.
joint attention: When two people attend to the same object or event at the same time.
kangaroo care: Extensive skin-to-skin contact in early parenting; named so because newborn kangaroos spend an additional month in close contact with their mothers in her pouch.
kinetic (motion-based) cues: Depth information that stem from movement of the object or the observer.
Klinefelter's syndrome: A birth disorder in males wherein there are multiple X chromosomes (XXY as opposed to the normal XY).
labials: Sounds created by placing the tongue against the lips (e.g., /p/ and /b/).
labor: Involuntary uterine contractions, beginning at the top of the uterus muscle, that literally force the fetus through the vaginal canal.
language caregiving: Parent behaviors that subserve verbal communication with newborns, infants, and children and support all aspects of parenting and development.

learning: Acquiring and internalizing information.
limbic system: Brain structures that support emotions and memory.
linear perspective: Two lines that are known to be parallel in real life converge in a two-dimensional representation, yielding the perception of depth.
long-term memory: A function of memory that represents a limitless, permanent storehouse of knowledge.
longitudinal design: Repeated measurement of the same newborns, infants, or children over time.
looming: When an object moves directly toward us on a "hit path," its image on the retina expands and we normally move to avoid the impending collision. The reverse happens when an object moves away from us: The image on the retina contracts.
macrosystem: Environmental influences that are most distant from newborns, infants, or children, such as patterns of beliefs, values, and laws of the social class and culture in which babies grow up.
maintaining (maintenance): Experience preserves an already partially or fully developed structure or function; the absence of experience will result in loss of the structure or function.
masculinity/femininity: The extent to which a culture is competitive and achievement-oriented (masculine) versus cooperative and nurturant (feminine).
mass-to-specific: Directionality from large muscle groups to fine ones.
material caregiving: Parent behaviors that lead to provisioning and organizing newborns', infants', and children's home and local environments, including the number, variety, and composition of inanimate objects available to newborns, infants, and children; the level of ambient stimulation; the limits on physical freedom; and the overall physical features of newborns', infants', and children's experiences.
maternal gatekeeping: Activities that mothers engage in to limit others', particularly fathers', interactions with their newborns, infants, and children.
maternal serum alpha-fetoprotein (MSAFP): A noninvasive measure of fetal chromosomal structure.
meiosis: Complex changes in the reproductive cells of each parent that split so as to retain half the number of chromosomes present in the original cell.
mental representation: The ability to think about objects or people even in their absence.
mesoderm: Predifferentiation of the muscles, blood, and the circulatory system.
microcephaly: A smaller than normal head, often associated with cognitive impairment.
microsystem: Environmental influences that are most proximal to newborns, infants, and children, such as interpersonal relationship and patterns of activities that they experience in face-to-face settings.
mind-mindedness: Mothers' explicit use of mental state language to comment on their own infants' minds.
mirror neurons: Brain cells that are activated in a person while observing another person making an action.
monozygotic or monozygotic twins (MZ): Twins born from the same egg and fertilized by a single sperm.
Moro reflex: The tendency to swing the arms wide and bring them together again in the midline (as if around the body of a caregiver).
motion parallax: Objects that are closer seem to move faster in the field of vision than objects that are farther away.
multilingualism: Ability to speak and understand more than one language.
multimodal perception: When information about objects and events is available to different sensory modalities simultaneously.
myelin: A fatty substance that surrounds the axon of neurons and facilitates the speed of nerve conduction, rendering information transmission more efficient.

myelination: The process by which undeveloped neurons are wrapped in a sheath of myelin.

nativist: Philosophers and scientists who believe knowledge is present at birth.

natural experiments: A study using naturally occurring groupings of participants instead of assigning participants to different treatment conditions.

negative affectivity: Fear, sadness, frustration, discomfort, and the ability to lower one's own arousal or distress.

neonatal abstinence syndrome: Opioid-exposed newborns experience withdrawal symptoms and require longer hospital stays after birth.

Neonatal Behavioral Assessment Scale (NBAS): Test designed for newborns that evaluates their neurological functioning using 18 reflex items and newborns' interactional repertoire on 27 indices of information processing, motoric capacities, ability to control state, and response to stress.

neonatal intensive care unit (NICU): A special area of a hospital that provides care for critically ill or premature newborns.

neoteny: The prolongation of infancy, especially in human beings.

neurogenesis: Neural cell formation.

neuron: Core component of the nervous system composed of a cell body, nucleus, axon, and dendrites.

neurotransmitters: Neurochemicals that neurons use to communicate with each other.

niche: Physical, social, and environmental conditions and the interactions they foster.

niche picking: Preferring certain environments over others, especially those settings that best suit a behavioral style.

nominal insight: The realization that things have names.

nonshared environment: Environmental differences that act on individuals in the same situation or setting differently.

nonsymbolic (exploratory) play: Play that appears designed to extract information about objects.

normative development: Often characterized by a developmental function that reflects the changing status of newborns, infants, or children on some aspect of development across ages.

norms: The average for a population.

novelty responsiveness: The amount newborns attend to a novel stimulus relative to the familiar stimulus following habituation.

nucleus: Central part of the neuron that contains DNA.

nurturant caregiving: Parent behaviors that promote newborns', infants', or children's basic survival needs for protection, supervision, and sustenance.

object examining: A procedure used to test infants' and children's categorization, where participants' amount of time examining object(s) is recorded.

object permanence: Understanding that an object that is out of sight continues to exist.

observational learning: Learning by listening or watching.

occipital lobe: Region of the cortex that governs the processing of visual information.

operant conditioning: Learning that involves associations between actions and their consequences.

optic flow: Movement of stimulation on the retina as we move through the visual world.

ovum: An unfertilized egg (female gamete).

oxytocin: A hormone secreted by the pituitary gland which induces contractions and then labor; also plays a role in the regulation of social behavior.

palmar grasp: Newborns close their fingers when something touches their palm.

parietal lobe: Region of the cortex that governs the processing of temperature, taste, and touch and directs motor movements.

person permanence: The notion that people have a permanent existence independent of their immediate presence.

phenotype: Observed characteristics of the individual.

phonation: A stage of pre-speech vocalization that involves fussing, crying, sneezing, and burping.
phonemes: The smallest meaningful units of sound.
phonotactic learning: Understanding combinations of speech sounds that are allowed in a language.
physical caregiving: Parent behaviors that promote newborns', infants', and children's gross and fine psychomotor balance and movement through interactions, such as supporting them in an upright position on their laps.
physical circumstances: Environmental factors affecting how a child is reared.
placenta: Connects the body of the developing organism to the body of the mother and permits the exchange of nutrients and waste.
power distance: The extent to which a culture accepts unequal power in society.
predictability: The degree to which newborns', infants', and children's behaviors can be anticipated reliably from their own preceding behaviors or contextual events.
predictive validity: When a measure in one domain predicts a later performance in another domain.
pretend (symbolic) play: Play that is non-literal in quality.
primary circular reactions: Newborns' tendency to repeat chance discoveries involving the coordination of two actions.
primary emotions: Emotions that are deeply rooted in human biology that are either innate or very early developing.
primitive streak: The first stage in the development of the central nervous system.
productive or expressive language: Words that are spoken.
proprioception: The sense of the body in physical space.
prosody: Patterns of rhythm in speech.
prototypes: Best example of a category.
proximodistally: From the center of the body outward.
pruning: The elimination of unused synapses.
punishment: Negative consequence to an action that suppress the action.
pyramidal system: Controls precise, rapid, and skilled movements of the extremities.
qualitative change: Change in structure or organization.
quantitative change: Change in amount or degree.
quickening: Felt movement of fetus in utero, beginning around 4 months.
rapid eye movement (REM): A period during sleep when dreaming.
reactivity: The excitability or arousability of an individual's response systems.
readability: The definitiveness of infants', newborns', and children's behavioral signals.
recall: Retrieval that requires memory for a prior experience without the advantage of cues.
receptive language: Language comprehension.
receptors: Where sensory nerves come into contact with the external world, such as the eyes, ears, skin, nose, and taste buds.
reciprocity: Taking turns acting and reacting to an interactant's behavior.
recognition: Retrieval that requires that we remember having previously experienced whatever is to be remembered when contextual cues are provided.
redirecting: A way for mothers to regulate the focus of attention of newborns, infants, and children by changing their focus of attention to a different topic or object.
reference: The link between sounds or words and their meaning.
reflexes: Integrated and organized automatic stimulus–response behaviors.
regulatory capacity: The ability to direct attention, control behavior, and enjoy calm activities.
reinforcement: A reward that comes after a behavior that increases the likelihood of the behavior being repeated.

relational play: Play that brings together two unrelated objects with no indication of pretense.
reliability: Consistency in measurement of the same participant.
respiratory distress syndrome: A breathing disorder associated with preterm newborns.
responsiveness: Extent and quality of infant reactivity to stimulation.
reticular formation: A subcortical structure that regulates sleep/wake patterns.
retinopathy of prematurity: A disorder produced by excess oxygen that involves damage to the retinas, causing permanent blindness.
retrieval: Processes used to get information out of memory.
rooting: Response to stimulation around the mouth involving tracking, searching, and head redirection toward the source of stimulation.
rouge test: A test of self-recognition that involves placing a mark on the child's face, usually the nose or forehead, with a substance like rouge, and then watching the child's reaction when looking at their reflection in the mirror.
scaffolding: Informal teaching aids to learning.
scale errors: Engaging with miniature toy versions of cars, chairs, and slides as though they were the appropriate real sizes for them, such as sitting in a toy chair.
schemas: The signifiers or symbols that constitute mental life after the advent of representational abilities.
scheme: A way of perceiving or acting in the world.
secondary (self-conscious) emotions: Feelings of affect that depend on advanced developmental capacities, including cognition.
secondary circular reactions: Infants' repetition of movements that accidentally produce environmental events.
secure attachment: A type of attachment in which infants and children use their parents as a secure base from which they confidently engage with other people and explore the physical environment.
secure base: Use of trust in one's attachment figure for venturing farther afield and exploring the world beyond the dyad.
segmentation problem: Figuring out which elements of the continuous speech stream are words.
self-conscious (secondary) emotions: See *secondary (self-conscious) emotions*.
self-efficacy: Belief in one's abilities.
self-evaluative emotions: Emotions, such as embarrassment, hubris, pride, and shame, requiring an understanding of others' expectations and whether or not the expectations have been met.
self-regulation: Processes that modulate reactivity through approach, avoidance, inhibition, or attention.
sense of self: Understanding that one is separate from others.
sensitive parenting: Nurturant, attentive, responsive, nonrestrictive parental care.
sensitive period: A time during which the organism is especially vulnerable to external influences that alter or modify its structures or functions, often, although not always, in irreversible fashion.
sensory register: Memory that temporarily stores incoming sensory information.
separation anxiety: An unpleasant state of mental uneasiness, nervousness, or apprehension provoked in infants and children by separation or the threat of separation from an attachment figure.
sequential touching: A procedure to test infants' and children's categorization that involves presenting eight small three-dimensional models, four each belonging to two different categories, such as animals and vehicles.
shading: Depth information provided when contours of an object oriented away from a light source appear darker than contours oriented toward the light.

shared environment: The environment components that affect individuals similarly.

short-term (working) memory: Memory that has limited and momentary access to information where conscious cognition takes place. Includes the ability to remember and follow directions.

sleeper effect: An early experience may have no effect on the infant at the time, but that experience uniquely affects the infant at a later time point.

slow-to-warm-up temperament: Newborns, infants, and children who are negative in mood, slow to adapt, and withdraw from new situations.

social caregiving: Parent behaviors that include visual, verbal, affective, and physical activities that engage newborns, infants, and children in interpersonal exchanges, express affection, and involve social play as well as regulate affect and emotions.

social referencing: The deliberate search for information from other people to help clarify uncertain or ambiguous events.

socioeconomic status: The social standing or class of an individual or group.

somatic: A division of the nervous system comprised of voluntary conscious functions.

somesthetic system: A cortical system that regulates temperature, tactile, and positional information.

specificity principle: Specific experiences at specific times shape specific developmental outcomes in specific people in specific ways.

speech perception: Perceiving the features of a language.

stability: Consistency over time in the relative ranking of individuals in a group.

stage: In human development, a set of shared quantitative and qualitative characteristics which differ from those of another stage.

static monocular (pictorial) information: Depth information that is available when looking at a distance or with one eye without the observer or the object moving.

statistically normal: A distribution of scores that shows a pattern like a bell-shaped curve.

Strange Situation: An experimental protocol to study attachment; it is designed to expose infants and children to stress, which then elicits attachment behaviors.

structural perspectives: Define emotions in terms of their component processes.

structure: Physical components, such as the visual system or legs.

structure dependence: The idea that grammatical rules are defined over words and syntactic phrases (e.g., noun phrases).

subcortical structures: Noncortical structures in the brain that control state and arousal.

subjective contours: Extrapolating form or object edges where none is present.

sudden infant death syndrome (SIDS): The unexpected and unexplained death of a newborn or infant younger than 1 year of age.

sulci: Indentations in the cerebral cortex.

surfactin: A soapy substance that coats the lungs and facilitates the exchange of oxygen from the air.

subordinate categories: Subsumed under basic categories. Their instances or members are still discriminable, but they share many perceptual features, such as Siamese and Persian cats.

superordinate categories: The category level that has the greatest inclusiveness. Individual members of the category may not share much perceptual similarity, such as sharks and cows being included in the category of animals.

surgency: The aspect of emotional reactivity in which a person tends toward high levels of positive affect.

symbolic (pretend) play: A form of play that takes on more of a non-literal quality (e.g., using a stick as a gun).

symbolic (representational) play: Play that has a non-literal quality.

symbolic relations: Activities such as matching line drawings, scale models, or photographs to real objects.
synapses: Connections between axons and dendrites which aid in communication between neurons.
synaptogenesis: Formation of synapses.
syntax: Grammar or the rules for combining words into meaningful communications.
systems perspective: View of how structure supports function that suggests that the organization of the system as a whole reflects the activity of all different structures and functions and how they change as humans mature and gain new experiences.
tabula rasa: Means "blank slate"; refers to the idea that newborns come into the world with no preconceived knowledge and experiences contribute to knowledge.
temperament: Individual differences in behavioral functioning that tend to be biological in origin and stable over time.
temporal features: Descriptors of temperament that include the speed with which behaviors begin after stimulation (latency), how rapidly they escalate (rise time), how long they last (duration), and how slowly they go away (decay or recovery).
temporal lobe: Region of the cortex that governs the processing of auditory information and language comprehension and production.
tertiary circular reactions: Intentionally repeating an accidental event by systematically and deliberately varying the manner in which the event was initiated.
texture gradients: Depth information provided when elements of a textured surface gradually reduce in size.
theory of mind: The ability to attribute mental states – beliefs, intents, desires, pretending, knowledge – to oneself and others and to understand that others have beliefs, intents, desires, pretending, and knowledge that differ from one's own.
transaction (transaction framework): In development, when characteristics of the individual shape and are shaped by experience and environment across time.
transitional probabilities: The statistical likelihood of a sound or word following a prior sound or word.
trisomy 21: A genetic disorder resulting from having an extra chromosome; also known as Down syndrome.
true experiments: Random assignment of participants to conditions and the high level of control over their experiences.
turn-taking: The alternation of individuals in normal interaction or conversation.
Turner's syndrome: A female birth disorder where the female has only one X chromosome (as opposed to the normal XX).
trust: In attachment theory, it is the idea that caregivers can be trusted to respond to one's needs.
ultrasound imaging: A noninvasive fetal assessment wherein sounds are passed into the pregnant woman's body from a probe applied to the abdominal skin and pulses that are reflected back are used to map structures within the body.
umbilical cord: The connecting structure between the mother and the fetus that contains channels which allow the exchange of nutrients and waste.
uncertainty avoidance: The extent to which members of a culture are threatened by novel, surprising, or unknown situations.
unconditioned response: A concept from classical conditioning; automatic response to the unconditioned stimulus.
unconditioned stimulus: A concept from classical conditioning; a stimulus which elicits a response in the absence of any learning or conditioning.
universal grammar: The assertion that aspects of syntax are innate.

vagal tone: A reflection of heart rate changes mediated by the vagus nerve and controlled by the parasympathetic branch of the autonomic nervous system.
validity: When measurements measure what they are supposed to measure.
velars: Sounds created at the roof of the mouth (e.g., /k/ and /g/).
ventricles: Cavities in the brain that produce and store cerebrospinal fluid.
video deficit: The inability to learn from video or digital stimuli.
viewpoint invariance: The understanding that an object viewed from different perspectives is the same object.
visual acuity: Resolution of detail.
visual cliff: An experimental technique used to assess depth perception in crawling infants.
violation of expectation paradigm: An experimental method wherein newborns or infants are shown an impossible event (such as two objects occupying the same space at the same time) and their attention is monitored.
vocal play (expansion): A stage of pre-speech vocalization that involves the appearance of syllable-like productions with long vowels.
voicing: When a speaker produces different frequencies of sound waves at slightly different times.
working memory: Memory that has limited and momentary access to information, and it is where conscious cognition takes place. Includes the ability to remember and follow directions.
zone of proximal development: The difference between infants' and children's spontaneous performance on a task without guidance and performance on a task with guidance.
zygote: The prenatal organism from approximately conception to 2 weeks.

References

Aboagye, R. G., Ahinkorah, B. O., Seidu, A. A., Frimpong, J. B., Archer, A. G., Adu, C., Hagan, J. E., Amu, H., & Yaya, S. (2022). Birth weight and nutritional status of children under five in sub-Saharan Africa. *Plos One, 17*(6), e0269279. https://doi.org/10.1371/journal.pone.0269279

Abramovitch, R., Corter, C., & Lando, B. (1979). Sibling interaction in the home. *Child Development, 50*, 997–1003. https://doi.org/10.2307/1129325

Academy of Nutrition and Dietetics. (2019). *Healthy weight during pregnancy*. https://www.eatright.org/health/pregnancy/prenatal-nutrition/healthy-weight-during-pregnancy

Adolph, K. E., Cole, W. G., Komati, M., Garciaguirre, J. S., Badaly, D., Lingeman, J. M., Chan, G. L. Y., & Sotsky, R. B. (2012). How do you learn to walk? Thousands of steps and dozens of falls per day. *Psychological Science, 23*(11), 1387–1394. https://doi.org/10.1177/0956797612446346

Adolph, K. E., & Hospodar, C. M. (2025). Motor development. In M. H. Bornstein & M. E. Lamb (Eds.), *Developmental science: An advanced textbook* (8th ed., pp. 234–269). Psychology Press.

Adolph, K. E., Karasik, L. B., & Tamis-LeMonda, C. S. (2010). Motor skills. In M. H. Bornstein (Ed.), *Handbook of cultural development science, Vol. 1: Domains of development across cultures* (pp. 61–88). Taylor and Francis.

Ahnert, L. (2021). Attachment to childcare providers. In R. A. Thompson, J. A. Simpson, & L. J. Berlin (Eds.), *Attachment: The fundamental questions* (pp. 31–38). Guilford Press.

Ahnert, L., Eckstein-Madry, T., Datler, W., Deichmann, F., & Piskernik, B. (2022). Stress during transition from home to public childcare. *Applied Developmental Science, 27*(4), 320–335. https://doi.org/10.1080/10888691.2022.2070168

Ainsworth, M. (1967). *Infancy in Uganda*. Johns Hopkins University Press.

Ainsworth, M. D. S. (1973). The development of infant-mother attachment. In B. M. Caldwell & H. N. Ricciuti (Eds.), *Review of child development research* (Vol. 3, pp. 135–143). University of Chicago Press.

Ainsworth, M. D. S., & Wittig, B. A. (1969). Attachment and exploratory behavior of one-year-olds in a strange situation. In B. M. Foss (Ed.), *Determinants of infant behavior* (Vol. 4, pp. 111–136). Routledge Methuen.

Alfirevic, Z., Navaratnam, K., & Mujezinovic, F. (2017). Amniocentesis and chorionic villus sampling for prenatal diagnosis. *Cochrane Database of Systematic Reviews*, (9). https://doi.org/10.1002/14651858.CD003252.pub2

Allam, M. D., Marlier, L., & Schaal, B. (2006). Learning at the breast: Preference formation for an artificial scent and its attraction against the odor of maternal milk. *Infant Behavior and Development, 29*, 308–321. https://doi.org/10.1016/j.infbeh.2005.12.008

AL-Gubory, K. H. (2014). Environmental pollutants and lifestyle factors induce oxidative stress and poor prenatal development. *Reproductive BioMedicine Online, 29*, 17–31. https://doi.org/10.1016/j.rbmo.2014.03.002

American Academy of Pediatrics. (2016). Media and young minds. *Pediatrics, 138*(5), e20162591. https://doi.org/10.1542/peds.2016-2591

American Academy of Pediatrics. (2024). *Safe sleep*. https://www.aap.org/en/patient-care/safe-sleep/?srsltid=AfmBOopamQVmQbog2sXVJj0_Cxe2OBTaxnzyyUFtSvc8ZcNLgsexrbU

Amir, D., & Bornstein, M. H. (2025). Cross-cultural developmental research. In M. H. Bornstein & M. E. Lamb (Eds.), *Developmental science: An advanced textbook* (8th ed., pp. 35–80). Psychology Press.

Anderson, S. E., & Whitaker, R. C. (2011). Attachment security and obesity in US preschool-aged children. *Archives of Pediatrics & Adolescent Medicine, 165*, 235–242. https://doi.org/10.1001/archpediatrics.2010.292

Apgar, V. A. (1953). Proposal for a new method of evaluation of the newborn infant. *Anesthesia and Analgesia, Current Researches, 22*, 260.

Aral, N. (2020). *Handbook of prenatal, postnatal, and early childhood development*. Medical Information Science Reference/IGI Global.

Archer, J. (2006). Testosterone and human aggression: An evaluation of the challenge hypothesis. *Neuroscience and Biobehavioral Review, 30*, 219–345. https://doi.org/10.1016/j.neubiorev.2004.12.007

Archer, K., Wood, E., & De Pasquale, D. (2021). Examining joint parent-child interactions involving infants and toddlers when introducing mobile technology. *Infant Behavior and Development, 63*, 101568. https://doi.org/10.1016/j.infbeh.2021.101568

Arredondo, M. M., Aslin, R. N., Zhang, M., & Werker, J. F. (2022). Attentional orienting abilities in bilinguals: Evidence from a large infant sample. *Infant Behavior and Development, 66*, 101683. https://doi.org/10.1016/j.infbeh.2021.101683

Arterberry, M. E., & Bornstein, M. H. (2001). Three-month-old infants' categorization of animals and vehicles based on static and dynamic attributes. *Journal of Experimental Child Psychology, 80*, 333–346. https://doi.org/10.1006/jecp.2001.2637

Arterberry, M. E., & Bornstein, M. H. (2024). *Development in infancy* (6th ed.). Routledge/Taylor & Francis Group.

Arterberry, M. E., Hespos, S. J., & Herth, R. A. (2018). Integration of thought and action: Arm weights facilitate search accuracy in 24-month-old children. *Infancy, 23*(2), 173–193. https://doi.org/10.1111/infa.12208

Arterberry, M. E., Hespos, S. J., Walsh, C. E., & Daniels, C. A. (2020). Integration of thought and action continued: Scale errors and categorization in toddlers. *Infancy, 25*, 851–870. https://doi.org/10.1111/infa.12364

Arterberry, M. E., & Kellman, P. J. (2016). *Development of perception in infancy: The cradle of knowledge revisited*. Oxford University Press.

Asok, A., Bernard, K., Roth, T. L., Rosen, J. B., & Dozier, M. (2013). Parental responsiveness moderates the association between early-life stress and reduced telomere length. *Development and Psychopathology, 25*(3), 577–585. https://doi.org/10.1017/S0954579413000011

Aviles, A. I., & Zeifman, D. M. (2021). Casting a wider net. In R. A. Thompson, J. A. Simpson, & L. J. Berlin (Eds.), *Attachment: The fundamental questions* (pp. 53–59). Guilford Press.

Aylward, G. P. (2005). Neurodevelopmental outcomes of infants born prematurely. *Journal of Developmental and Behavioral Pediatrics, 26*, 427–440. https://doi.org/10.1097/00004703-200512000-00008

Badiee, Z., Asghari, M., & Mohammadizadeh, M. (2013). The calming effect of maternal breast milk odor on premature infants. *Pediatrics & Neonatology, 54*(5), 322–325. https://doi.org/10.1016/j.pedneo.2013.04.004

Bahrick, L. E., & Lickliter, R. (2012). The role of intersensory redundancy in early perceptual, cognitive, and social development. In A. Bremner, D. J. Lewkowicz, & C. Spence (Eds.), *Multisensory development* (pp. 183–205). Oxford University Press.

Baillargeon, R., Spelke, E. S., & Wasserman, S. (1985). Object permanence in 5-month-old infants. *Cognition, 20,* 191–208. https://doi.org/10.1016/0010–0277(85)90008–3

Baker, S. T., Gjersoe, N. L., Sibielska-Woch, K., Leslie, A. M., & Hood, B. M. (2011). Inhibitory control interacts with core knowledge in toddlers' manual search for an occluded object. *Developmental Science, 14*(2), 270–279. https://doi.org/10.1111/j.1467–7687.2010.00972.x

Bandstra, E. S., Morrow, C. M., Mansorr, E., & Accornero, V. H. (2010). Prenatal drug exposure: Infant and toddler outcomes. *Journal of Addictive Diseases, 29,* 245–258. https://doi.org/10.1080/10550881003684871

Barbosa, M., Beeghly, M., Moreira, J., Tronick, E., & Fuertes, M. (2018). Robust stability and physiological correlates of infants' patterns of regulatory behavior in the still-face paradigm at 3 and 9 months. *Developmental Psychology, 54*(11), 2032. https://doi.org/10.1037/dev0000616

Barr, R., Kirkorian, H., Coyne, S. & Radesky, J. (2024). *Early Childhood and Digital Media*. In M. H. Bornstein (Series Editor), *Cambridge Elements in Child Development*. Cambridge University Press. https://doi.org/10.1017/9781108885751

Barr, R., Zack, E., Garcia, A., & Muentener, P. (2008). Infants' attention and responsiveness to television increases with prior exposure and parental interaction. *Infancy, 13,* 30–56. https://doi.org/10.1080/15250000701779378

Barrett, K. C., & Campos, J. J. (1987). Perspectives on emotional development II: A functionalist approach to emotions. In J. D. Osofsky (Ed.), *Handbook of infant development* (2nd ed., pp. 555–578). Wiley.

Barry, E. S. (2019). Co-sleeping as a proximal context for infant development: The importance of physical touch. *Infant Behavior and Development, 57,* 101385. https://doi.org/10.1016/j.infbeh.2019.101385

Bauman, B., Ko, J., Cox, S., D'Angelo, D., Warner, L., Folger, S., Tevendale, H., Coy, K., Harrison, L., & Barfield, W. (2020). *Vital signs: Postpartum depressive symptoms and provider discussions about perinatal depression – United States, 2018*. https://www.cdc.gov/mmwr/volumes/69/wr/mm6919a2.htm?s_cid=mm6919a2_w#suggestedcitation

Bayley, N. (1933). *Bayley scales of infant development* (2nd ed., manual). Psychological Corporation.

Beck, C. T. (2006). Postpartum depression: It isn't just the blues. *American Journal of Nursing, 106*(5), 40–51. https://doi.org/10.1097/00000446-200605000-00020

Behrman, R. E., & Butler, A. S. (2007). *Preterm birth: Causes, consequences, and prevention*. National Academies Press.

Belsky, J., & Barends, N. (2002). Personality and parenting. In M. H. Bornstein (Ed.), *Handbook of parenting: Status and social ecology of parenting* (Vol. 3, pp. 415–438). Erlbaum.

Belsky, J., Vandell, D. L., Burchinal, M., K. Clarke-Stewart, McCartney, K., Owne, M. T., & NICHD Early Child Care Research Network. (2007). Are there long-term effects of early child care? *Child Development, 78,* 681–701. https://doi.org/10.1111/j.1467–8624.2007.01021.x

Benenson, J. F., Tennyson, R., & Wrangham, R. W. (2011). Male more than female infants imitate propulsive motion. *Cognition, 121,* 262–267. https://doi.org/10.1016/j.cognition.2011.07.006

Berger, S. E., & Moore, C. T. (2021). A time series analysis of the relation between motor skill acquisition and sleep in infancy. *Infant Behavior and Development, 65,* 101654. https://doi.org/10.1016/j.infbeh.2021.101654

Berger, S. E., & Scher, A. (2017). Naps improve new walkers' locomotor problem solving. *Journal of Experimental Child Psychology, 162,* 292–300. https://doi.org/10.1016/j.jecp.2017.04.021

Berger, S. E., Theuring, C., & Adolph, K. E. (2007). How and when infants learn to climb stairs. *Infant Behavior and Development, 30*, 36–49. https://doi.org/10.1016/j.infbeh.2006.11.002

Bergmann, O., Spalding, K. L., & Frisén, J. (2015). Adult neurogenesis in humans. *Cold Spring Harbor Perspectives in Biology, 7*(7), a018994. https://doi.org/10.1101/cshperspect.a018994

Bernard, K., Frost, A., Jelinek, C., & Dozier, M. (2019b). Secure attachment predicts lower body mass index in young children with histories of child protective services involvement. *Pediatric Obesity, 14*(7), e12510. https://doi.org/10.1111/ijpo.12510

Bernard, K., Hostinar, C. E., & Dozier, M. (2019a). Longitudinal associations between attachment quality in infancy, C-reactive protein in early childhood, and BMI in middle childhood: Preliminary evidence from a CPS-referred sample. *Attachment & Human Development, 21*(1), 5–22. https://doi.org/10.1080/14616734.2018.1541513

Bernard, K., Peloso, E., Laurenceau, J. P., Zhang, Z., & Dozier, M. (2015). Examining change in cortisol patterns during the 10-week transition to a new child-care setting. *Child Development, 86*(2), 456–471. https://doi.org/10.1111/cdev.12304

Berthier, N. E., DeBlois, S., Poirier, C. R., Novak, M. A., & Clifton, R. K. (2000). Where's the ball? Two-and three-year-olds reason about unseen events. *Developmental Psychology, 36*(3), 394–401. https://doi.org/10.1037/0012-1649.36.3.394

Bhatt, R. S., Bertin, E., Hayden, A., & Reed, A. (2005). Face perception in infancy: Developmental changes in the use of different kinds of relational information. *Child Development, 76*, 169–181. https://doi.org/10.1111/j.1467–8624.2005.00837.x

Bick, J., & Dozier, M. (2013). The effectiveness of an attachment-based intervention in promoting foster mothers' sensitivity toward foster infants. *Infant Mental Health Journal, 34*(2), 95–103. https://doi.org/10.1002/imhj.21373

Bigelow, A. E., Power, M., & Dadgar, H. (2023). Maternal mind-mindedness over infants' first three months. *Infant Behavior and Development, 72*, 101864. https://doi.org/10.1016/j.infbeh.2023.101864

Biringen, Z., Derscheid, D., Vliegen, N., Closson, L., & Easterbrooks, M. A. (2014). Emotional availability (EA): Theoretical background, empirical research using the EA scales, and clinical applications. *Developmental Review, 34*(2), 114–167. https://doi.org/10.1016/j.dr.2014.01.002

Bizzego, A., Gabrieli, G., Bornstein, M. H., Deater-Deckard, K., Lansford, J. E., Bradley, R. H., Costa, M., & Esposito, G. (2021). Predictors of contemporary under-5 child mortality in low- and middle-income countries: A machine learning approach. *International Journal of Environmental Research and Public Health, 18*, 1315. https://doi.org/10.3390/ijerph18031315

Bjorklund, D. (2020). Child development in evolutionary perspective. In M. H. Bornstein (Ed.), *Cambridge elements in child development*. Cambridge University Press. https://doi.org/10.1017/9781108866187

Blass, E. M., Ganchrow, J. R., & Steiner, J. E. (1984). Classical conditioning in newborn humans 2–48 hours of age. *Infant Behavior and Development, 7*, 223–235. https://doi.org/10.1016/S0163–6383(84)80060–0

Boe, J. L., & Woods, R. J. (2018). Parents' influence on infants' gender-typed toy preferences. *Sex Roles, 79*(5), 358–373. https://doi.org/10.1007/s11199-017-0858-4

Boggess, T., & Risher, W. C. (2022). Clinical and basic research investigations into the long-term effects of prenatal opioid exposure on brain development. *Journal of Neuroscience Research, 100*(1), 396–409. http://doi.org/10.1002/jnr.24642

Bohr, Y. (2010). Transnational infancy: A new context for attachment and the need for better models. *Child Development Perspectives, 4*, 189–196.

Bornstein, M. H. (1989). Sensitive periods in development: Structural characteristics and causal interpretations. *Psychological Bulletin, 105*, 179–197. https://doi.org/10.1037/0033–2909.105.2.179

Bornstein, M. H. (2007). On the significance of social relationships in the development of children's earliest symbolic play: An ecological perspective. In A. Göncü & S. Gaskins (Eds.), *Play and development: Evolutionary, sociocultural, and functional perspectives* (pp. 101–129). Erlbaum.

Bornstein, M. H. (2009). Toward a model of culture↔parent↔child transactions. In A. Sameroff (Ed.), *The transactional model of development: How children and contexts shape each other* (pp. 139–161). American Psychological Association.

Bornstein, M. H. (2013). Parenting X gender X culture X time. In W. B. Wilcox & K. K. Kline (Eds.), *Gender and parenthood: Biological and social scientific perspectives* (pp. 91–119). Columbia University Press.

Bornstein, M. H. (2015). Emergence and early development of color vision and color perception. In A. Elliot, M. Fairchild, & A. Franklin (Eds.), *Handbook of color psychology* (pp. 149–179). Cambridge University Press.

Bornstein, M. H. (2019a). "It's about time!" Ecological systems, transaction, and specificity as key developmental principles in children's changing worlds. In R. D. Parke & G. H. Elder (Eds.), *Children in changing worlds: Sociocultural and temporal perspectives* (pp. 277–286). Cambridge University Press.

Bornstein, M. H. (2019b). Parenting infants. In M. H. Bornstein (Ed.), *Handbook of parenting, Vol. 1. Children and parenting* (3th ed., pp. 3–55). Routledge.

Bornstein, M. H. (Ed.). (2022). *Parenting, infancy, culture: Specificity and commonality in Argentina, Belgium, Israel, Italy, and the United States*. Routledge.

Bornstein, M. H. (2024). Parenting science and emotion regulation: Principles, effects, determinants, and supports. In I. Roskam, J. Gross, & M. Mikolajczak (Eds.), *Emotion regulation and parenting* (pp. 3–32). Cambridge University Press.

Bornstein, M. H., & Arterberry, M. E. (2003). Recognition, categorization, and apperception of the facial expression of smiling by 5-month-old infants. *Developmental Science, 6*, 585–599. https://doi.org/10.1111/1467–7687.00314

Bornstein, M. H., & Arterberry, M. E. (2010). The development of object categorization in young children: Hierarchical inclusiveness, age, perceptual attribute and group versus individual analyses. *Developmental Psychology, 46*, 350–365. https://doi.org/10.1037/a0018411

Bornstein, M. H., Arterberry, M. E., & Mash, C. (2004a). Long-term memory for an emotional interpersonal interaction occurring at 5 months of age. *Infancy, 6*, 407–416.

Bornstein, M. H., Arterberry, M. E., & Mash, C. (2025). Perceptual development. In M. H. Bornstein & M. E. Lamb (Eds.), *Developmental science: An advanced textbook* (pp. 270–320). Routledge.

Bornstein, M. H., & Bradley, R. H. (Eds.). (2003). *Socioeconomic status, parenting, and child development*. Erlbaum.

Bornstein, M. H., & Colombo, J. (2012). Infant cognitive functioning and mental development. In S. Pauen (Ed.), *Early childhood development and later achievement* (pp. 118–147). Cambridge University Press.

Bornstein, M. H., Cote, L. R., Haynes, O. M., Suwalsky, J. T. D., & Bakeman, R. (2012a). Modalities of infant-mother interaction in Japanese, Japanese American immigrant, and European American dyads. *Child Development, 83*, 2073–2088. https://doi.org/10.1111/j.1467–8624.2012.01822.x

Bornstein, M. H., Cote, L. R., Maital, S., Painter, K., Park, S.-Y., Pascual, L., Pêcheux, M.-G., Ruel, J., Venuti, P., & Vyt, A. (2004b). Cross-linguistic analysis of vocabulary in young children: Spanish, Dutch, French, Hebrew, Italian, Korean, and American English. *Child Development, 75*(4), 1115–1139. https://doi.org/10.1111/j.1467–8624.2004.00729.x

Bornstein, M. H., DiPietro, J. A., Hahn, C. H., Painter, K. M., Haynes, O. M., & Costigan, K. A. (2002). Prenatal cardiac function and postnatal cognitive development: An exploratory study. *Infancy, 3*, 475–494.

Bornstein, M. H., Gaughran, J. M., & Seguí, I. (1991). Multimethod assessment of infant temperament: Mother questionnaire and mother and observer reports evaluated and compared at five months using the infant temperament measure. *International Journal of Behavioral Development, 14*, 131–151. https://doi.org/10.1177/016502549101400202

Bornstein, M. H., Gini, M., Putnick, D. L., Haynes, O. M., Painter, K. M., & Suwalsky, J. T. D. (2006). Short-term reliability and continuity of emotional availability in mother–child dyads across contexts of observation. *Infancy, 10*, 1–16. https://doi.org/10.1207/s15327078in1001_1

Bornstein, M. H., Hahn, C., & Haynes, O. M. (2011). Maternal personality, parenting cognitions, and parenting practices. *Developmental Psychology, 47*, 658–675. https://doi.org/10.1037/a0023181

Bornstein, M. H., Hahn, C.-S., Putnick, D., & Pearson, R. (2019a) Stability of child temperament: Multiple moderation by child and mother characteristics. *British Journal of Developmental Psychology, 37*, 51–67. https://doi.org/10.1111/bjdp.12253

Bornstein, M. H., Kessen, W., & Weiskopf, S. (1976a). The categories of hue in infancy. *Science, 191*, 201–202. https://doi.org/10.1126/science.1246610

Bornstein, M. H., Kessen, W., & Weiskopf, S. (1976b). Color vision and hue categorization in young human infants. *Journal of Experimental Psychology: Human Perception and Performance, 2*, 115–129. https://doi.org/10.1037/0096–1523.2.1.115

Bornstein, M. H., Kotler, J. A., & Lansford, J. E. (2022a). The future of parenting programs: An introduction. *Parenting: Science and Practice, 22*, 189–275. https://doi.org/10.1080/15295192.2022.2086808

Bornstein, M. H., Manian, N., & Henry, L. M. (2022b). Clinically depressed and typically developing mother-infant dyads: Domain base rates and correspondences, relationship contingencies and attunement. *Infancy, 26*(6), 877–900. https://doi.org/10.1111/infa.12427

Bornstein, M. H., & Putnick, D. L. (2012). Stability of language in childhood: A multiage, multidomain, multimeasure, and multisource study. *Developmental Psychology, 48*, 477–491. https://doi.org/10.1037/a0025889

Bornstein, M. H., Putnick, D. L., & Esposito, G. (2017a). Continuity and stability in development. *Child Development Perspectives, 11*, 113–119. https://doi.org/10.1111/cdep.12221

Bornstein, M. H., Putnick, D. L., & Esposito, G. (2022c). The nature and structure of mothers' parenting their infants. *Parenting: Science and Practice, 22*(2), 83–127. https://doi.org/10.1080/15295192.2022.2057799

Bornstein, M. H., Putnick, D. L., Gartstein, M. A., Hahn, C.-S., Auestad, N., & O'Connor, D. L. (2015). Infant temperament: Stability by age, gender, birth order, term status, and socioeconomic status. *Child Development, 86*, 844–863. https://doi.org/10.1111/cdev.12367

Bornstein, M. H., Putnick, D. L., Lansford, J. E., Deater-Deckard, K., & Bradley, R. (2016). Gender in low- and middle-income countries. *Monographs of the Society for Research in Child Development, 81*. https://doi.org/10.1111/mono.12229

Bornstein, M. H., Putnick, D. L., Rigo, P., Esposito, G., Swain, J. E., Suwalsky, J. T. D., Su, X., Du, X., Cote, L. R., De Pisapia, N., & Venuti, P. (2017b). The neurobiology of culturally common maternal responses to infant cry. *Proceedings of the National Academy of Sciences, 114*(45), E9465–E9473. https://doi.org/10.1073/pnas.1712022114

Bornstein, M. H., Putnick, D. L., & Suwalsky, J. T. (2019b). Mother–infant interactions with firstborns and secondborns: A within-family study of European Americans. *Infant Behavior and Development, 55*, 100–111. https://doi.org/10.1016/j.infbeh.2019.03.009

Bornstein, M. H., Rothenberg, W. A., & Putnick, D. L. (2022). Cognitive and socioemotional caregiving, national development, and child development in 51 low- and middle-income countries. In M. H. Bornstein, W. A. Rothenberg, A. Bizzego, R. H. Bradley, K. Deater-Deckard, G. Esposito, J. E. Lansford, D. L. Putnick, & S. Zietz (Eds.), *Parenting and child development in low- and middle-income countries* (pp. 79–127). Routledge.

Bornstein, M. H., Suwalsky, J. T., & Breakstone, D. A. (2012b). Emotional relationships between mothers and infants: Knowns, unknowns, and unknown unknowns. *Development and Psychopathology, 24*(1), 113–123. https://doi.org/10.1017/S0954579411000708

Bornstein, M. H., & Tamis-LeMonda, C. S. (2007). Infants at play: Development, functions, and partners. In A. Slater & M. Lewis (Eds.), *Introduction to infant development* (2th ed., pp. 253–269). Oxford University Press.

Bouchard, T. J., Lykken, D. T., McGue, M., Segal, N. L., & Tellegen, A. (1990). Sources of human psychological differences: The Minnesota study of twins reared apart. *Science, 250*(4978), 223–228. https://doi.org/10.1126/science.2218526

Bower, T. G. R. (1977). *A primer of infant development*. Freeman.

Bowker, J. C., Rubin, K. H., McDonald, K. L., Mulvey, K. L., Güroğlu, B., Nishina, A., & Chen, X. (2025). Peer relationships. In M. H. Bornstein & M. E. Lamb (Eds.), *Developmental science* (pp. 558–598). Routledge.

Bowlby, J. (1969). *Attachment and loss: Attachment* (2nd ed., Vol. 1). Basic Books.

Boysson-Bardies, B., Sagart, L., & Durand, C. (1984). Discernible differences in the babbling of infants according to target language. *Journal of Child Language, 11*(1), 1–15. https://doi.org/10.1017/S0305000900005559

Bradley, R. H. (2010). *Handbook of cultural developmental science*. Psychology Press.

Bradley, R. H., & Rothenberg, W. A. (2022). Children's physical home environment, national development, and child development in 51 low- and middle-income countries. In M. H. Bornstein, W. A. Rothenberg, A. Bizzego, R. H. Bradley, K. Deater-Deckard, G. Esposito, J. E. Lansford, D. L. Putnick, & S. Zietz (Eds.), *Parenting and child development in low and middle income countries* (pp. 160–209). Taylor and Francis. https://doi.org/10.4324/9781003044925-5

Bradley-Johnson, S., Johnson, C. M., Swanson, J., & Jackson, A. (2004). Exploratory behavior: A comparison of infants who are congenitally blind and infants who are sighted. *Journal of Visual Impairment and Blindness, 98*, 496–502. https://doi.org/10.1177/0145482X0409800805

Brazelton, T. B., Nugent, J. K., & Lester, B. M. (1987). Neonatal behavioral assessment scale. In J. D. Osofsky (Ed.), *Handbook of infant development* (2nd ed., pp. 780–817). Wiley.

Bremner, J. G., Slater, A. M., Johnson, S. P., Mason, U. C., & Spring, J. (2012). Illusory contour figures are perceived as occluding contours by 4-month-old infants. *Developmental Psychology, 48*(2), 398–405. https://doi.org/10.1037/a0024922

Bribiescas, R. G. (2001). Reproductive ecology and life history of the human male. *American Journal of Physical Anthropology, 44*, 148–176. https://doi.org/10.1002/ajpa.10025

Bridgett, D. J., Gartstein, M. A., Putnam, S. P., Lance, K. O., Iddins, E., Waits, R., VanVleet, J., & Lee, L. (2011). Emerging effortful control in toddlerhood: The role of infant orienting/regulation, maternal effortful control, and maternal time spent in caregiving activities. *Infant Behavior and Development, 34*, 189–199. https://doi.org/10.1016/j.infbeh.2010.12.008

Bridgett, D. J., Gartstein, M. A., Putnam, S. P., McKay, T., Iddins, E., Robertson, C., Ramsay, K., & Rittmueller, A. (2009). Maternal and contextual influences and the effect of temperament development during infancy on parenting in toddlerhood. *Infant Behavior & Development, 32*, 103–116. https://doi.org/10.1016/j.infbeh.2008.10.007

Broderick, A. V., & Neiderhiser, J. M. (2019). Genetics and parenting. In M. H. Bornstein (Ed.), *Handbook of parenting, Vol. 2: Biology and ecology of parenting* (3rd ed., pp. 123–165). Routledge.

Bronfenbrenner, U. (1961). The changing American child. *Journal of Social Issues, 17*, 6–18. https://doi.org/10.1111/j.1540-4560.1961.tb01659.x

Brown, G. L., Mangelsdorf, S. C., Neff, C., Shigeto, A., Aytuglu, A., & Thomas, C. R. (2022). Infant attachment configurations with mothers and fathers: Implications for triadic interaction quality and children's parental preferences. *Early Childhood Research Quarterly, 58*, 155–164. https://doi.org/10.1016/j.ecresq.2021.09.004

Brownell, C. A., Lemerise, E. A., Pelphrey, K. A., & Roisman, G. I. (2015). Measuring socioemotional development. In M. E. Lamb & R. M. Lerner (Eds.), *Handbook of child psychology and developmental science: Socioemotional processes* (Vol. 3, 7th ed., pp. 11–56). Wiley.

Brubaker, C. J., Schmithorst, V. J., Haynes, E. N., Deitrick, K. N., Egelhoff, J. C., Lindquist, D. M., Lanphear, B. P., & Cecil, K. M. (2009). Altered myelination and axonal integrity in adults with childhood lead exposure: A diffusion tensor imaging study. *NeuroToxicology, 30*, 867–875. https://doi.org/10.1016/j.neuro.2009.07.007

Burchinal, M., Magnuson, K., Powell, D., & Hong, S. S. (2015). Early childcare and education. In M. H. Bornstein, T. Leventhal, & R. M. Lerner (Eds.), *Handbook of child psychology and developmental science: Ecological settings and processes*. (Vol. 4, 7th ed., pp. 223–267). Wiley.

Burchinal, M., Whitaker, A. A., & Jenkins, J. M. (2023). The promise and purpose of early care and education. *Child Development Perspectives, 16*, 134–140. https://psycnet.apa.org/doi/10.1111/cdep.12463

Burns, T. C., & Verfaillie, C. M. (2015). From mice to mind: Strategies and progress in translating neuroregeneration. *European Journal of Pharmacology, 759*, 90–100. https://doi.org/10.1016/j.ejphar.2015.03.041

Buss, A. H., & Plomin, R. (1984). *Temperament: Early developing personality traits*. Erlbaum.

Cabrera, N. J., Karberg, E., Malin, J. L., & Aldoney, D. (2017). The magic of play: Low-income mothers' and fathers' playfulness and children's emotion regulation and vocabulary skills. *Infant Mental Health Journal, 38*(6), 757–771. https://doi.org/10.1002/imhj.21682

Calabrese, E. J., & Baldwin L. A. (2003). Toxicology rethinks its central belief. *Nature, 421*(6924), 691–692. https://doi.org/10.1038/421691a

Calkins, S. D., Howse, R. B., & Philippot, P. (2004). Individual differences in self-regulation: Implications for childhood adjustment. In P. Philippot & R. S. Feldman (Eds.), *The regulation of emotion* (pp. 307–332). Psychology Press.

Caller, P. (2020). A cultural linguistics approach to the "discovery of childhood" in sixteenth and seventeenth century Britain. *Token: A Journal of English Linguistics, 10*, 181–204.

Campanella, J., & Rovee-Collier, C. (2005). Latent learning and deferred imitation at 3 months. *Infancy, 7*, 243–262. https://doi.org/10.1207/s15327078in0703_2

Camras, L. A. (2022). *Emotional development across the lifespan*. Guilford Press.

Camras, L. A., Oster, H., Bakeman, R., Meng, Z., Ujiie, T., & Campos, J. J. (2007). Do infants show distinct facial expressions for fear and anger? Emotional expression in 11-month-old European American, Chinese, and Japanese infants. *Infancy, 11*, 131–155. https://doi.org/10.1111/j.1532–7078.2007.tb00219.x

Caputo, C., Wood, E., & Jabbour, L. (2016). Impact of fetal alcohol exposure on body systems: A systematic review. *Birth Defects Research Part C: Embryo Today: Reviews, 108*(2), 174–180. https://doi.org/10.1002/bdrc.21129

Cardenas, S. I., Morris, A. R., Marshall, N., Aviv, E. C., Marinez Garcia, M., Sellery, P., & Saxbe, D. E. (2022). Fathers matter from the start: The role of expectant fathers in child development. *Child Development Perspectives, 16*, 54–59.

Carlson, L. M., & Vora, N. L. (2017). Prenatal diagnosis: Screening and diagnostic tools. *Obstetrics and Gynecology Clinics of North America, 44*(2), 245–256. https://doi.org/10.1016/j.ogc.2017.02.004

Carr, A., & Dempster, T. (2021). Parent-child interactions during joint engagement with touchscreen technology: A comparison of younger versus older toddlers. *Infant Behavior and Development, 64*, 101587. https://doi.org/10.1016/j.infbeh.2021.101587

Casler, K., Eshleman, A., Greene, K., & Terziyan, T. (2011). Children's scale errors with tools. *Developmental Psychology, 47*(3), 857–866. https://doi.org/10.1037/a0021174

Cassidy, J. (2021). In the service of protection from threat: Attachment and internal working models. In R. A. Thompson, J. A. Simpson, & L. J. Berlin (Eds.), *Attachment: The fundamental questions* (pp. 103–110). Guilford Press.

Cavazos-Rehg, P. A., Krauss, M. J., Spitznagel, E. L., Bommarito, K., Madden, T., Olsen, M. A., Subramaniam, H., Peipert, J. F., & Bierut, L. J. (2015). Maternal age and risk of labor and delivery complications. *Maternal and Child Health Journal, 19*(6), 1202–1211. https://doi.org/10.1007/s10995-014-1624-7

Centers for Disease Control. (2000). *Growth charts*. https://www.cdc.gov/growthcharts/
Centers for Disease Control. (2023, June 3). *Important milestones: Your child by three years*. https://www.cdc.gov/ncbddd/actearly/milestones/index.html
Centers for Disease Control. (2024, May 15). *Symptoms of depression among women*. https://www.cdc.gov/reproductive-health/depression/
Cerezo, M. A., Sierra-García, P., Pons-Salvador, G., & Trenado, R. M. (2017). Parental and infant gender factors in parent–infant interaction: State-space dynamic analysis. *Frontiers in Psychology*, *8*, 1724. https://doi.org/10.3389/fpsyg.2017.01724
Cernoch, J. M., & Porter, R. H. (1985). Recognition of maternal auxiliary odors by infants. *Child Development*, *56*, 1593–1598. https://doi.org/10.2307/1130478
Champagne, F. A. (2018). Epigenetics. In M. H. Bornstein (Ed.), *Encyclopedia of lifespan human development* (Vol. 2, pp. 759–762). Sage.
Chassin, L., Hussong, A. M., Rothenberg, W. A., & Sternberg, A. (2019). Parenting and substance use disorder. In M. H. Bornstein (Ed.), *Handbook of parenting, Vol. 4: Social conditions and applied parenting* (3rd ed., pp. 483–516). Routledge.
Cheffins, T., Chan A., Haan E. A., Ranieri, E., Ryall, R. G., Keane, R. J., Scott, H., Gjerde, M., Nguyen, A. M., Ford, J. H., & Sykes, S. (2000). The impact of maternal serum screening on the birth prevalence of Down's syndrome and the use of amniocentesis and chorionic villus sampling in South Australia. *BJOG: An International Journal of Obstetrics and Gynaecology*, *107*, 1453–1459. https://doi.org/10.1111/j.1471–0528.2000.tb11668.x
Chen, X., & Schmidt, L. A. (2015). Temperament and personality. In M. E. Lamb & R. M. Lerner (Eds.), *Handbook of child psychology and developmental science: Socioemotional processes* (Vol. 3, 7th ed., pp. 152–200). Wiley.
Chen, Y., Keen, R., Rosander, K., & von Hofsten, C. (2010). Movement planning reflects skill level and age changes in toddlers. *Child Development*, *81*, 1846–1858. https://doi.org/10.1111/j.1467–8624.2010.01514.x
Cheraghi, P., Poorolajal, J., Hazavehi, S. M. M., & Rezapur-Shahkolai, F. (2014). Effect of educating mothers on injury prevention among children aged <5 years using the health belief model: A randomized controlled trial. *Public Health*, *128*(9), 825–830. https://doi.org/10.1016/j.puhe.2014.06.017
Chick, K. A., Heilman-Houser, R. A., & Hunter, M. W. (2002). The impact of child care on gender role development and gender stereotypes. *Early Childhood Education Journal*, *29*, 149–154. https://doi.org/10.1023/A:1014528424032
Chomsky, N. (1965). *Aspects of the theory of syntax*. MIT Press.
Chronis-Tuscano, A., Degnan, K. A., Pine, D. S., Perez-Edgar, K., Henderson, H. A., Diaz, Y., Raggi, V. L., & Fox, N. A. (2009). Stable early maternal report of behavioral inhibition predicts lifetime social anxiety disorder in adolescence. *American Academy of Child and Adolescent Psychiatry*, *48*, 1–8. https://doi.org/10.1097/CHI.0b013e3181ae09df
Clark, R. E. (2004). The classical origins of Pavlov's conditioning. *Integrative Physiological & Behavioral Science*, *39*, 279–294. https://doi.org/10.1007/BF02734167
Clearfield, M. W., & Nelson, N. M. (2006). Sex differences in mothers' speech and play behavior with 6-, 9-, and 14-month-old infants. *Sex Roles*, *54*, 127–137. https://doi.org/10.1007/s11199-005-8874-1
Coall, D. A., Callan, A. C., Sartori, J., & Chisholm, J. S. (2019). Prenatal parenting. In M. H. Bornstein (Ed.), *Handbook of parenting, Vol. 2: Biology and ecology of parenting* (3rd ed., pp. 166–219). Routledge.
Cohen, L. B., & Cashon, C. H. (2006). Infant cognition. In D. Kuhn & R. S. Siegler (Eds.), W. Damon (Series Ed.), *Handbook of child psychology: Cognition, perception, and language* (6th ed., Vol. 2, pp. 214–251). Wiley.
Cohn, J. F., Ambadar, Z., & Ekman, P. (2007). Observer-based measurement of facial expression with the facial action coding system. In J. A. Coan & J. J. B. Allen (Eds.), *The handbook of emotion elicitation and assessment* (pp. 203–221). Oxford University Press.

Cole, W. G., Lingeman, J. M., & Adolph, K. E. (2012). Go naked: Diapers affect infant walking. *Developmental Science, 15*, 783–790. https://doi.org/10.1111/j.1467–7687.2012.01169.x

Collis, R. E., & Davis, H. (2010). Analgesia in labour: Induction and maintenance. *Obstetric Anaesthesia, 11*, 266–269. https://doi.org/10.1016/j.mpaic.2010.04.002

Conrad, R. (1998). Darwin's baby and baby's Darwin: Mutual recognition in observational research. *Human Development, 41*, 47–64. https://doi.org/10.1159/000022568

Cooray, N., Sun, S. L., Adams, S., Keay, L., Nassar, N., & Brown, J. (2022). Exploring infant fall events using online parenting discussion forums: Infodemiology study. *JMIR Pediatrics and Parenting, 5*(2), e34413. https://doi.org/10.2196/34413

Corbetta, D., DiMercurio, A., Weiner, R. F., Connell, J. P., & Clark, M. (2018). How perception and action fosters exploration and selection in infant skill acquisition. In J. M. Plumert (Ed.), *Studying the perception-action system as a model system for understanding development* (Vol. 55, pp. 1–29). Elsevier.

Craton, L. G., & Yonas, A. (1990). The role of motion in infants' perception of occlusion. In L. G. Craton & A. Yonas (Eds.), *The development of attention: Research and theory* (pp. 21–46). Elsevier. https://doi.org/10.1016/S0166–4115(08)60449–5

Crnic, K., & Lin, B. (2021). Depression in children's lives. In M. H. Bornstein (Ed.), *Cambridge elements in child development*. Cambridge University Press. https://doi.org/10.1017/9781108887144

Crnic, K. A., & Coburn, S. S. (2019). Stress and parenting. In M. H. Bornstein (Ed.), *Handbook of parenting, Vol. 4: Social conditions and applied parenting* (3rd ed., pp. 421–448). Routledge.

Cycyk, L. M., & De Anda, S. (2021). Media exposure and language experience: Examining associations from home observations in Mexican immigrant families in the US. *Infant Behavior and Development, 63*, 101554. https://doi.org/10.1016/j.infbeh.2021.101554

Dahlke, J. D., & Chauhan, S. P. (2025). *Caesarean section delivery*. Cambridge University Press.

Dao, H., Mofenson, L. M., Ekpini R., Gilkas, C. F, Barnhart, M., Bolu, O., & Shaffer, N. (2007). International recommendations on antiretroviral drugs for treatment of HIV-infected women and prevention of mother-to-child transmission in resource-limited settings: 2006 update. *American Journal of Obstetrics and Gynecology, 3*, S42–S55. https://doi.org/10.1016/j.ajog.2007.03.001

Darwin, C. (1965). *The expression of the emotions in man and animals*. Murray. (Original work published 1872)

Davis, J., Redshaw, J., Suddendorf, T., Nielsen, M., Kennedy-Constantini, S., Oostenbroek, J., & Slaughter, V. (2021). Does neonatal imitation exist? Insights from a meta-analysis of 336 effect sizes. *Psychological Science, 16*, 1373–1397. https://doi.org/10.1177/1745691620959834

Dean, S. V., Lassi, Z. S., Imam, A. M., & Bhutta, Z. A. (2014). Preconception care: Nutritional risks and interventions. *Reproductive Health, 11*, 1–15. https://doi.org/10.1186/1742-4755-11-S3-S3

DeCasper, A. J., & Spence, M. J. (1986). Prenatal maternal speech influences newborns' perception of speech sounds. *Infant Behavior and Development, 9*(2), 133–150. https://doi.org/10.1016/0163–6383(86)90025–1

Décarie, T. G. (1969). A study of the mental and emotional development of the thalidomide child. In B. M. Foss (Ed.), *Determinants of infant behavior* (Vol. 4). Methuen.

de Haan, M. (2015). Neuroscientific methods with children. In W. F. Overton, P. C. Molenaar, & R. M. Lerner (Eds.), *Handbook of child psychology and developmental science: Theory and method* (Vol. 1, 7th ed., pp. 683–712). Wiley.

De Haan, M., Dummonthiel, I., & Johnson, M. H. (2023). *Developmental cognitive neuroscience – an introduction* (5th ed.). Wiley-Blackwell.

de Houwer, A. (2021). *Bilingual development in childhood*. Cambridge University Press.

Del Giudice, M., Manera, V., & Keysers, C. (2009). Programmed to learn? The ontogeny of mirror neurons. *Developmental Science, 12*, 350–363. https://doi.org/10.1111/j.1467–7687.2008.00783.x

DeLoache, J. S. (2004). Becoming symbol-minded. *Trends in Cognitive Sciences, 8*(2), 66–70. https://doi.org/10.1016/j.tics.2003.12.004

DeLoache, J. S. (2011). Early development of the understanding and use of symbolic artifacts. In U. Goswami (Ed.), *The Wiley-Blackwell handbook of childhood cognitive development* (pp. 312–336). Wiley-Blackwell.

DeLoache, J. S., Chiong, C. Sherman, K., Islam, N., Vanderborght, M., Troseht, G. L. Strouse, G. A., & O'Doherty, K. (2010). Do babies learn from baby media? *Psychological Science, 21*, 157–1574. https://doi.org/10.1177/0956797610384145

DeLoache, J. S., LoBue, V., Vanderborght, M., & Chiong, C. (2013). On the validity and robustness of the scale error phenomenon in early childhood. *Infant Behavior and Development, 36*(1), 63–70. https://doi.org/10.1016/j.infbeh.2012.10.007

De Marco, P. D., Merello, E., Cama, A., Kibar, Z., & Capra, V. (2011). Human neural tube defects: Genetic causes and prevention. *Biofactors, 37*, 261–268. https://doi.org/10.1002/biof.170

DeMasi, A., Horger, M. N., Allia, A. M., Scher, A., & Berger, S. E. (2021). Nap timing makes a difference: Sleeping sooner rather than later after learning improves infants' locomotor problem solving. *Infant Behavior and Development, 65*, 101652. https://doi.org/10.1016/j.infbeh.2021.101652

Dennis, W., & Dennis, M. G. (1940). The effect of cradling practices upon the onset of walking in Hopi children. *Journal of Genetic Psychology, 56*, 77–86. https://doi.org/10.1080/00221325.1991.9914713

Desmarais, E., Brown, K., Campbell, K., French, B. F., Putnam, S. P., Casalin, S., Linhares, M. B. M., Lecannelier, F., Wang, Z., Raikkonen, K., Heinonen, K., Tuovinen, S., Montirosso, R., Provenzi, L., Park, S.-Y., Han, S.-Y., Lee, E. G., Huitron, B., de Weerth, C., Beijers, R., & Gartstein, M. A. (2021). Links between television exposure and toddler dysregulation: Does culture matter? *Infant Behavior and Development, 63*, 101557. https://doi.org/10.1016/j.infbeh.2021.101557

Deuber, C., & Terhaar, M. (2011). Hyperoxia in very preterm infants: A systematic review of the literature. *Journal of Perinatal and Neonatal Nursing, 25*, 268–274. https://doi.org/10.1097/JPN.0b013e318226ee2c

Dias, C. C., Costa, R., Pinto, M. P., & Figueiredo, B. (2021). The infant behavior questionnaire – revised: Psychometric properties at 2 weeks, 3, 6, and 12 months of life. *Early Human Development, 153*, 105290. https://doi.org/10.1016/j.earlhumdev.2020.105290

DiCorcia, J. A., Snidman, N., Sravish, A. V., & Tronick, E. (2016). Evaluating the nature of the still-face effect in the double face-to-face still-face paradigm using different comparison groups. *Infancy, 21*(3), 332–352. https://doi.org/10.1111/infa.12123

DiPietro, J. A., Bornstein, M. H., Costigan, K. A., Pressman, E. K., Hahn, C.-S., Painter, K. M., Smith, B. A., & Yi, L. J. (2002). What does fetal movement predict about behavior during the first two years of life? *Developmental Psychobiology, 40*, 358–371. https://doi.org/10.1002/dev.10025

DiPietro, J. A., Hodgson, D. M., Costigan, K. A., & Johnson, T. R. B. (1996). Fetal antecedents of infant temperament. *Child Development, 67*, 2568–2583. https://doi.org/10.1111/j.1467-8624.1996.tb01875.x

DiPietro, J. A., Hopkins, J., Costigan, K. A., Voegtline, K. M., Brakke, K., & Sandman, C. A. (2015). Studies in fetal behavior: Revisited, renewed, and reimagined. *Monographs of the Society for Research in Child Development, 80*(3), 1–151. http://www.jstor.org/stable/43773573

DiPietro, J. A., Kivlighan, K. T., Costigan, K. A., Rubin, S. E., Shiffler, D. E., Henderson, J., & Pillion, J. P. (2010). Prenatal antecedents of newborn neurological maturation. *Child Development, 81*, 115–130. https://doi.org/10.1111/j.1467–8624.2009.01384.x

Ding, W.-P., Li, N., & Chen, M. (2020). Ultrasound screening of fetal anomalies at 11–13+6 weeks. *Maternal-Fetal Medicine, 2*(3), 175–180. https://doi.org/10.1097/FM9.0000000000000045

Dinkel, D., & Snyder, K. (2020). Exploring gender differences in infant motor development related to parent's promotion of play. *Infant Behavior and Development, 59*, 101440. https://doi.org/10.1016/j.infbeh.2020.101440

Doktorchik, C., Premji, S., Slater, D., Williamson, T., Tough, S., & Patten, S. (2018). Patterns of change in anxiety and depression during pregnancy predict preterm birth. *Journal of Affective Disorders, 227*, 71–78. https://doi.org/10.1016/j.jad.2017.10.001

Dondi, M., Messinger, D., Colle, M., Tabasso, A., Simion, F., Barba, B. D., & Fogel, A. (2007). A new perspective on neonatal smiling: Differences between the judgments of expert coders and naïve observers. *Infancy, 12*, 235–255. https://doi.org/10.1111/j.1532–7078.2007.tb00242.x

Dozier, M., Roben, C. K., Caron, E. B., Hoye, J., & Bernard, K. (2018). Attachment and biobehavioral catch-up: An evidence-based intervention for vulnerable infants and their families. *Psychotherapy Research, 28*(1), 18–29. https://doi.org/10.1080/10503307.2016.1229873

Drugli, M. B., Solheim, E., Lydersen, S., Moe, V., Smith, L., & Berg-Nielsen, T. S. (2018). Elevated cortisol levels in Norwegian toddlers in childcare. *Early Child Development and Care, 188*(12), 1684–1695. https://doi.org/10.1080/03004430.2016.1278368

Dubowitz, L., & Dubowitz, V. (1981). The neurological assessment of the preterm and full term newborn infant. *Clinics in Developmental Medicine, 79*. Spastics International Medical Publications.

Dukes, D., Samson, A. C., & Walle, E. A. (2022). *The Oxford handbook of emotional development*. Oxford University Press.

Dunbar, A. S., Leerkes, E. M., Coard, S. I., Supple, A. J., & Calkins, S. (2017). An integrative conceptual model of parental racial/ethnic and emotion socialization and links to children's social-emotional development among African American parents. *Child Development Perspectives, 11*(1), 16–22. https://doi.org/10.1111/cdep.12218

Dynia, J. M., Dore, R. A., Bates, R. A., & Justice, L. M. (2021). Media exposure and language for toddlers from low-income homes. *Infant Behavior and Development, 63*, 101542. https://doi.org/10.1016/j.infbeh.2021.101542

Dzwilewski, K. L., & Schantz, S. L. (2015). Prenatal chemical exposures and child language development. *Journal of Communication Disorders, 57*, 41–65. https://doi.org/10.1016/j.jcomdis.2015.07.002

East, P. L. (2010). Children's provision of family caregiving: Benefit or burden?. *Child Development Perspectives, 4*, 55–61. https://doi.org/10.1111/j.1750-8606.2009.00118.x

Easterbrooks, M. A., & Biringen, Z. (2000). Guest editors' introduction to the special issue: Mapping the terrain of emotional availability and attachment. *Attachment & Human Development, 2*(2), 123–129. https://doi.org/10.1080/14616730050085518

Easterbrooks, M. A., Katze, R. C., & Menon, M. (2019). Adolescent parenting. In M. H. Bornstein (Ed.), *Handbook of parenting, Vol. 3: Being and becoming a parent* (3rd ed., pp. 199–231). Routledge.

Eimas, P. D., Siqueland, E. R., Jusczyk, P., & Vigorito, J. (1971). Speech perception in infants. *Science, 171*, 303–306. https://doi.org/10.1126/science.171.3968.303

Else-Quest, N. M., Hyde, J. S., Goldsmith, H. H., & Van Hulle, C. A. (2006). Gender differences in temperament: A meta-analysis. *Psychological Bulletin, 132*, 33–72. https://doi.org/10.1037/0033–2909.132.1.33

Emde, R. N. (2000). Next steps in emotional availability research. *Attachment & Human Development, 2*, 242–248. http://doi.org/10.1080/14616730050085590

Erbeli, F., Rice, M., & Paracchini, S. (2022). Insights into dyslexia genetics research from the last two decades. *Brain Sciences, 12*(1), 27. https://doi.org/10.3390/brainsci12010027

Esposito, G., & Bornstein, M. H. (2019). Parenting and infant cry. *Parenting: Science and Practice, 19*(1–2), 1–4. https://www.tandfonline.com/toc/hpar20/19/1–2

Esposito, G., Nakazawa, J., Venuti, P., & Bornstein, M. H. (2013). Componential deconstruction of infant distress vocalizations via tree-based models: A study of cry in autism spectrum disorder and typical development. *Research in Developmental Disabilities, 34*, 2717–2724. https://doi.org/10.1016/j.ridd.2013.05.036

Evans, G. W., & Kim, P. (2013). Childhood poverty, chronic stress, self-regulation, and coping. *Child Development Perspectives*, *7*, 43–48.

Eyler, F. D., Behnke, M., Garvan, C. W., Woods, N. S., Wobie, K., & Conlon, M. (2001). Newborn evaluations of toxicity and withdrawal related to prenatal cocaine exposure. *Neurotoxicology and Teratology*, *23*, 399–411. https://doi.org/10.1016/S0892–0362(01)00166–0

Fagot, B. I., Rogers, C. S., & Leinbach, M. D. (2000). Theories of gender and socialization. In T. Eckes & H. M. Trautner (Eds.), *The developmental social psychology of gender* (pp. 65–89). Erlbaum.

Fanning, K. (2021). What about the babies? A critical review of infants' and toddlers' absence in homelessness scholarship. *Infant Behavior and Development*, *64*, 101625. https://doi.org/10.1016/j.infbeh.2021.101625

Fantz, R. L., Ordy, J. M., & Udelf, M. S. (1962). Maturation of pattern vision in infants during the first six months. *Journal of Comparative and Physiological Psychology*, *55*, 907–917. https://doi.org/10.1037/h0044173

Farr, A. C., Kleinschmidt, T., Yarlagadda, P., & Mengersen, K. (2012). Wayfinding: A simple concept, a complex process. *Transport Reviews*, *32*(6), 715–743. https://doi.org/10.1080/01441647.2012.712555

Farroni, T., Csibra, G., Simion, F., & Johnson, M. H. (2002). Eye contact detection in humans from birth. *Proceedings of the National Academy of Sciences*, *99*, 9602–9605. https://doi.org/10.1073/pnas.152159999

Fein, G. G. (1991). The self-building potential of pretend play, or 'I got a fish, all by myself'. In M. Woodhead, R. Carr, & P. Light (Eds.), *Becoming a person* (pp. 328–346). Routledge.

Feinberg, M. E., McHale, S. M., & Whiteman, S. D. (2019). Parenting siblings. In M. H. Bornstein (Ed.), *Handbook of parenting, Vol. 1: Children and parenting* (3rd ed., pp. 219–258). Routledge.

Feldman, R. (2019). The social neuroendocrinology of human parenting. In M. H. Bornstein (Ed.), *Handbook of parenting, Vol. 2: Biology and ecology of parenting* (3rd ed., pp. 220–249). Routledge.

Feldman, R., & Greenbaum, C. W. (1997). Affect regulation and synchrony in mother-infant play as precursors to the development of symbolic competence. *Infant Mental Health Journal*, *18*, 4–23. https://doi.org/10.1002/(SICI)1097–0355(199721)18:1<4::AID-IMHJ2>3.0.CO;2-R

Ferguson, K. T., & Casasola, M. (2015). Are you an animal too? US and Malawian infants' categorization of plastic and wooden animal replicas. *Infancy*, *20*, 189–207. https://doi.org/10.1111/infa.12069

Fernald, A., Marchman, V. A., & Weisleder, A. (2013). SES differences in language processing skill and vocabulary are evident at 18 months. *Developmental Science*, *16*, 234–248. https://doi.org/10.1111/desc.12019

Fernandez-Baizan, C., Arias, J. L., & Mendez, M. (2021). Spatial orientation assessment in preschool children: Egocentric and allocentric frameworks. *Applied Neuropsychology: Child*, *10*(2), 171–193. https://doi.org/10.1080/21622965.2019.1630278

Field, T., Field, T., Cullen, C., Largie, S., Diego, M., Schanberg, S., & Kuhn, C. (2008). Lavender bath oil reduces stress and crying and enhances sleep in very young infants. *Early Human Development*, *84*(6), 399–401. https://doi.org/10.1016/j.earlhumdev.2007.10.008

Fifer, W. P., Byrd, D. L., Kaku, M., Eigsti, I. M., Isler, J. R., Grose-Fifer, J., Tarullo, A. R., & Balsam, P. D. (2010). Newborn infants learn during sleep. *Proceedings of the National Academy of Sciences*, *107*(22), 10320–10323. https://doi.org/10.1073/pnas.1005061107

Flavell, J. H. (2020). *The developmental psychology of Jean Piaget*. Barakaldo Books.

Foley, S., Hughes, C., & Fink, E. (2022). Expectant mothers' not fathers' mind-mindedness predicts infant, mother, and father conversational turns at 7 months. *Infancy*, *27*(6), 1091–1103. https://doi.org/10.1111/infa.12498

Franklin, A., & Davies, I. R. L. (2004). New evidence for infant colour categories. *British Journal of Developmental Psychology*, *22*, 349–377. https://doi.org/10.1348/0261510041552738

French, T., & French, K. (2016). *Juniper: The girl who was born too soon*. Little, Brown Spark.

Friend, M., Smolak, E., Liu, Y., Poulin-Dubois, D., & Zesiger, P. (2018). A cross-language study of decontextualized vocabulary comprehension in toddlerhood and kindergarten readiness. *Developmental Psychology, 54*, 1317. https://doi.org/10.1037/dev0000514

Gagne, J. R., & Goldsmith, H. H. (2011). A longitudinal analysis of anger and inhibitory control in twins from 12 to 36 months of age. *Developmental Science, 14*, 112–124. https://doi.org/10.1111/j.1467-7687.2010.00969.x

Gallese, V., & Rochat, M. (2013). The evolution of motor cognition: Its role in the development of social cognition and implications for autistic spectrum disorder. In M. Legerstee, D. W. Haley, & M. H. Bornstein (Eds.), *The infant mind: Origins of the social brain* (pp. 19–47). Guilford Press.

Galluccio, L., & Rovee-Collier, C. (2006). Nonuniform effects of reinstatement within the time window. *Learning and Motivation, 37*, 1–17. https://doi.org/10.1016/j.lmot.2005.01.002

Gandhi, T. K., Singh, A. K., Swami, P., Ganesh, S., & Sinha, P. (2017). Emergence of categorical face perception after extended early-onset blindness. *Proceedings of the National Academy of Sciences, 114*(23), 6139–6143. https://doi.org/10.1073/pnas.1616050114

Ganong, L., Coleman, M., & Russell, L. (2015). Children in diverse families. In M. H. Bornstein & T. Leventhal (Eds.), *Handbook of child psychology and developmental science: Ecological settings and processes in developmental systems* (7th ed., Vol. 4, pp. 133–174). Wiley.

Gao, M., Speck, B., Ostlund, B., Neff, D., Shakiba, N., Vlisides-Henry, R. D., Kaliush, P. R., Molina, N. C., Thomas, L., Raby, K. L., Crowell, S. E., & Conradt, E. (2022). Developmental foundations of physiological dynamics among mother–infant dyads: The role of newborn neurobehavior. *Child Development*. https://doi.org/10.1111/cdev.13769

Gao, W., Zhu, H., Giovanello, K. S., Smith, J. K., Shen, D., Gilmore, J. H., & Lin, W. (2009). Evidence on the emergence of the brain's default network from 2-week-old to 2-year-old healthy pediatric subjects. *Proceedings of the National Academy of Sciences USA, 106*, 6790–6795. https://doi.org/10.1073/pnas.0811221106

Gartstein, M. A., & Putnam, S. P. (2019). *Toddlers, parents, and culture: Findings from the joint effort toddler temperament consortium*. Routledge.

Gartstein, M. A., Putnick, D. L., Kwak, K., Hahn, C.-S., & Bornstein, M. H. (2015). Stability of temperament in South Korean infants from 6 to 12 to 18 months: Moderation by age, gender, and birth order. *Infant Behavior and Development, 40*, 103–107. https://doi.org/10.1016/j.infbeh.2015.05.002

Gartstein, M. A., & Rothbart, M. K. (2003). Studying infant temperament via the revised infant behavior questionnaire. *Infant Behavior and Development, 26*(1), 64–86. https://doi.org/10.1016/S0163-6383(02)00169-8

Gattis, M. (2019). Parenting children born preterm. In M. H. Bornstein (Ed.), *Handbook of parenting, Vol. 1: Children and parenting* (3rd ed., pp. 424–466). Routledge.

Gauvain, M. (2022). *Cognitive development in infancy and childhood. Cambridge elements in child development series* (M. H. Bornstein, Series Ed.). Cambridge University Press. https://doi.org/10.1017/9781108955676

Geangu, E., Benga, O., Stahl, D., & Striano, T. (2010). Contagious crying beyond the first days of life. *Infant Behavior and Development, 33*, 279–288. https://doi.org/10.1016/j.infbeh.2010.03.004

Geangu, E., Benga, O., Stahl, D., & Striano, T. (2011). Individual differences in infants' emotional resonance to a peer in distress: Self-other awareness and emotion regulation. *Social Development, 20*, 450–470. https://doi.org/10.1111/j.1467-9507.2010.00596.x

George, C., Kaplan, N., & Main, M. (1984). *An adult attachment interview* [Unpublished manuscript]. University of California at Berkeley, Department of Psychology.

Gesell, A. L. (1945). *The embryology of behavior*. Harper and Row.

Gesell, A. L. (1954). The ontogenesis of infant behavior. In L. Carmichael (Ed.), *Manual of child psychology* (2nd ed.). Wiley.

Gettler, L. T., McDade, T. W., & Kuzawa, C. W. (2011). Cortisol and testosterone in Filipino young adult men: Evidence for co-regulation of both hormones by fatherhood and relationship status. *American Journal of Human Biology, 23*(5), 609–620. https://doi.org/10.1002/ajhb.21187

Gibson, E. J., & Walk, R. D. (1960). The "visual cliff". *Scientific American, 202*, 64–71. https://www.jstor.org/stable/24940447

Gibson, J. J. (1979). *The ecological approach to visual perception*. Houghton Mifflin.

Goldin-Meadow, S. (2006). Nonverbal communication: The hand's role in talking and thinking. In W. Damon, D. Kuhn, & R. Siegler (Eds.), *The handbook of child psychology: Cognition, perception, and language* (6th ed., pp. 336–369). Wiley.

Goldschmidt, L., Richardson, G. A., Willford, J., & Day, N. L. (2008). Prenatal marijuana exposure and intelligence test performance at age 6. *Journal of American Academy of Child and Adolescent Psychiatry, 47*, 254–263. https://doi.org/10.1097/CHI.0b013e318160b3f0

Goldstein, M. H., & Schwade, J. A. (2008). Social feedback to infants' babbling facilitates rapid phonological learning. *Psychological Science, 19*, 515–523. https://doi.org/10.1111/j.1467-9280.2008.02117.x

Golombok, S. (2020). *Parenting: What really counts*. Psychology Press.

Gosdin, L. K. (2022). Alcohol consumption and binge drinking during pregnancy among adults aged 18–49 years – United States, 2018–2020. *MMWR. Morbidity and Mortality Weekly Report, 71*. https://doi.org/10.15585/mmwr.mm7101a2

Gottlieb, G., Wahlsten, D., & Lickliter, R. (2006). The significance of biology for human development: A developmental psychobiological systems view. In G. Gottlieb, D. Wahlsten, & R. Lickliter (Eds.), *Handbook of child psychology: Theoretical models of human development* (6th ed., Vol. 1, pp. 210–257). John Wiley & Sons.

Goubet, N., Rattaz, C., Pierrat, V., Allemann, E., Bullinger, A., & Lequien, P. (2002). Olfactory familiarization and discrimination in preterm and full-term newborns. *Infancy, 3*, 53–76. https://doi.org/10.1207/S15327078IN0301_3

Goubet, N., Strasbaugh, K., & Chesney, J. (2007). Familiarity breeds content? Soothing effect of a familiar odor on full-term newborns. *Journal of Developmental and Behavioral Pediatrics, 28*, 189–194. https://doi.org/10.1097/dbp.0b013e31802d0b8d

Gouin, K., Murphy, K., & Shah, P. S. (2011). Effects of cocaine use during pregnancy on low birthweight and preterm birth: Systematic review and meta analysis. *American Journal of Obstetrics and Gynecology, 204*, 340. https://doi.org/10.1016/j.ajog.2010.11.013

Granat, A., Gadassi, R., Gilboa-Schechtman, E., & Feldman, R. (2017). Maternal depression and anxiety, social synchrony, and infant regulation of negative and positive emotions. *Emotion, 17*(1), 11–27. https://doi.org/10.1037/emo0000204

Granqvist, P., Sroufe, L. A., Dozier, M., Hesse, E., Steele, M., van IJzendoorn, M., Solomon, J., Schuengel, C., Fearon, P., Bakermans-Kranenberg, M., Steele, H., Cassidy, J., Carlson, E., Madigan, S., Jacobvitz, D., Foster, S., Behrens, K., Rifkin-Graboi, A., Gribneau, N., Spangler, G., . . . Duschinsky, R. (2017). Disorganized attachment in infancy: A review of the phenomenon and its implications for clinicians and policy-makers. *Attachment & Human Development, 19*, 534–558. https://doi.org/10.1080/14616734.2017.1354040

Graziano, P., & Derefinko, K. (2013). Cardiac vagal control and children's adaptive functioning: A meta-analysis. *Biological Psychology, 94*, 22–37. https://doi.org/10.1016/j.biopsycho.2013.04.011

Greenough, W. T., Black, J. E., & Wallace, C. S. (2002). Experience and brain development. In W. T. Greenough, J. E. Black, & C. S. Wallace (Eds.), *Brain development and cognition* (pp. 186–216). Blackwell Publishing.

Grewen, K. M., Girdler, S. S., Amico, J., & Light, K. C. (2005). Effects of partner support on resting oxytocin, cortisol, norepinephrine, and blood pressure before and after warm partner contact. *Psychosomatic Medicine, 67*, 531–538. https://doi.org/10.1097/01.psy.0000170341.88395.47

Grisham, L. M., Rankin, L., Maurer, J. A., Gephart, S. M., & Bell, A. F. (2023). Scoping review of biological and behavioral effects of babywearing on mothers and infants. *Journal of Obstetric, Gynecologic, and Neonatal Nursing, 52,* 191–201. https://doi.org/10.1016/j.jogn.2022.12.008

Groh, A. M., Fearon, R. P., van IJzendoorn, M. H., Bakermans-Kranenburg, M. J., & Roisman, G. I. (2017). Attachment in the early life course: Meta-analytic evidence for its role in socioemotional development. *Child Development Perspectives, 11,* 70–76. https://doi.org/10.1111/cdep.12213

Groh, A. M., Roisman, G. I., van IJzendoorn, Bakermans-Kranenburg, M. J., & Fearon, R. P. (2012). The significance of insecure and disorganized attachment for children's internalizing symptoms: A meta-analytic study. *Child Development, 83,* 591–610. https://doi.org/10.1111/j.1467–8624.2011.01711.x

Gronqvist, H., Brodd, K. S., & von Hofsten, C. (2011). Reaching strategies of very preterm infants at 8 months corrected age. *Experimental Brain Research, 209,* 225–233. https://doi.org/10.1007/s00221-011-2538-x

Groome, L. J., Swiber, M. J., Holland, S. B., Bentz, L. S., Atterbury, J. L., & Trimm III, F. R. (1999). Spontaneous motor activity in the perinatal infant before and after birth: Stability in individual differences. *Developmental Psychobiology, 35,* 15–24. https://doi.org/10.1002/(SICI)1098–2302(199907)35:1<15::AID-DEV3>3.0.CO;2-U

Grzyb, B. J., Cangelosi, A., Cattani, A., & Floccia, C. (2019). Children's scale errors: A by-product of lexical development? *Developmental Science, 22,* e12741. https://doi.org/10.1111/desc.12741

Guedes, M., & Canavarro, M. C. (2015). Personal competencies, social resources, and psychosocial adjustment of primiparous women of advanced maternal age and their partners. *Infant Mental Health Journal, 36,* 506–521. https://doi.org/10.1002/imhj.21528

Gunn, J. K. L., Rosales, C. B., Center, K. E., Nuñez, A., Gibson, S. J., Christ, C., & Ehiri, J. E. (2016). Prenatal exposure to cannabis and maternal and child health outcomes: A systematic review and meta-analysis. *BMJ Open, 6.* https://doi.org/10.1136/bmjopen-2015–009986

Hackshaw, A., Rodeck, C., & Boniface, S. (2011). Maternal smoking in pregnancy and birth defects: A systematic review based on 173,687 malformed cases and 11.7 million controls. *Human Reproduction Update, 17,* 589–604. https://doi.org/10.1093/humupd/dmr022

Hagihara, H., Ishibashi, M., Moriguchi, Y., & Shinya, Y. (2024). Large-scale data decipher children's scale errors: A meta-analytic approach using the zero-inflated Poisson models. *Developmental Science, 27*(4), e13499. https://doi.org/10.1111/desc.13499

Hamer, J., Tamblyn, J., Castleman, J., & Morris, R. K. (2025). *Multiple pregnancy*. Cambridge University Press.

Hane, A., & Fox, N. A. (2006). Ordinary variations in maternal caregiving influence human infants' stress reactivity. *Psychological Science, 17,* 550–556. https://doi.org/10.1111/j.1467–9280.2006.01742.x

Harlow, H. F. (1960). Primary affectional patterns in primates. *American Journal of Orthopsychiatry, 30,* 676–684. https://doi.org/10.1111/j.1939–0025.1960.tb02085.x

Harlow, H. F., & Zimmermann, R. R. (1959). Affectional responses in the infant monkey. *Science, 130,* 421–432.

Harris, P. L. (2022). *Children's Imagination.* In M. H. Bornstein (Series Editor), *Cambridge Elements in Child Development.* Cambridge University Press. doi:10.1017/9781009128216

Hasselmann, M. H., Werneck, G. L., & Silva, C. V. (2008). Symptoms of postpartum depression and early interruption of exclusive breastfeeding in the first two months of life. *Cad Saude Publica, 24,* S341–S352. https://doi.org/10.1590/S0102–311X2008001400019

Hebb, D. O. (1949). *The organization of behavior: A neuropsychology theory.* Wiley.

Heckman, J. J. (2006). Skill formation and the economics of investing in disadvantaged children. *Science, 312,* 1900–1902. https://doi.org/10.1126/science.1128898

Heckman, J. J. (2007). The economics, technology, and neuroscience of human capability formation. *Proceedings of the National Academy of Sciences, 104*, 13250–13255. https://doi.org/10.1073/pnas.0701362104

Heckman, J. J. (2011). The American family in black and white: A post-racial strategy for improving skills to promote equality. *IZA Discussion Paper*, #5495.

Hedenbro, M., & Rydelius, P. (2014). Early interaction between infants and their parents predicts social competence at the age of four. *Acta Paediatrica, 103*, 268–274. https://doi.org/10.1111/apa.12512

Heller, N. A. (2021). Infant media use: A harm reduction approach. *Infant Behavior and Development, 64*, 101610. https://doi.org/10.1016/j.infbeh.2021.101610

Hensch, T. K., & Bilimoria, P. M. (2012). Re-opening windows: Manipulating critical periods for brain development. In *Cerebrum: The Dana forum on brain science*. Dana Foundation.

Herbert, J., Gross, J., & Hayne, J. (2007). Crawling is associated with more flexible memory retrieval by 9-month-old infants. *Developmental Science, 10*, 183–189. https://doi.org/10.1111/j.1467-7687.2007.00548.x

Hernández-Martínez, C., Canals Sans, J., & Fernández-Ballart, J. (2011). Parents' perceptions of their neonates and their relation to infant development. *Child: Care, Health and Development, 37*(4), 484–492.

Hertenstein, M. J., & Campos, J. J. (2004). The retention effects of an adults' emotional displays on infant behavior. *Child Development, 75*, 595–613. https://doi.org/10.1111/j.1467-8624.2004.00695.x

Hess, C. R., Teti, D. M., & Hussey-Gardner, B. (2004). Self-efficacy and parenting of high-risk infants: The moderating role of parent knowledge of infant development. *Applied Developmental Psychology, 25*, 423–437. https://doi.org/10.1016/j.appdev.2004.06.002

Hezelgrave, N. L., & Shennan, A. (2025). *Spontaneous preterm labour and birth (Including preterm pre-labour rupture of membranes)*. Cambridge University Press.

Hill, M. M., Gangi, D., Miller, M., Rafi, S. M., & Ozonoff, S. (2020). Screen time in 36-month-olds at increased likelihood for ASD and ADHD. *Infant Behavior and Development, 61*, 101484. https://doi.org/10.1016/j.infbeh.2020.101484

Hinde, R. A., & Stevenson-Hinde, J. (1973). *Constraints on learning: Limitations and predispositions*. Academic Press.

Hoff, E. (2015). Language development. In M. H. Bornstein & M. E. Lamb (Eds.), *Developmental science: An advanced textbook* (7th ed., pp. 443–490). Psychology Press.

Hoff, E., Core, C., Place, S., Rumiche, R., Señor, M., & Parra, M. (2012). Dual language exposure and early bilingual development. *Journal of Child Language, 39*(1), 1–27. https://doi.org/10.1017/S0305000910000759

Hoff, E., & Laursen, B. (2019). Socioeconomic status and parenting. In M. H. Bornstein (Ed.), *Handbook of parenting, Vol. 2: Biology and ecology of parenting* (3rd ed., pp. 421–447). Routledge.

Hofstede, G. (2011). Dimensionalizing cultures: The Hofstede model in context. *Online Readings in Psychology and Culture, 2*, 8. https://doi.org/10.9707/2307-0919.1014

Holden, G. W., & Smith, M. M. (2019). Parenting cognitions. In M. H. Bornstein (Ed.), *Handbook of parenting, Vol. 3: Being and becoming a parent* (3rd ed., pp. 681–721). Routledge.

Holt, C., Gentilleau, C., Gemmill, A. W., & Milgrom, J. (2021). Improving the mother-infant relationship following postnatal depression: A randomised controlled trial of a brief intervention (HUGS). *Archives of Women's Mental Health, 24*(6), 913–923. https://doi.org/10.1007/s00737-021-01116-5

Hornik, R., Risenhoover, N., & Gunnar, M. (1987). The effects of maternal positive, neutral and negative affective communications on infant responses to new toys. *Child Development, 58*, 937–944. https://doi.org/10.2307/1130534

Howe, M. L. (2015). Memory development. In L. S. Liben, U. Müller, & R. M. Lerner (Eds.), *Handbook of child psychology and developmental science: Cognitive processes* (Vol. 2, 7th ed., pp. 203–249). Wiley.

Hsu, V. C. (2010). Time windows in retention over the first year-and-a-half of life: Spacing effects. *Developmental Psychobiology*, *52*, 764–774. https://doi.org/10.1002/dev.20472

Hughes, C., Foley, S., Browne, W., McHarg, G., & Devine, R. T. (2023). Developmental links between executive function and emotion regulation in early toddlerhood. *Infant Behavior and Development*, *71*, 101782. https://doi.org/10.1016/j.infbeh.2022.101782

Hunley, S. B., & Hahn, E. R. (2016). Labels affect preschoolers' tool-based scale errors. *Journal of Experimental Child Psychology*, *151*, 40–50. https://doi.org/10.1016/j.jecp.2016.01.007

Hyde, J. S. (2014). Gender similarities and differences. *Annual Review of Psychology*, *65*, 373–398. https://doi.org/10.1146/annurev-psych-010213–115057

Illamola, S. M., Amaeze, O. U., Krepkova, L. V., Birnbaum, A. K., Karanam, A., Job, K. M., Bortnikova, V. V., Sherwin, C. M. T., & Enioutina, E. Y. (2020). Use of herbal medicine by pregnant women: What physicians need to know. *Frontiers in Pharmacology*, *10*, 1483. https://doi.org/10.3389/fphar.2019.01483

Ishii, N., Kono, Y., Yonemoto, N., Kusuda, S., Fujimura, M., & Neonatal Research Network, Japan. (2013). Outcomes of infants born at 22 and 23 weeks' gestation. *Pediatrics*, *132*, 62–71. https://doi.org/10.1542/peds.2012–2857

Izard, C. E. (2007). Basic emotions, natural kinds, emotion schemas, and a new paradigm. *Perspectives on Psychological Science*, *2*, 260–280. https://doi.org/10.1111/j.1745–6916.2007.00044.x

Jackson, I. R., & Sirois, S. (2022). But that's possible! Infants, pupils, and impossible events. *Infant Behavior and Development*, *67*, 101710. https://doi.org/10.1016/j.infbeh.2022.101710

Jacobson, J. L., & Jacobson, S. W. (1994). The effects of perinatal exposure to polychlorinated biphenyls and related contaminants. In H. L. Needleman & D. Bellinger (Eds.), *Prenatal exposure to toxicants: Developmental consequences* (pp. 130–147). Johns Hopkins University Press.

Jacobson, S. W., Jacobson, J. L., Stanton, M. E., Meintjes, E. M., & Molteno, C. D. (2011). Biobehavioral markers of adverse effect in fetal alcohol spectrum disorders. *Neuropsychological Review*, *21*, 148–166. https://doi.org/10.1007/s11065-011-9169-7

Jadva, V., Hines, M., & Golombok, S. (2010). Infants' preferences for toys, colors, and shapes: Sex differences and similarities. *Archives of Sexual Behavior*, *39*, 1261–1273. https://doi.org/10.1007/s10508-010-9618-z

Jakobson, R. (1968). *Child language, aphasia, and phonological universals*. Mouton.

Janssen, A. E. J., Koeck, R. M., Essers, R., Cao, P., van Dijk, W., Drüsedau, M., Meekels, J., Yaldiz, B., van de Vorst, M., de Koning, B., Hellebrekers, D. M. E. I., Stevens, S. J. C., Ming Sun, S., Heijligers, M., de Munnik, S. A., van Uum, C. M. J., Achten, J., Hamers, L., Naghdi, M., Vissers, L. E. L. M., . . . Zamani Esteki, M. (2024). Clinical-grade whole genome sequencing-based haplarithmisis enables all forms of preimplantation genetic testing. *Nature Communications*, *15*(1), 7164. https://doi.org/10.1038/s41467-024-51508-1

Jiang, M. J., & Rosengren, K. S. (2018). Action errors: A window into the early development of perception-action system. *Advances in Child Development*, *55*, 145–171. https://doi.org/10.1016/bs.acdb.2018.04.002

Johansson, M., Fenwick, J., & Premberg, Å. (2015). A meta-synthesis of fathers' experiences of their partner's labour and the birth of their baby. *Midwifery*, *31*, 9–18. https://doi.org/10.1016/j.midw.2014.05.005

Johnson, M. H., Dziurawiec, S., Ellis, H., & Morton, J. (1991). Newborns' preferential tracking of face-like stimuli and its subsequent decline. *Cognition*, *40*, 1–19. https://doi.org/10.1016/0010-0277(91)90045-6

Johnson, M. H. (2011). *Developmental cognitive neuroscience* (3rd ed.). Wiley-Blackwell.

Johnson, M. H. (2025). Developmental neuroscience, psychophysiology, and genetics. In M. H. Bornstein & M. E. Lamb (Eds.), *Developmental science: An advanced textbook* (8th ed., pp. 193–233). Psychology Press.

Johnson, S. C., Dweck, C. S., Chen, F. S., Stern, H. L., Ok, S., & Barth, M. (2010). At the intersection of social and cognitive development: Internal working models of attachment in infancy. *Cognitive Science, 34*, 807–825. https://doi.org/10.1111/j.1551–6709.2010.01112.x

Johnson, S. K., Klimstra, T. A., & Lerner, R. M. (2025). Concepts and theories of human development. In M. H. Bornstein & M. E. Lamb (Eds.), *Developmental science: An advanced textbook* (pp. 3–34). Routledge.

Johnson, S. P., & Hannon, E. E. (2015). Perceptual development. In L. S. Liben, U. Müller, & R. M. Lerner (Eds.), *Handbook of child psychology and developmental science: Cognitive processes* (7th ed., vol. 2, pp. 63–112). Wiley.

Jones, E. J., Pascalis, O., Eacott, M. J., & Herbert, J. S. (2011). Visual recognition memory across contexts. *Developmental Science, 14*, 136–147. https://doi.org/10.1111/j.1467–7687.2010.00964.x

Jung, M., & Fouts, H. N. (2011). Multiple caregivers' touch interactions with young children among the Bofi foragers in Central Africa. *International Journal of Psychology, 46*, 24–32. https://doi.org/10.1080/00207594.2010.507766

Kagan, J. (2007). *What is emotion? History, measures, and meanings*. Yale University Press.

Kagan, J. (2010). Temperaments as sets of preparedness. In B. M. Lester & J. D. Sparrow (Eds.), *Nurturing children and families: Building on the legacy of T. Berry Brazelton* (pp. 164–173). Wiley-Blackwell.

Kagan, J., & Snidman, N. (2009). *The long shadow of temperament*. Belknap.

Kahrs, B. A., & Lockman, J. J. (2014). Tool using. *Child Development Perspectives, 8*, 231–236.

Karasik, L. B., Adolph, K. E., Tamis-LeMonda, C. S., & Zuckerman, A. L. (2012). Carry on: Spontaneous object carrying in 13-month-old crawling and walking infants. *Developmental Psychology, 48*, 389–397. https://doi.org/10.1037/a0026040

Karasik, L. B., Kuchirko, Y. A., Dodojonova, R. M., & Elison, J. T. (2022). Comparison of US and Tajik infants' time in containment devices. *Infant and Child Development, 31*(4), e2340. https://doi.org/10.1002/icd.2340

Karasik, L. B., & Robinson, S. R. (2022). Milestones or millstones: How standard assessments mask cultural variation and misinform policies aimed at early childhood development. *Policy Insights from the Behavioral and Brain Sciences, 9*(1), 57–64. https://doi.org/10.1177/23727322211068546

Karasik, L. B., Tamis-LeMonda, C. S., Ossmy, O., & Adolph, K. E. (2018). The ties that bind: Cradling in Tajikistan. *Plos One, 13*(10), e0204428. https://doi.org/10.1371/journal.pone.0204428

Kavšek, M. J. (2002). The perception of static subjective contours in infancy. *Child Development, 73*(2), 331–344. https://www.jstor.org/stable/3696361

Kavšek, M., & Bornstein, M. H. (2010). Visual habituation and dishabituation in preterm infants: A review and meta-analysis. *Research in Developmental Disabilities, 31*(5), 951–975. https://doi.org/10.1016/j.ridd.2010.04.016

Kavšek, M., & Braun, S. (2018). Infants perceive three-dimensional subjective contours. *Perception, 47*(12), 1153–1165. https://doi.org/10.1177/0301006618811051

Keen, R. (2003). Representation of objects and events: Why do infants look so smart and toddlers look so dumb? *Current Directions in Psychological Science, 12*, 79–83. https://doi.org/10.1111/1467–8721.01234

Keen, R. (2011). The development of problem solving in young children: A critical cognitive skill. *Annual Review of Psychology, 62*, 1–21. https://doi.org/10.1146/annurev.psych.031809.130730

Keller, H., & Lamm, B. (2005). Parenting as the expression of sociohistorical time: The case of German individualisation. *International Journal of Behavioral Development, 29*, 238–246. https://doi.org/10.1080/01650250544000026

Kerig, P. K. (2019). Parenting and family systems. In M. H. Bornstein (Ed.), *Handbook of parenting, Vol. 3: Being and becoming a parent* (3rd ed., pp. 3–35). Routledge.

Kessen, W., Haith, M. M., & Salapatek, P. H. (1970). Human infancy: A bibliography and guide. In P. Mussen (Ed.), *Carmichael's manual of child psychology*. Wiley.

Khashan, A. S., Baker, P. N., & Kenny, L. C. (2010). Preterm birth and reduced birthweight in first and second teenage pregnancies: A register-based cohort study. *BMC Pregnancy Childbirth, 10*, 36. https://doi.org/10.1186/1471-2393-10-36

Kim, G., & Kwak, K. (2010). Uncertainty matters: Impact of stimulus ambiguity on infant social referencing. *Infant and Child Development, 20*, 449–462. https://doi.org/10.1002/icd.708

Klein, R. G. (2011). Temperament: Half a century in the journal. *Journal of the American Academy of Child & Adolescent Psychiatry, 50*, 1090–1092. https://doi.org/10.1016/j.jaac.2010.07.013

Klingberg, T. (2008). White matter maturation and cognitive development during childhood. In C. A. Nelson & M. Lucianna (Eds.), *Handbook of developmental cognitive neuroscience* (2nd ed., pp. 237–244). MIT Press.

Klingelhöfer, D., Braun, M., Quarcoo, D., Brüggmann, D., & Groneberg, D. A. (2021). Epidemiological influences and requirements of global childhood obesity research. *Obesity Facts, 14*(4), 382–396. https://doi.org/10.1159/000516777

Kobayashi, M., Otsuka, Y., Nakato, E., Kanazawa, S., Yamaguchi, M. K., & Kakigi, R. (2011). Do infants represent the face in a viewpoint-invariant manner? Neural adaptation study as measured by near-infrared spectroscopy. *Frontiers in Human Neuroscience, 5*, Article 153. https://doi.org/10.3389/fnhum.2011.00153

Koffka, K. (1935). *Principles of Gestalt psychology*. Harcourt, Brace.

Köhler, W. (1929). *Gestalt psychology*. Liveright.

Konishi, H., Karsten, A., & Vallotton, C. D. (2018). Toddlers' use of gesture and speech in service of emotion regulation during distressing routines. *Infant Mental Health Journal, 39*(6), 730–750. https://doi.org/10.1002/imhj.21740

Korzeniowski, C., Ison, M. S., & Difabio de Anglat, H. (2021). A summary of the developmental trajectory of executive functions from birth to adulthood. In P. A. Gargiulo & H. L. M. Arroyo (Eds.), *Psychiatry and neuroscience update: From epistemology to clinical psychiatry* (Vol. IV, pp. 459–473). Springer.

Kramer, L., & Hamilton, T. N. (2019). Sibling caregiving. In M. H. Bornstein (Ed.), *Handbook of parenting, Vol. 3: Being and becoming a parent* (3rd ed., pp. 372–408). Routledge.

Krasotkina, A., Götz, A., Höhle, B., & Schwarzer, G. (2021). Perceptual narrowing in face-and speech-perception domains in infancy: A longitudinal approach. *Infant Behavior and Development, 64*, 101607. https://doi.org/10.1016/j.infbeh.2021.101607

Kretch, K. S., & Adolph, K. E. (2013). Cliff or step? Posture-specific learning at the edge of a drop-off. *Child Development, 84*, 226–240. https://doi.org/10.1111/j.1467–8624.2012.01842.x

Kristen, S., Sodian, B., Thoermer, C., & Perst, H. (2011). Infants' joint attention skills predict toddlers' emerging mental state language. *Developmental Psychology, 47*, 1207–1219. https://doi.org/10.1037/a0024808

Ladd, G. W., & Kochenderfer-Ladd, B. (2019). Parents and children's peer relationships. In M. H. Bornstein (Ed.), *Handbook of parenting, Vol. 5: The practice of parenting* (3rd ed., pp. 278–316). Routledge.

LaGasse, L. L., Neal, A. R., & Lester, B. M. (2005). Assessment of infant cry: Acoustic cry analysis and parental perception. *Mental Retardation and Developmental Disabilities Research Reviews, 11*, 83–93. https://doi.org/10.1002/mrdd.20050

Lagattuta, K. H., & Thompson, R. A. (2007). The development of self-conscious emotions: Cognitive processes and social influences. In J. L. Tracy, R. W. Robins, & J. P. Tangney (Eds.), *The self-conscious emotions: Theory and research* (pp. 91–113). Guilford Press.

Lahat, A., Benson, B. E., Pine, D. S., Fox, N. A., & Ernst, M. (2018). Neural responses to reward in childhood: Relations to early behavioral inhibition and social anxiety. *Social Cognitive and Affective Neuroscience, 13*(3), 281–289. https://doi.org/10.1093/scan/nsw122

LaMaestra, S., Kisby, G. E., Micale, R. T., Johnson, J., Kow, Y. W., Bao, G., Sheppard, C., Stanfield, S., Tran, H., Woltjer, R. L., D'Agostini, F., Steele, V. E., & De Flora, S. (2011). Cigarette smoke induces DNA damage and alters base-excision repair and tau levels in the brain of neonatal mice. *Toxicological Sciences, 123*, 471–479. https://doi.org/10.1093/toxsci/kfr187

Lambert, B. L., & Bauer, C. R. (2012). Developmental and behavioral consequences of prenatal cocaine exposure: A review. *Journal of Perinatology, 32*(11), 819–828. https://doi.org/10.1038/jp.2012.90

Lamm, B., Gudi, H., Fassbender, I., Freitag, C., Graf, F., Goertz, C., Spangler, S., Teubert, M., Knopf, M., Lohaus, A., Schwarzer, G., & Keller, H. (2015). Rural NSO and German middle-class mothers' interaction with their 3-and 6-month-old infants: A longitudinal cross-cultural analysis. *Journal of Family Psychology, 29*(4), 649–655. https://doi.org/10.1037/fam0000100

Lau, E. X., Rapee, R. M., & Coplan, R. J. (2017). Combining child social skills training with a parent early intervention program for inhibited preschool children. *Journal of Anxiety Disorders, 51*, 32–38. https://doi.org/10.1016/j.janxdis.2017.08.007

Lavelli, M., & Fogel, A. (2013). Interdyad differences in early mother-infant face-to-face communication: Real-time dynamics and developmental pathways. *Developmental Psychology, 49*, 2257–2271. https://doi.org/10.1037/a0032268

Learmonth, A. E., Newcombe, N. S., & Huttenlocher, J. (2001). Toddlers' use of metric information and landmarks to reorient. *Journal of Experimental Child Psychology, 80*(3), 225–244. https://doi.org/10.1006/jecp.2001.2635

Lebel, C., Roussotte, F., & Sowell, E. R. (2011). Imaging the impact of prenatal alcohol exposure on the structure of the developing human brain. *Neuropsychological Review, 21*, 102–118. https://doi.org/10.1007/s11065-011-9163-0

Lee, C. C., Jhang, Y., Relyea, G., Chen, L. M., & Oller, D. K. (2018). Babbling development as seen in canonical babbling ratios: A naturalistic evaluation of all-day recordings. *Infant Behavior and Development, 50*, 140–153. https://doi.org/10.1016/j.infbeh.2017.12.002

Leerkes, E. M., & Qu, J. (2019). Families with infants and young children. In B. H. Fiese, M. Celano, K. Deater-Deckard, E. N. Jouriles, & M. A. Whisman (Eds.), *APA handbook of contemporary family psychology: Foundations, methods, and contemporary issues across the lifespan* (Vol. 1, pp. 575–591). American Psychological Association.

Lemerise, E. A., & Dodge, K. A. (2000). The development of anger and hostile interactions. In M. Lewis & J. M. Haviland-Jones (Eds.), *Handbook of emotions* (2nd ed., pp. 594–606). Guilford Press.

Lengua, L. J., Gartstein, M. A., Zhou, Q., Colder, C. R., & Jacques, D. T. (2024). Temperament and child development in context. In M. H. Bornstein (Series Ed.), *Cambridge elements in child development.* Cambridge University Press.

Leppanen, J. M. (2011). Neural and developmental bases of the ability to recognize social signals of emotion. *Emotion Review, 3*, 179–188. https://doi.org/10.1177/1754073910387942

Lerner, R. M. (2018). *Concepts and theories of human development* (4th ed.). Routledge.

Leve, L. D., Neiderhiser, J. M., Scaramella, L. V., & Reiss, D. (2010). The early growth and development study: Using the prospective adoption design to examine genotype–environment interplay. *Behavior Genetics, 40*(3), 306–314. https://doi.org/10.1007/s10519-010-9353-1

Lewis, M. (2014). *The rise of consciousness and the development of emotional life.* Guilford Press.

Lewis, M. (2015). Emotional development and consciousness. In W. F. Overton, P. C. M. Molenaar, & R. M. Lerner (Eds.), *Handbook of child psychology and developmental science: Theory and method* (Vol. 1, 7th ed., pp. 407–451). Wiley.

Lewis, M. (2022). The self-conscious emotions. In *The encyclopedia on early childhood development*. https://www.child-encyclopedia.com/emotions/according-experts/self-conscious-emotions

Lewis, M., Alessandri, S. M., & Sullivan, M. W. (1992). Differences in shame and pride as a function of children's gender and task difficulty. *Child Development, 63*(3), 630–638. https://doi.org/10.2307/1131351

Lewis, S. N., West, A. F., Stein, A., Malmberg, L., Bethell, K., Barnes, J., Sylva, K., Leach, P., & The Families, Children and Child Care (FCCC) Project Team. (2008). A comparison of father-infant interaction between primary and non-primary care giving fathers. *Child: Care, Health, and Development, 35*, 199–207. https://doi.org/10.1111/j.1365–2214.2008.00913.x

Libertus, K., & Needham, A. (2011). Reaching experience increases face preference in 3-month-old infants. *Developmental Science, 14*, 1355–1364. https://doi.org/10.1111/j.1467–7687.2011.01084.x

Liebschutz, J. M., Crooks, D., Rose-Jacobs, R., Cabral, H. J., Heeren, T. C., Gerteis, J., Appugliese, D. P., Heymann, O. D., Lange, A. V., & Frank, D. A. (2015). Prenatal substance exposure: What predicts behavioral resilience by early adolescence? *Psychology of Addictive Behaviors, 29*(2), 329. https://psycnet.apa.org/doi/10.1037/adb0000082

Lillard, A. S. (2015). The development of play. In L. S. Liben, U. Müller, & R. M. Lerner (Eds.), *Handbook of child psychology and developmental science: Cognitive processes* (Vol. 2, 7th ed., pp. 425–468). Wiley.

Lind, T., Raby, K. L., Caron, E. B., Roben, C. K., & Dozier, M. (2017). Enhancing executive functioning among toddlers in foster care with an attachment-based intervention. *Development and Psychopathology, 29*(2), 575–586. https://doi.org/10.1017/S0954579417000190

Liu, C., Li, J., Chen, C., Wu, H., Yuan, L., & Yu, G. (2021). Individual pride and collective pride: Differences between Chinese and American corpora. *Frontiers in Psychology, 12*, 513779. https://doi.org/10.3389/fpsyg.2021.513779

Lockman, J. J., & Kahrs, B. A. (2017). New insights into the development of human tool use. *Current Directions in Psychological Science, 26*(4), 330–334. https://doi.org/10.1177/0963721417692035

López, B. G. (2020). Incorporating language brokering experiences into bilingualism research: An examination of informal translation practices. *Language and Linguistics Compass, 14*(1), e12361. https://doi.org/10.1111/lnc3.12361

Lorenz, K. (1970). *Studies in animal and human behavior* (R. Martin, Trans.). Methuen. (Original work published 1935)

Love, J. M., Harrison, L., Sagi-Schwartz, A., van IJzendoorn, M. A., Ross, C., Ungerer, J., Raikes, H., Brady-Smith, C., Boller, K., Brookes-Gunn, J., Constantine, J., Kisker, E. E., Paulsell, D., & Chazan-Cohen, R. (2003). Child-care quality matters: How conclusions may vary with context. *Child Development, 74*, 1021–1033. https://doi.org/10.1111/1467–8624.00584

Lucassen, N., Tharner, A., van IJzendoorn, M. H., Bakermans-Kranenburg, M. J., Volling, B. L., Verhulst, F. C., Lambregtse-Van den Berg, M. P., & Tiemeier, H. (2011). The association between paternal sensitivity and infant-father attachment security: A meta-analysis of three decades of research. *Journal of Family Psychology, 25*, 986–992. https://doi.org/10.1037/a0025855

Luke, B., & Brown, M. B. (2007). Elevated risks of pregnancy complications and adverse outcomes with increasing maternal age. *Human Reproduction, 22*, 1264–1272. https://doi.org/10.1093/humrep/del522

Lynn, F. A., Alderdice, F. A., Crealey, G. E., & McElnay, J. C. (2011). Associations between maternal characteristics and pregnancy-related stress among low-risk mothers: An observational cross-sectional study. *International Journal of Nursing Studies, 48*, 620–627. https://doi.org/10.1016/j.ijnurstu.2010.10.002

MacMillan, C. (2023, March 16). Epidurals during childbirth: What every woman should know. *Yale Medicine*.

MacPhee, D., & Prendergast, S. (2019). Room for improvement: Girls' and boys' home environments are still gendered. *Sex Roles, 80*(5), 332–346.

MacWhinney, B. (2010). Language development. In W. F. Overton & R. M. Lerner (Eds.), *The handbook of life-span development, Vol 1: Cognition biology, and methods* (pp. 467–508). Wiley. https://doi.org/10.1002/9780470880166.hlsd001014

MacWhinney, B. (2015). Language development. In L. S. Liben, U. Muller, & R. M. Lerner (Eds.), *Handbook of child psychology and developmental science: Cognitive processes* (Vol. 2, 7th ed., pp. 296–338). Wiley.

MacWhinney, B. (2019). Neuroemergentism: Levels and constraints. *Journal of Neurolinguistics, 49*, 232–234. https://doi.org/10.1016/j.jneuroling. 2018.04.002

Main, M., & Cassidy, J. (1988). Categories of response to reunion with a parent at age six: Predictable from infant attachment classifications and stable over a one-month period. *Developmental Psychology, 24*, 415–426. https://doi.org/10.1037/0012–1649.24.3.415

Main, M., & Solomon, J. (1991). Procedure for identifying infants as disorganized/disoriented during the Ainsworth Strange Situation. In M. Greensberg, D. Ciccetti, & E. M. Cummings (Eds.), *Attachment during the preschool years: Theory, research, and intervention*. University of Chicago Press.

Majdandžlć, M. (2017). Commentary on fathers'play: Measurement, conceptualization, culture, and connections with child development. *Infant Mental Health Journal, 38*(6), 789–794. https://doi.org/10.1002/imhj.21677

Majorano, M., & D'Odorico, L. (2011). The transition into ambient language: A longitudinal study of babbling and first word production of Italian children. *First Language, 31*(1), 47–66. https://doi.org/10.1177/0142723709359239

Malatesta, C. Z., Grigoryev, P., Lamb, C., Albin, M., & Culver, C. (1986). Emotion, socialization and expressive development in preterm and full term infants. *Child Development, 57*, 316–330. https://doi.org/10.2307/1130587

Malatesta, C. Z., & Haviland, J. M. (1982). Learning display rules: The socialization of emotion expression in infancy. *Child Development, 53*, 991–1003. https://www.jstor.org/stable/1129139

Mandler, J. M., Fivush, R., & Reznick, J. S. (1987). The development of contextual categories. *Cognitive Development, 2*, 339–354. https://doi.org/10.1016/S0885–2014(87)80012–6

Mangalindan, D. M. J., & Schmuckler, M. A. (2017). To cue or not to cue: Toddlers' use of beacons and associative cues in object-displacement tasks. *Infancy, 22*(5), 713–731. https://doi.org/10.1111/infa.12178

Manian, N., & Bornstein, M. H. (2009). Dynamics of emotion in infants of clinically depressed and nondepressed mothers. *Journal of Child Psychology and Psychiatry, 50*, 1410–1418. https://doi.org/10.1111/j.1469–7610.2009.02166.x

Mantis, I., Mercuri, M., Stack, D. M., & Field, T. M. (2019). Depressed and non-depressed mothers' touching during social interactions with their infants. *Developmental Cognitive Neuroscience, 35*, 57–65. https://doi.org/10.1016/j.dcn.2018.01.005

March of Dimes. (2021). *Delivery method*. https://www.marchofdimes.org/peristats/data?lev=1&obj=1&reg=99&slev=1&stop=355&top=8

March of Dimes. (2025). *Vaginal birth after Cesarean deliveries: United States, 2018–2023*. National Center for Health Statistics, final natality data. Retrieved January 19, 2025, from www.marchofdimesorg/peristats

Marin, M. M., Rapisardi, G., & Tani, F. (2015). Two-day-old newborn infants recognise their mother by her axillary odour. *Acta Paediatrica, 104*(3), 237–240. https://doi.org/10.1111/apa.12905

Marinelli, K. A., Ball, H. L., McKenna, J. J., & Blair, P. S. (2019). An integrated analysis of maternal-infant sleep, breastfeeding, and sudden infant death syndrome research supporting a balanced discourse. *Journal of Human Lactation, 35*(3), 510–520. https://doi.org/10.1177/0890334419851797

Marshall, P. J., & Meltzoff, A. N. (2014). Neural mirroring mechanisms and imitation in human infants. *Philosophical Transactions of the Royal Society B: Biological Sciences, 369*(1644), 20130620. https://doi.org/10.1098/rstb.2013.0620

Mascolo, M., Fischer, K. W., & Li, J. (2003). Dynamic development of component systems of emotions: Pride, shame, and guilt in China and the United States. In R. J. Davidson, K. Scherer, & H. H. Goldsmith (Eds.), *Handbook of affective science* (pp. 375–408). Oxford University Press.

Mash, C., Arterberry, M. E., & Bornstein, M. H. (2007). Mechanisms of object recognition in 5-month-old infants. *Infancy, 12*, 31–43. https://doi.org/10.1111/j.1532-7078.2007.tb00232.x

Mash, C., & Bornstein, M. H. (2012). Five-month-olds' categorization of novel objects: Tasks and measure dependence. *Infancy, 17*, 179–197. https://doi.org/10.1111/j.1532-7078.2011.00076.x

Mash, C., Bornstein, M. H., & Arterberry, M. A. (2013). Brain dynamics in young infants' recognition of faces. *NeuroReport, 24*, 359–363. https://doi.org/10.1097/WNR.0b013e32835f6828

Maughan, B., Rowe, R., & Murray, J. (2018). Family poverty and structure. In J. E. Lochman & W. Matthys (Eds.), *The Wiley handbook of disruptive and impulse-control disorders* (pp. 257–274). Wiley Blackwell.

Maurer, D., Gibson, L. C., & Spector, F. (2013). Synesthesia in infants and very young children. In J. Simner & E. M. Hubbard (Eds.), *Oxford handbook of synesthesia* (pp. 46–63). Oxford University Press.

Mayo Clinic. (2022). *Postpartum depression*. https://www.mayoclinic.org/diseases-conditions/postpartum-depression/symptoms-causes/syc-20376617

McCall, R. B., & Groark, C. J. (2015). Research on institutionalized children: Implications for international child welfare practitioners and policymakers. *International Perspectives in Psychology, 4*(2), 142–159. https://doi.org/10.1037/ipp0000033

McHale, J. P., & Sirotkin, Y. S. (2019). Coparenting in diverse family systems. In M. H. Bornstein (Ed.), *Handbook of parenting, Vol. 3: Being and becoming a parent* (3rd ed., pp. 137–166). Routledge.

McKenna, J. J., & Gettler, L. T. (2016). There is no such thing as infant sleep, there is no such thing as breastfeeding, there is only breastsleeping. *Acta Paediatrica, 105*(1), 17–21. https://doi.org/10.1111/apa.13161

McLaughlin, K. A., Sheridan, M. A., Tibu, F., Fox, N. A., Zeanah, C. H., & Nelson III, C. A. (2015). Causal effects of the early caregiving environment on development of stress response systems in children. *Proceedings of the National Academy of Sciences, 112*(18), 5637–5642. https://doi.org/10.1073/pnas.1423363112

McRae, K., & Shiota, M. (2017). Biological and physiological aspects of emotion regulation. In C. A. Essau, S. LeBlanc, & T. H. Ollendick (Eds.), *Emotion regulation and psychopathology in children and adolescents* (pp. 43–59). Oxford University Press. https://doi.org/10.1093/med:psych/9780198765844.003.0003

Mead, M., & MacGregor, F. C. (1951). *Growth and culture*. Putnam.

Mehler, J., Nespor, M., & Pena, M. (2008). What infants know and what they have to learn about language. *European Review, 16*, 429–444. https://doi.org/10.1017/S1062798708000392

Meins, E., Fernyhough, C., Arnott, B., Turner, M., & Leekham, S. (2011). Mother- versus infant-centered correlates of maternal mind-mindedness in the first year of life. *Infancy, 16*, 137–165. https://doi.org/10.1111/j.1532-7078.2010.00039.x

Meins, E., Fernyhough, C., de Rosnay, M., Arnott, B., Leekham, S., & Turner, M. (2012). Mind-mindedness as a multidimensional construct: Appropriate and nonattuned mind-related comments independently predict infant-mother attachment in a socially diverse sample. *Infancy, 17*, 393–415. https://doi.org/10.1111/j.1532-7078.2011.00087.x

Meltzoff, A. N., & Marshall, P. J. (2018). Human infant imitation as a social survival circuit. *Current Opinion in Behavioral Sciences, 24*, 130–136. https://doi.org/10.1016/j.cobeha.2018.09.006

Meltzoff, A. N., & Moore, M. K. (1977). Imitation of facial and manual gestures by human neonates. *Science, 198*, 75–78. https://www.science.org/doi/10.1126/science.198.4312.75

Mennella, J. A., & Bobowski, N. K. (2015). The sweetness and bitterness of childhood: Insights from basic research on taste preferences. *Physiology & Behavior, 152*, 502–507. https://doi.org/10.1016/j.physbeh.2015.05.015

Mercuri, M., Stack, D. M., De France, K., & Jean, A. D. L. (2022). An intensive longitudinal investigation of maternal and infant touching patterns across context and throughout the first 9-months of life. *Infant Mental Health Journal, 44*, 495–512. https://doi.org/10.1002/imhj.22070

Mesman, J., Van IJzendoorn, H., & Sagi-Schwartz, A. (2016). Cross-cultural patterns of attachment. In A. Sagi-Schwartz (Ed.), *Handbook of attachment: Theory, research, and clinical applications* (pp. 852–877). Academia.

Mezzacappa, E., Buckner, J. C., & Earls, F. (2011). Prenatal cigarette exposure and infant learning stimulation as predictors of cognitive control in childhood. *Developmental Science, 14*, 881–891. https://doi.org/10.1111/j.1467–7687.2011.01038.x

Mills, K. L., Siegmund, K. D., Tamnes, C. K., Ferschmann, L., Wierenga, L. M., Bos, M. G., Luna, B., Li, C., & Herting, M. M. (2021). Inter-individual variability in structural brain development from late childhood to young adulthood. *NeuroImage, 242*, 118450.

Moller, A. P. (2003). The evolution of monogramy: Mating relationships, parental care, and sexual selection. In C. Boesch (Ed.), *Monogamy: Mating strategies and partnerships in birds, humans, and other mammals* (pp. 29–41). Cambridge University Press.

Mondloch, C. J., Segalowitz, S. J., Lewis, T. L., Dywan, J., Le Grand, R., & Maurer, D. (2013). The effect of early visual deprivation on the development of face detection. *Developmental Science, 16*(5), 728–742. https://doi.org/10.1111/desc.12065

Mondschein, E. R., Adolph, K. E., & Tamis-LeMonda, C. S. (2000). Gender bias in mothers' expectations about infant crawling. *Journal of Experimental Child Psychology, 77*, 304–316. https://doi.org/10.1006/jecp.2000.2597

Moore, D. G. (2012). Understanding of human motion, form and levels of meaning: Evidence from the perception of human point-light displays by infants and people with autism. In V. Slaughter & C. A. Brownell (Eds.), *Early development of body representations* (pp. 122–145). Cambridge University Press.

Mora, R., Crippa, B., Cervoni, E., Santomauro, V., & Guastini, L. (2012). Acoustic features of voice in patients with severe hearing loss. *Journal of Otolaryngology – Head and Neck Surgery, 4*, 8–13; 22498262. https://doi.org/10.2310/7070.2011.110150

Morales, S., & Fox, N. A. (2019). A neuroscience perspective on emotional development. In V. LoBue, K. Pérez-Edgar, & K. A. Buss (Eds.), *Handbook of emotional development* (pp. 57–81). Springer.

Morgan, R., & Rochat, P. (1997). Intermodal calibration of the body in early infancy. *Ecological Psychology, 9*, 1–23. https://doi.org/10.1207/s15326969eco0901_1

Mosca, F., Colnaghi, M., & Fumagalli, M. (2011). BPD: Old and new problems. *Journal of Maternal-Fetal & Neonatal Medicine, 24*, 80–82. https://doi.org/10.3109/14767058.2011.607675

Motlagh, M. G., Sukhodolsky, D. G., Landeros-Weisenberger, A., Katsovich, L., Thompson, N., Scahill, L., King, R. A., Peterson, B. S., Schultz, R. T., & Leckman, J. F. (2011). Adverse effects of heavy prenatal maternal smoking on attentional control in children with ADHD. *Journal of Attention Disorders, 15*, 593–603. https://doi.org/10.1177/1087054710374576

Mulligan, C. S., Adams, S., Tzioumi, D., & Brown, J. (2017). Injury from falls in infants under one year. *Journal of Paediatrics and Child Health*, *53*(8), 754–760. https://doi.org/10.1111/jpc.13568

Mumme, D. L., & Fernald, A. (2003). The infant as onlooker: Learning from emotional reactions observed in a televised scenario. *Child Development*, *74*, 221–237. https://doi.org/10.1111/1467-8624.00532

Muraskas, J., DeGregoris, L., Rusciolelli, C., & Sajous, C. (2012). Preterm birth of extremely low birth weight infants. In J. C. Morrison (Ed.), *Preterm birth-mother and child* (pp. 263–274). InTechOpen.

Mushi, S. (2002). Acquisition of multiple languages among children of immigrant families: Parents' role in the home-school language pendulum. *Early Child Development and Care*, *172*(5), 517–530. https://doi.org/10.1080/03004430214546

Myers, M. M., Burtchen, N., Retamar, M. O., Lucchini, M., & Fifer, W. P. (2018). Neonatal monitoring: Prediction of autonomic regulation at 1 month from newborn assessments. In J. R. Duncan & R. W. Byard (Eds.), *SIDS sudden infant and early childhood death: The past, the present, and the future* (pp. 431–448). University Adelaide Press.

Narea, M., Arriagada, V., & Allel, K. (2020). Center-based care in toddlerhood and child cognitive outcomes in Chile: The moderating role of family socio-economic status. *Early Education and Development*, *31*(2), 218–233. https://doi.org/10.1080/10409289.2019.1626191

Nath, S., Pearson, R. M., Moran, P., Pawlby, S., Molyneaux, E., Challacombe, F. L., & Howard, L. M. (2019). The association between prenatal maternal anxiety disorders and postpartum perceived and observed mother-infant relationship quality. *Journal of Anxiety Disorders*, *68*, 102148. https://doi.org/10.1016/j.janxdis.2019.102148

National Center for Education Statistics. (2021). *Early childhood program participation: 2019* (NCES 2020–075REV). https://nces.ed.gov/fastfacts/display.asp?id=4

Nawrot, E., & Nawrot, M. (2013). The role of eye movements in depth from motion parallax during infancy. *Journal of Vision*, *13*(14), 1–13. https://doi.org/10.1167/13.14.15

Needham, A. W. (2016). *Learning about objects in infancy*. Routledge.

Needleman, H. L., & Bellinger, D. (1991). The health effects of low level exposure to lead. *Annual Review of Public Health*, *12*(1), 111–140. https://doi.org/10.1146/annurev.pu.12.050191.000551

Newman, C. G. (1985). Teratogen update: Clinical aspects of thalidomide embryopathy: A continuing preoccupation. *Teratology*, *32*, 133–144. https://doi.org/10.1002/tera.1420320118

Newman, R. S., & Hussain, I. (2006). Changes in preference for infant-directed speech in low and moderate noise by 4.5- to 13-month-olds. *Infancy*, *10*(1), 61–76. https://doi.org/10.1207/s15327078in1001_4

Ng, M., Dai, X., Cogen, R. M., Abdelmasseh, M., Abdollahi, A., Abdullahi, A., Aboagye, R. G., Abukhadijah, H. J., Adeyeoluwa, T. E., Afolabi, A. A., Ahmad, D., Ahmad, N., Ahmed, A., Ahmed, S. A., Akkaif, M. A., Akrami, A. E., Al Hasan, S. M., Al Ta'ani, O., Alahdab, F., . . . Khan, M. S. (2024). National-level and state-level prevalence of overweight and obesity among children, adolescents, and adults in the USA, 1990–2021, and forecasts up to 2050. *The Lancet*, *404*, 2278–2298. https://doi.org/10.1016/S0140-6736(24)01548-4

Niedenthal, P. M., & Ric, F. (2017). *Psychology of emotion*. Psychology Press.

Noll, L. M., & Harding, C. G. (2003). The relationship of mother-child interaction and the child's development of symbolic play. *Infant Mental Health Journal*, *24*, 557–570. https://doi.org/10.1002/imhj.10071

Numan, M. (2006). Hypothalamic neural circuits regulating maternal responsiveness toward infants. *Behavioral and Cognitive Neuroscience Reviews*, *5*, 163–190. https://doi.org/10.1177/1534582306288790

Nunes, M. L., & Costa da Costa, J. (2010). Sleep and epilepsy in neonates. *Sleep Medicine*, *11*, 665–673. https://doi.org/10.1016/j.sleep.2009.10.009

Oakes, L., M., Madole, K. L., & Cohen, L. B. (1991). Infants' object examining: Habituation and categorization, *Cognitive Development*, *6*, 377–392. https://doi.org/10.1016/0885–2014(91)90045-F

Oates, J., Lewis, C., & Lamb, M. E. (2005). Parenting and attachment. In J. Oates, C. Lewis, & M. E. Lamb (Eds.), *Children's personal and social development* (pp. 12–51). Blackwell Publishing.

Oga, E. A., Mark, K., & Coleman-Cowger, V. H. (2018). Cigarette smoking status and substance use in pregnancy. *Maternal and Child Health Journal*, *22*(10), 1477–1483. https://doi.org/10.1007/s10995-018-2543-9

Ogren, M., Kaplan, B., Peng, Y., Johnson, K. L., & Johnson, S. P. (2019). Motion or emotion: Infants discriminate emotional biological motion based on low-level visual information. *Infant Behavior and Development*, *57*, 101324. https://doi.org/10.1016/j.infbeh.2019.04.006

Oller, J. (2000). Language and its normal processing. *Modern Language Journal*, *84*, 302–303.

Onishi, K. H., Baillargeon, R., & Leslie, A. M. (2007). 15-month-old infants detect violations in pretend scenarios. *Acta Psychologica*, *124*, 106–128. https://doi.org/10.1016/j.actpsy.2006.09.009

Oostenbroek, J., Suddendorf, T., Nielsen, M., Redshaw, J., Kennedy-Costantini, S., Davis, J., Clark, J., & Slaughter, V. (2016). Comprehensive longitudinal study challenges the existence of neonatal imitation in humans. *Current Biology*, *26*(10), 1334–1338. https://doi.org/10.1016/j.cub.2016.03.047

Ornoy, A., Daka, L., Goldzweig, G., Gil, Y., Mjen, L., Levit, S., Shufman, Emi., Bar-Hamburger, R., & Greenbaum, C. W. (2010). Neurodevelopmental and psychological assessment of adolescents born to drug-addicted parents: Effects of SES and adoption. *Child Abuse and Neglect*, *34*, 354–368. https://doi.org/10.1016/j.chiabu.2009.09.012

Oster, H. (2005). The repertoire of infant facial expressions: An ontogenetic perspective. In J. Nadel & D. Muir (Eds.), *Emotional development: Recent research advances* (pp. 261–292). Oxford University Press.

Out, D., Pieper, Bakermans-Kranenburg, M. J., Zeskind, P. S., & van IJzendoorn, M. H. (2010). Intended sensitive and harsh caregiving responses to infant crying: The role of cry pitch and perceived urgency in an adult twin sample. *Child Abuse and Neglect*, *34*, 863–873. https://doi.org/10.1016/j.chiabu.2010.05.003

Palazzi, A., Filippa, M., Meschini, R., & Piccinini, C. A. (2021). Music therapy enhances preterm infant's signs of engagement and sustains maternal singing in the NICU. *Infant Behavior and Development*, *64*, 101596. https://doi.org/10.1016/j.infbeh.2021.101596

Palomo-Gómez, R., Rúger-Navarrete, A., Antúnez-Calvente, I., Vázquez-Lara, J. M., Rodríguez-Díaz, L., Gómez-Salgado, J., Riesco-González, F. J., Vázquez-Lara, M. D., Muñoz-Vela, F. J., & Fernández-Carrasco, F. J. (2024). Prenatal stress as a risk factor for maternal-foetal morbidity: A longitudinal study. *Healthcare*, *12*, 312. https://doi.org/10.3390/healthcare12030312

Pampers. (2023, January 29). *Baby proofing your house: Checklist and tips*. https://www.pampers.com/en-us/baby/parenting-life/article/baby-proofing-your-home

Papoušek, H., & Bernstein, P. (1969). Basic cognitive functions in the pre-verbal period of infancy. *Acta Nervosa Superior*, *11*, 285–286.

Parithathvi, A., Choudhari, N., & Dsouza, H. S. (2024). Prenatal and early life lead exposure induced neurotoxicity. *Human & Experimental Toxicology*, *43*, 09603271241285523. https://doi.org/10.1177/09603271241285523

Park, Y., & Casasola, M. (2015). Plain or decorated? Object visual features matter in infant spatial categorization. *Journal of Experimental Child Psychology*, *140*, 105–119. https://doi.org/10.1016/j.jecp.2015.07.002

Parke, R. D., & Cookston, J. T. (2019). Fathers and families. In M. H. Bornstein (Ed.), *Handbook of parenting, Vol. 3: Being and becoming a parent* (3rd ed., pp. 64–136). Routledge.

Partanen, E., & Virtala, P. (2017). Prenatal sensory development. In B. Hopkins, E. Geangu, & S. Linkenauger (Eds.), *The Cambridge encyclopedia of child development* (pp. 231–241). Cambridge University Press.

Patel, S., Gaylord, S., & Fagen, J. (2013). Generalization of deferred imitation in 6-, 9-, and 12-month-old infants using visual and auditory contexts. *Infant Behavior and Development, 36*(1), 25–31. https://doi.org/10.1016/j.infbeh.2012.09.006

Pathak, R., Mustafa, M. D., Ahmed, T., Ahmed, R. S., Tripathi, A. K., Guleria, K., & Banerjee, B. D. (2011). Intrauterine growth retardation: Association with organochlorine pesticide residue levels and oxidative stress markers. *Reproductive Toxicology, 31*, 534–539. https://doi.org/10.1016/j.reprotox.2011.02.007

Patra, J., Bakker, R., Irving, H., Jaddoe, V. W. V., Malini, S., & Rehm, J. (2011). Dose-response relationship between alcohol consumption before and during pregnancy and the risks of low birthweight, preterm birth and small for gestational age (SGA) – a systematic review and meta-analysis. *BJOG – An International Journal of Obstetrics and Gynaecology, 118*, 1411–1421. https://doi.org/10.1111/j.1471–0528.2011.03050.x

Patterson, C. J. (2019). Lesbian and gay parenthood. In M. H. Bornstein (Ed.), *Handbook of parenting* (pp. 345–371). Routledge.

Pavlyshyn, H., & Sarapuk, I. (2023). Skin-to-skin contact – An effective intervention on pain and stress reduction in preterm infants. *Frontiers in Pediatrics, 11*, 1148946. https://doi.org/10.3389/fped.2023.1148946

Paz, N. C., Sanchez, S. E., Huaman, L. E., Chang, G. D., Pacora, P. N., Garcia, P. J., Ananth, C. V., Qiu, C., & Williams, M. A. (2011). Risk of placental abruption in relation to maternal depression, anxiety, and stress symptoms. *Journal of Affective Disorders, 130*, 280–284. https://doi.org/10.1016/j.jad.2010.07.024

Pearson, R. M., Heron, J., Melotti, R., Joinson, C., Stein, A., Ramchandani, P. G., & Evans, J. (2011). The association between observed nonverbal maternal responses at 12 months and later infant development at 18 months and IQ at 4 years: A longitudinal study. *Infant Behavior and Development, 34*, 525–533. https://doi.org/10.1016/j.infbeh.2011.07.003

Pelaez, M., & Monlux, K. (2017). Operant conditioning methodologies to investigate infant learning. *European Journal of Behavior Analysis, 18*(2), 212–241. https://doi.org/10.1080/15021149.2017.1412633

Peyvandi, F., Garagiola, I., & Mortarino, M. (2011). Prenatal diagnosis and preimplantation genetic diagnosis: Novel technologies and state of the art PDG in different regions of the world. *Haemophilia, 17*, 14–17. https://doi.org/10.1111/j.1365–2516.2011.02559.x

Piaget, J. (1952). *The origins of intelligence in children*. W.W. Norton.

Piaget, J. (1954). *The construction of reality in the child*. Basic Books. (Original work published 1937)

Piaget, J. (1962). The relation of affectivity to intelligence in the mental development of the child. *Bulletin of the Menninger Clinic, 26*, 129–137.

Pino, O. (2016). Fetal memory: The effects of prenatal auditory experience on human development. *BAOJ Medical and Nursing, 2*(4), 2. https://doi.org/10.24947/baojmn/2/2/120

Pinquart, M., Feußner, C., & Ahnert, L. (2013). Meta-analytic evidence for stability in attachments from infancy to early adulthood. *Attachment & Human Development, 15*(2), 189–218. https://doi.org/10.1080/14616734.2013.746257

Planalp, E. M., Van Hulle, C., Gagne, J. R., & Goldsmith, H. H. (2017). The infant version of the laboratory temperament assessment battery (Lab-TAB): Measurement properties and implications for concepts of temperament. *Frontiers in Psychology, 8*, Article 846. https://doi.org/10.3389/fpsyg.2017.00846

Planalp, E. M., Van Hulle, C. A., & Goldsmith, H. H. (2019). Parenting in context: Marital adjustment, parent affect, and child temperament in complex families. *Journal of Family Psychology, 33*(5), 532–541. https://doi.org/10.1037/fam0000511

Plomin, R. (2018). *Blueprint: How DNA makes us who we are*. MIT Press.

Plomin, R., Haworth, C. M., Meaburn, E. L., Price, T. S., Wellcome Trust Case Control Consortium 2, & Davis, O. S. (2013). Common DNA markers can account for more than half of the genetic influence on cognitive abilities. *Psychological Science, 24*(4), 562–568. https://doi.org/10.1177/0956797612457952

Porges, S. W. (2011). *The polyvagal theory: Neurophysiological foundations of emotions, attachment, communication, and self-regulation*. W.W. Norton.

Porter, R. H., Bologh, R. D., & Makin, J. W. (1988). Olfactory influences on mother-infant interactions. In C. Rovee-Collier & L. P. Lipsitt (Eds.), *Advances in infancy research* (Vol. 5, pp. 39–69). Ablex.

Porter, R. H., & Winberg, J. (1999). Unique salience of maternal breast odors for newborn infants. *Neuroscience and Biobehavioral Reviews, 23*, 439–449. https://doi.org/10.1016/S0149–7634(98)00044-X

Poulin-Dubois, D. (2023). Bilingualism in development: The good, the bad and the unknown. In G. Luk, J. A. E. Anderson, & J. Grundy (Eds.), *Understanding language and cognition through bilingualism: In honor of Ellen Bialystok* (pp. 142–168). John Benjamins.

Pruden, S. M., Levine, S. C., & Huttenlocher, J. (2011). Children's spatial thinking: Does talk about the spatial world matter? *Developmental Science, 14*, 1417–1430. https://doi.org/10.1111/j.1467–7687.2011.01088.x

Putnam, S. P., & Gartstein, M. A. (2017). Aggregate temperament scores from multiple countries: Associations with aggregate personality traits, cultural dimensions, and allelic frequency. *Journal of Research in Personality, 67*, 157–170. https://doi.org/10.1016/j.jrp.2016.07.009

Putnam, S. P., Sehic, E., French, B., Gartstein, M. A., Lira Luttges, B., & 486 Additional Partners in the Global Temperament Project. (2024). The global temperament project: Parent-reported temperament in infants, toddlers, and children from 59 nations. *Developmental Psychology, 60*(5), 916–941. https://doi.org/10.1037/dev0001732

Putnick, D. L., Trinh, M. H., Sundaram, R., Bell, E. M., Ghassabian, A., Robinson, S. L., & Yeung, E. (2023). Displacement of peer play by screen time: Associations with toddler development. *Pediatric Research, 93*(5), 1425–1431. https://doi.org/10.1038/s41390-022-02261-y

Quinn, P. C. (2004). Development of subordinate-level categorization in 3- to 7-month-old infants. *Child Development, 75*, 886–899. https://doi.org/10.1111/j.1467–8624.2004.00712.x

Quinn, P. C. (2011). Born to categorize. In U. Goswami (Ed.), *The Wiley-Blackwell handbook of childhood cognitive development* (2nd ed., pp. 129–152). Wiley-Blackwell.

Quinn, P. C., Doran, M. M., Reiss, J. E., & Hoffman, J. E. (2010). Neural markers of subordinate-level categorization in 6- to 7-month-old infants. *Developmental Science, 13*, 499–507. https://doi.org/10.1111/j.1467–7687.2009.00903.x

Raby, K. L., Fraley, R. C., & Roisman, G. I. (2021). Categorical or dimensional measures of attachment? Insights from factor-analytic and taxometric research. In R. A. Thompson, J. A. Simpson, & L. J. Berlin (Eds.), *Attachment: The fundamental questions* (pp. 70–77). Guilford Press.

Raby, K. L., Freedman, E., Yarger, H. A., Lind, T., & Dozier, M. (2019). Enhancing the language development of toddlers in foster care by promoting foster parents' sensitivity: Results from a randomized controlled trial. *Developmental Science, 22*(2), e12753 https://doi.org/10.1111/desc.12753

Rakison, D. H., & Oakes, L. M. (Eds.). (2003). *Early category and concept development: Making sense of the blooming buzzing confusion*. Oxford University Press.

Ramírez, N. F., Hippe, D. S., & Shapiro, N. T. (2021). Exposure to electronic media between 6 and 24 months of age: An exploratory study. *Infant Behavior and Development, 63*, 101549. https://doi.org/10.1016/j.infbeh.2021.101549

Rauh, H., Ziegenhain, T., Müller, B., & Wijnroks, L. (2000). Stability and change in infant-mother attachment in the second year of life: Relations to parenting quality and varying degrees of day-care experience. In P. M. Crittenden & A. H. Claussen (Eds.), *The organization of attachment relationships: Maturation, culture, and context* (pp. 251–276). Cambridge University Press.

Ravn, I. H., Smith, L., Lindemann, R., Smedy, N. A., Kyno, N. M., Bunch, E. H., & Sandvik, L. (2011). Effect of intervention on social interaction between mothers and preterm infants at 12 months of age: A randomized controlled trial. *Infant Behavior and Development, 34*, 215–225. https://doi.org/10.1016/j.infbeh.2010.11.004

Ray, E., & Heyes, C. (2011). Imitation in infancy: The wealth of the stimulus. *Developmental Science, 14*(1), 92–105. https://doi.org/10.1111/j.1467–7687.2010.00961.x

Reby, D., Levréro, F., Gustafsson, E., & Mathevon, N. (2016). Sex stereotypes influence adults' perception of babies' cries. *BMC Psychology, 4*(1), 1–12. https://doi.org/10.1186/s40359-016-0123-6

Reddy, U. M., Davis, J. M., Ren, Z., & Greene, M. F. (2017). Opioid use in pregnancy, neonatal abstinence syndrome, and childhood outcomes: Executive summary of a joint workshop by the Eunice Kennedy Shriver National Institute of Child Health and Human Development, American College of Obstetricians and Gynecologists, American Academy of Pediatrics, Society for Maternal-Fetal Medicine, Centers for Disease Control and Prevention, and the March of Dimes Foundation. *Obstetrics & Gynecology, 130*(1), 10–28. https://doi.org/10.1097/AOG.0000000000002054

Reeb-Sutherland, B. C., Fifer, W. P., Byrd, D. L., Hammock, E. A., Levitt, P., & Fox, N. A. (2011). One-month-old human infants learn about the social world while they sleep. *Developmental Science, 14*(5), 1134–1141. https://doi.org/10.1111/j.1467–7687.2011.01062.x

Repacholi, B. M., Meltzoff, A. N., Toub, T. S., & Ruba, A. L. (2016). Infants' generalizations about other people's emotions: Foundations for trait-like attributions. *Developmental Psychology, 52*(3), 364–378. https://doi.org/10.1037/dev0000097

Reynolds, G. D., Courage, M. L., & Richards, J. E. (2013). The development of attention. In D. Reisberg (Ed.), *Oxford handbook of cognitive psychology* (pp. 1000–1013). Oxford University Press.

Reynolds, G. D., & Romano, A. C. (2016). The development of attention systems and working memory in infancy. *Frontiers in Systems Neuroscience, 10*, Article 15. https://doi.org/10.3389/fnsys.2016.00015

Rhea, S. A., Bricker, J. B., Wadsworth, S. J., & Corley, R. P. (2013). The Colorado adoption project. *Twin Research and Human Genetics, 16*(1), 358–365. https://doi.org/10.1017/thg.2012.109

Rideout, V. J., & Hamel, E. (2006). *The media family: Electronic media in the lives of infants, toddlers, preschoolers, and their parents*. Kaiser Family Foundation.

Righetti-Veltema, M., Conne-Perréard, E., Bousquet, A., & Manzano, J. (2002). Postpartum depression and mother–infant relationship at 3 months old. *Journal of Affective Disorders, 70*(3), 291–306. https://doi.org/10.1016/S0165–0327(01)00367–6

Rigo, P., Esposito, G., Bornstein, M. H., De Pisapia, N., Manzardo, C., & Venuti, P. (2019). Brain processes in mothers and nulliparous women in response to cry in different situational contexts: A default mode network study. *Parenting, 19*(1–2), 69–85. https://doi.org/10.1080/15295192.2019.1555430

Rivkees, S. A. (2003). Developing circadian rhythms in infants. *Pediatrics, 112*, 373–381. https://doi.org/10.1542/peds.112.2.373

Rivkees, S. A., & Hao, H. P. (2000). Developing circadian rhythmicity. *Seminars in Perinatology, 24*, 232–242. https://doi.org/10.1053/sper.2000.8598

Rochat, P. (2019). Self-unity as ground zero of learning and development. *Frontiers in Psychology, 10*, Article 414. https://doi.org/10.3389/fpsyg.2019.00414

Rochat, P., & Hespos, S. J. (1997). Differential rooting response by neonates: Evidence for an early sense of self. *Early Development and Parenting, 6*, 105–112. https://doi.org/10.1002/(SICI)1099-0917(199709/12)6:3/4<105::AID-EDP150>3.0.CO;2-U

Rodkey, E. N. (2015). The visual cliff's forgotten menagerie: Rats, goats, babies, and myth-making in the history of psychology. *Journal of the History of the Behavioral Sciences*, *51*(2), 113–140. https://doi.org/10.1002/jhbs.21712

Rogoff, B. (2003). *The cultural nature of human development*. Oxford University Press.

Rogoff, B. (2014). Learning by observing and pitching in to family and community endeavors: An orientation. *Human Development*, *57*(2–3), 69–81. https://doi.org/10.1159/000356757

Roisman, G. I., & Groh, A. M. (2011). Attachment theory and research in developmental psychology: An overview and appreciative critique. In M. K. Underwood & L. H. Rosen (Eds.), *Social development: Relationships in infancy, childhood, and adolescence* (pp. 101–126). Guilford Press.

Roisman, G. I., & Groh, A. M. (2021). The legacy of early attachments: Past, present, future. In R. A. Thompson, J. A. Simpson, & L. J. Berlin (Eds.), *Attachment: The fundamental questions* (pp. 187–194). Guilford Press.

Roopnarine, J. L., Fouts, H. N., Lamb, M. E., & Lewis-Elligan, T. Y. (2005). Mothers' and fathers' behaviors toward their 3- to 4-month-old infants in lower, middle, and upper socioeconomic African American families. *Developmental Psychology*, *41*, 723–732. https://doi.org/10.1037/0012-1649.41.5.723

Rose, S. A., Feldman, J. F., Jankowski, J. J., & Van Rossem, R. (2011). Basic information processing abilities at 11 years account for deficits in IQ associated with preterm birth. *Intelligence*, *39*(4), 198–209. https://doi.org/10.1016/j.intell.2011.03.003.

Rothbart, M. K. (1981). Measurement of temperament in infancy. *Child Development*, *52*(2), 569–578. https://doi.org/10.2307/1129176

Rothbart, M. K. (2011). *Becoming who we are: Temperament and personality in development*. Guilford Press.

Rothbart, M. K., & Bates, J. E. (2006). Temperament. In W. Damon, R. Lerner, & N. Eisenberg (Eds.), *Handbook of child psychology, Vol. 3. Social, emotional, and personality development* (6th ed., pp. 99–166). Wiley.

Rovee-Collier, C., & Cuevas, K. (2009). The development of infant memory. In M. L. Courage & N. Cowan (Eds.), *The development of memory in infancy and childhood* (2nd ed., pp. 11–41). Psychology Press.

Rovee-Collier, C., & Giles, A. (2010). Why a neuromaturational model of memory fails: Exuberant learning in infancy. *Behavioural Processes*, *83*, 197–206. https://doi.org/10.1016/j.beproc.2009.11.013

Saffran, J. R. (2020). Statistical language learning in infancy. *Child Development Perspectives*, *14*(1), 49–54. https://doi.org/10.1111/cdep.12355

Sagi, A., & Hoffman, M. L. (1976). Empathetic distress in the newborn. *Developmental Psychology*, *12*, 175–176. https://psycnet.apa.org/doi/10.1037/0012-1649.12.2.175

Sameroff, A. (2009). The transactional model. In A. Sameroff (Ed.), *The transactional model of development: How children and contexts shape each other* (pp. 3–21). American Psychological Association.

Sameroff, A. J. (2014). A dialectic integration of development for the study of psychopathology. In M. Lewis & K. D. Rudolph (Eds.), *Handbook of developmental psychopathology* (3rd ed., pp. 25–43). Springer.

Sann, C., & Streri, A. (2008). Inter-manual transfer of object texture and shape in human neonates. *Neuropsychologia*, *46*(2), 698–703. https://doi.org/10.1016/j.neuropsychologia.2007.09.014

Satterfield-Nash, A., Kotzky, K., Allen, J., Bertolli, J., Moore, C. A., Pereira, I. O., Pessoa, A., Melo, F., Santelli, A. C. F. e. S., Boyle, C. A., & & Peacock, G. (2017). Health and development at age 19–24 months of 19 children who were born with microcephaly and laboratory evidence of congenital Zika virus infection during the 2015 Zika virus outbreak – Brazil, 2017. *Morbidity and Mortality Weekly Report*, *66*(49), 1347–1351. https://doi.org/10.15585/mmwr.mm6649a2

Scaff, C., & Cristia, A. (2025). Language development. In M. H. Bornstein & M. E. Lamb (Eds.), *Developmental science: An advanced textbook* (pp. 362–406). Routledge.

Scarr, S. (1993). Biological and cultural diversity: The legacy of Darwin for development. *Child Development, 64*(5), 1333–1353. https://doi.org/10.2307/1131538

Scher, M. S., Ludington-Hoe, S., Kaffashi, F., Johnson, M. W., Holditch-Davis, D., & Loparo, K. A. (2009). Neurophysiologic assessment of brain maturation after an 8-week trial of skin-to-skin contact on preterm infants. *Clinical Neurophysiology, 120,* 1812–1818. https://doi.org/10.1016/j.clinph.2009.08.004

Scherling, D. (1994). Prenatal cocaine exposure and childhood psychopathology: A developmental analysis. *American Journal of Orthopsychiatry, 64,* 9–19. https://doi.org/10.1037/h0079494

Schmitow, C., & Stenberg, G. (2013). Social referencing in 10-month-old infants. *European Journal of Developmental Psychology, 10*(5), 533–545. https://doi.org/10.1080/17405629.2013.763473

Schmuckler, M. A., & Jewell, D. T. (2007). Infants' visual-proprioceptive intermodal perception with imperfect contingency information. *Developmental Psychobiology, 49*(4), 387–398. https://doi.org/10.1002/dev.20214

Schofield, Z., & Schofield, Z. (2025). *Mental health disorders in pregnancy and the early postpartum.* Cambridge University Press.

Schoppe-Sullivan, S. J., & Kübra Aytaç-DiCarlo, F. (Eds.). (2025). *Parental gatekeeping.* Routledge.

Schuengel, C., & Oosterman, M. (2019). Parenting self-efficacy. In M. H. Bornstein (Ed.), *Handbook of parenting, Vol. 3: Being and becoming a parent* (3rd ed., pp. 654–681). Routledge.

Schwartz, A. N., Campos, J. J., & Baisel, E. J. (1973). The visual cliff: Cardiac and behavioral responses on the deep and shallow sides of five and nine months of age. *Journal of Experimental Child Psychology, 15,* 86–99. https://doi.org/10.1016/0022–0965(73)90133–1

Schwartz, C. E., Wright, C. I., Shin, L. M., Kagan, J., & Rauch, S. (2003). Inhibited and uninhibited infants "grown up": Adult amygdala response to novelty. *Science, 300,* 1952–1953. https://doi.org/10.1126/science.1083703

Schwilling, D., Vogeser, M., Kirchhoff, F., Schwaiblmair, F., Boulesteix, A. L., Schulze, A., & Flemmer, A. W. (2015). Live music reduces stress levels in very low-birthweight infants. *Acta Paediatrica, 104*(4), 360–367. https://doi.org/10.1111/apa.12913

Seavey, C. A, Katz, P. A., & Zalk, S. R. (1975). Baby X: The effect of gender labels on adult responses to infants. *Sex Roles, 1,* 103–109.

Seligman, M. E. P. (1970). On the generality of the laws of learning. *Psychological Review, 77,* 406–418. https://psycnet.apa.org/doi/10.1037/h0029790

Shah, P. E., Fonagy, P., & Strathearn, L. (2010). Is attachment transmitted across generations? The plot thickens. *Clinical Child Psychology and Psychiatry, 15,* 329–345. https://doi.org/10.1177/1359104510365449

Shammas, M. A. (2011). Telomeres, lifestyle, cancer, and aging. *Current Opinion in Clinical Nutrition & Metabolic Care, 14*(1), 28–34. https://doi.org/10.1097/MCO.0b013e32834121b1

Shannon, J. D., Tamis-LeMonda, C. S., & Margolin, A. (2005). Father involvement in infancy: Influences of past and current relationships. *Infancy, 8,* 21–41. https://doi.org/10.1207/s15327078in0801_2

Shaw, P., Greenstein, D., Lerch, J., Clasen, L., Lenroot, R., Gogtay, N., Evans, A., & Rapoort, J. (2006). Intellectual ability and cortical development in children and adolescents. *Nature, 440,* 676–679. https://doi.org/10.1038/nature04513

Shim, S.-S. (2014). Chorionic villus sampling. *Journal of Genetic Medicine, 11*(2), 43–48. https://doi.org/10.5734/JGM.2014.11.2.43

Shin, M., Choi, Y., & Mazuka, R. (2018). Development of fricative sound perception in Korean infants: The role of language experience and infants' initial sensitivity. *Plos One, 13*(6), e0199045. https://doi.org/10.1371/journal.pone.0199045

Shinskey, J. L., & Munakata, Y. (2003). Are infants in the dark about hidden objects? *Developmental Science, 6*, 272–282. https://doi.org/10.1111/1467–7687.00283

Shonkoff, J. P., & Phillips, D. A. (2000). *From neurons to neighborhoods: The science of early childhood development*. National Academies Press.

Sidorowicz, L. S., & Lunney, G. S, (1980). Baby X revisited. *Sex Roles, 6*, 67–73. https://doi.org/10.1007/BF00288362

Silva, C. S., Lima, M. C., Sequeira-de-Andrade, L. A., Oliveira, J. S., Monteiro, J. S., Lima, N. M., Santos, R. M. A. B., & Lira, P. I. C. (2017). Association between postpartum depression and the practice of exclusive breastfeeding in the first three months of life. *Journal of Pediatrics (Rio J), 93*, 356–64. 10.1016/j.jped.2016.08.005

Silventoinen, K., Jelenkovic, A., Yokoyama, Y., Sund, R., Sugawara, M., Tanaka, M., Matsumoto, S., Bogl, L. H., Freitas, D. L., Maia, J. A., Hjelmborg, J. v. B., Aaltonen, S., Piirtola, M., Latvala, A., Calais-Ferreira, L., Oliveira, V. C., Ferreira, P. H., Ji, F., Ning, F., . . . Kaprio, J. (2019). The CODATwins project: The current status and recent findings of collaborative project of development of anthropometrical measures in twins. *Twin Research and Human Genetics, 22*(6), 800–808. https://doi.org/10.1017/thg.2019.35

Simion, F., & Giorgio, E. D. (2015). Face perception and processing in early infancy: Inborn predispositions and developmental changes. *Frontiers in Psychology, 6*, Article 969. https://doi.org/10.3389/fpsyg.2015.00969

Simpson, J. L. (2012). Invasive procedures for prenatal diagnosis: Any future left? *Best Practice & Research Clinical Obstetrics & Gynaecology, 26*(5), 625–638. https://doi.org/10.1016/j.bpobgyn.2012.05.007

Skelton, A. E., & Franklin, A. (2020). Infants look longer at colours that adults like when colours are highly saturated. *Psychonomic Bulletin & Review, 27*(1), 78–85. https://doi.org/10.3758/s13423-019-01688-5

Skinner, B. F. (1957). *Verbal behavior*. Appleton-Century-Crofts.

Slaughter, V. (2020). Foundations of imitation. In J. Decety (Ed.), *The social brain: A developmental perspective* (pp. 89–106). MIT Press.

Slomian, J., Honvo, G., Emonts, P., Reginster, J.-Y., & Bruyère, O. (2019). Consequences of maternal postpartum depression: A systematic review of maternal and infant outcomes. *Women's Health, 15*. https://doi.org/10.1177/1745506519844044

Smith, P. K., & Roopnarine, J. L. (2019). *The Cambridge handbook of play: Developmental and disciplinary perspectives*. Cambridge University Press.

Smolak, E., De Anda, S., Enriquez, B., Poulin-Dubois, D., & Friend, M. (2020). Code-switching in young bilingual toddlers: A longitudinal, cross-language investigation. *Bilingualism: Language and Cognition, 23*(3), 500–518. https://doi.org/10.1017/S1366728919000257

Sobelweski, J., & King, V. (2005). The importance of the coparental relationship for non-residential fathers' ties to children. *Journal of Marriage and Family, 67*, 1196–1212. https://doi.org/10.1111/j.1741–3737.2005.00210.x

Sohr-Preston, S. L., Scaramella, L. V., Martin, M. J., Neppl, T. K., Ontai, L., & Conger, R. (2013). Parental socioeconomic status, communication, and children's vocabulary development: A third-generation test of the family investment model. *Child Development, 84*(3), 1046–1062. https://doi.org/10.1111/cdev.12023

Sommer, K., Redshaw, J., Slaughter, V., Wiles, J., & Nielsen, M. (2021). The early ontogeny of infants' imitation of on screen humans and robots. *Infant Behavior and Development, 64*, 101614. https://doi.org/10.1016/j.infbeh.2021.101614

Song, L., Tamis-LeMonda, C. S., Yoshikawa, H., Kahana-Kalman, R., & Wu, I. (2012). Language experiences and vocabulary development in Dominican and Mexican infants across the first 2 years. *Developmental Psychology, 48*, 1106–1123. https://doi.org/10.1037/a0026401

Soska, K. C., Adolph, K. E., & Johnson, S. P. (2010). Systems in development: Motor skill acquisition facilitates three-dimensional object completion. *Developmental Psychology, 46*, 129–138. https://doi.org/10.1037/a0014618

Southgate, V. (2020). Are infants altercentric? The other and the self in early social cognition. *Psychological Review, 127*(4), 505–523. https://doi.org/10.1037/rev0000182

Southgate, V., Johnson, M. H., El Karoui, I., & Csibra, G. (2010). Motor system activation reveals infants' on-line prediction of others' goals. *Psychological Science, 21*(3), 355–359. https://doi.org/10.1177/0956797610362058

Sparrow, J. (2013). Newborn behavior, parent-infant interaction, and developmental change processes: Research roots of developmental, relational, and systems-theory-based practice. *Journal of Child and Adolescent Psychiatric Nursing, 26*, 180–185. https://doi.org/10.1111/jcap.12047

Spelke, E. S. (2016). Core knowledge and conceptual change: A perspective on social cognition. In D. Barner & A. S. Baron (Eds.), *Core knowledge and conceptual change* (pp. 279–300). Oxford University Press.

Spelke, E. S., Breinlinger, K., Macomber, J., & Jacobson, K. (1992). Origins of knowledge. *Psychological Review, 99*, 605–632. https://psycnet.apa.org/doi/10.1037/0033–295X.99.4.605

Spelt, D. K. (1948). The conditioning of the human fetus in utero. *Journal of Experimental Psychology, 38*, 375–376. https://psycnet.apa.org/doi/10.1037/h0059632

Spinelli, M., Bornstein, M. H., Putnick, D. L., & Shah, P. E. (2022). Multimodal assessments of preterm temperament across the first year of life: Continuity, stability, and moderation by country of origin and infant age. *Infant Mental Health Journal, 43*, 287–299. https://doi.org/10.1002/imhj.21974

Spitz, R. A. (1965). *The first year of life*. International Universities Press.

Sravya, G., Kamlesh, C., Deepti, S., & Seema, Y. (2024). Advancements and applications of preimplantation genetic testing in in vitro fertilization: A comprehensive review. *Cureus, 16*(3), 57357. https://doi.org/10.7759/cureus.57357

Sroufe, L. A. (2017). Attachment theory: A humanistic approach for research and practice across cultures. In S. Gojman-de-Millan, C. Herreman, & L. A. Sroufe (Eds.), *Attachment across clinical and cultural perspectives: A relational psychoanalytic approach* (pp. 3–29). Taylor & Francis Group. https://doi.org/10.4324/9781315658100

Sroufe, L. A. (2021). The legacy of the first 3 years. *Zero to Three, 41*(3). https://www.zerotothree.org/resource/journal/the-legacy-of-the-first-3-years/

Sroufe, L. A., Egeland, B., Carlson, E. A., & Collins, W. A. (2005). *The development of the person: The Minnesota study of risk and adaptation from birth to adulthood*. Guilford Press.

Staples, A. D., Hoyniak, C., McQuillan, M. E., Molfese, V., & Bates, J. E. (2021). Screen use before bedtime: Consequences for nighttime sleep in young children. *Infant Behavior and Development, 62*, 101522. https://doi.org/10.1016/j.infbeh.2020.101522

Steiner, J. E. (1977). Facial expressions of the neonate infant indicating the hedonics of food-related chemical stimuli. In J. M. Weiffenbach (Ed.), *Taste and development*. Department of Health, Education, and Welfare.

Steiner, J. E. (1979). Human facial expressions in response to taste and smell stimulation. In H. Reese & L. Lipsitt (Eds.), *Advances in child development and behavior* (Vol. 13, pp. 257–295). Academic Press.

Steiner, J. E., Glaser, D., Hawilo, M. E., & Berridge, K. C. (2001). Comparative expression of hedonic impact: Affective reactions to taste by human infants and other primates. *Neuroscience and Biobehavioral Reviews, 25*, 53–74. https://doi.org/10.1016/S0149–7634(00)00051–8

Stenberg, G. (2017). Does contingency in adults' responding influence 12-month-old infants' social referencing? *Infant Behavior and Development, 46*, 67–79. https://doi.org/10.1016/j.infbeh.2017.06.003

Stets, M., Stahl, D., & Reid, V. M. (2012). A meta-analysis investigating factors underlying attrition rates in infant ERP studies. *Developmental Neuropsychology*, *37*, 226–252. https://doi.org/10.1080/87565641.2012.654867

Stiles, J. (2008). *The fundamentals of brain development: Integrating nature and nurture*. Harvard.

Stiles, J., Brown, T. T., Haist, F., & Jernigan, T. L. (2015). Brain and cognitive development. In L. S. Liben & U. Müller (Eds.), *Handbook of child psychology and developmental science, Vol. 2: Cognitive processes* (7th ed., pp. 9–62). Wiley.

Stockdale, L. A., Porter, C. L., Coyne, S. M., Essig, L. W., Booth, M., Keenan-Kroff, S., & Schvaneveldt, E. (2020). Infants' response to a mobile phone modified still-face paradigm: Links to maternal behaviors and beliefs regarding technoference. *Infancy*, *25*(5), 571–592. https://doi.org/10.1111/infa.12342

Striano, T., & Vaish, A. (2006). Seven- to 9-month-old infants use facial expressions to interpret others' actions. *British Journal of Developmental Psychology*, *24*, 753–760. https://doi.org/10.1348/026151005X70319

Strouse, G. A., & Ganea, P. A. (2021). Learning to learn from video? 30-month-olds benefit from continued use of supportive scaffolding. *Infant Behavior and Development*, *64*, 101574. https://doi.org/10.1016/j.infbeh.2021.101574

Strouse, G. A., & Samson, J. E. (2021). Learning from video: A meta-analysis of the video deficit in children ages 0 to 6 years. *Child Development*, *92*(1), e20–e38. https://doi.org/10.1111/cdev.13429

Sturge-Apple, M. L., Toth, S. L., Suor, J. H., & Adams, T. R. (2019). Parental maltreatment. In M. H. Bornstein (Ed.), *Handbook of parenting, Vol. 4: Social conditions and applied parenting* (3rd ed., pp. 556–589). Routledge.

Sulpizio, S., Doi, H., Bornstein, M. H., Cui, J., Esposito, G., & Shinohara, K. (2018). fNIRS reveals enhanced brain activation to female (versus male) infant directed speech (relative to adult directed speech) in young human infants. *Infant Behavior and Development*, *52*, 89–96. https://doi.org/10.1016/j.infbeh.2018.05.009

Super, C. M., & Harkness, S. (2013). Culture and children's sleep. In A. R. Wolfson & H. E. Montgomery-Downs (Eds.), *The Oxford handbook of infant, child, and adolescent sleep and behavior* (pp. 81–98). Oxford University Press.

Suzigan, L., Silva, R., Guerra-Junior, G., Marini, S., & Maciel-Guerra, A. (2011). Social skills in women with Turner syndrome. *Scandinavian Journal of Psychology*, *52*, 440–447. https://doi.org/10.1111/j.1467–9450.2011.00887.x

Sweeney, J., & Bradbard, M. R. (1988). Mothers' and fathers' changing perceptions of their male and female infants over the course of pregnancy. *Journal of Genetic Psychology*, *149*, 393–404. https://doi.org/10.1080/00221325.1988.10532167

Szekely, E., Zusman, E. Z., Kandiyoti, A., Wazana, A., & Oberlander, T. F. (2025). Prenatal stress and child and adolescent development: Pathways, processes, and interventions. In M. H. Bornstein & P. E. Shah (Eds.), *APA handbook of pediatric psychology, developmental–behavioral pediatrics, and developmental science, Vol. 1: Developmental origins of risk and resilience* (pp. 139–158). American Psychological Association.

Takács, L., Abuaish, S., Kaňková, Š., Hill, M., Ullmann, J., Včelák, J., & Monk, C. (2024). Maternal negative affect in pregnancy predicts cytokine levels which in turn predict birth outcomes – a prospective longitudinal study in a low-risk population. *Journal of Affective Disorders*, *366*, 345–353. https://doi.org/10.1016/j.jad.2024.08.141

Tamis-LeMonda, C. S., & Kahana-Kalman, R. (2009). Mothers' views at the transition to a new baby: Variation across ethnic groups. *Parenting: Science and Practice*, *9*, 36–55. https://doi.org/10.1080/15295190802656745

Tamis-LeMonda, C. S., Kuchirko, Y., Escobar, K., & Bornstein, M. H. (2019). Language and play in parent-child interactions. In M. H. Bornstein (Ed.), *Handbook of parenting, Vol. 5: The practice of parenting* (3th ed., pp. 189–213). Routledge.

Tan, P., & Cole, P. M. (2019). Infant temperament and early self-regulation. In R. DelCarmen-Wiggins & A. S. Carter (Eds.), *The Oxford handbook of infant, toddler, and preschool mental health assessment* (pp. 175–223). Oxford University Press.
Tang, A., Crawford, H., Morales, S., Degnan, K. A., Pine, D. S., & Fox, N. A. (2020). Infant behavioral inhibition predicts personality and social outcomes three decades later. *Proceedings of the National Academy of Sciences, 117*(18), 9800–9807. https://doi.org/10.1073/pnas.1917376117
Teepe, R. C., Molenaar, I., Oostdam, R., Fukkink, R., & Verhoeven, L. (2017). Children's executive and social functioning and family context as predictors of preschool vocabulary. *Learning and Individual Differences, 57*, 1–8. https://doi.org/10.1016/j.lindif.2017.05.012
Teichner, G., Ames, E. W., & Kerig, P. K. (1997). The relation of infant crying and the sex of the infant to parents' perceptions of the infant and themselves. *Psychology: A Journal of Human Behavior, 34*, 59–60.
Tella, P., Piccolo, L. D. R., Rangel, M. L., Rohde, L. A., Polanczyk, G. V., Miguel, E. C., Grisi, S. J. F. E., Fleitlich-Bilyk, B., & Ferraro, A. A. (2018). Socioeconomic diversities and infant development at 6 to 9 months in a poverty area of São Paulo, Brazil. *Trends in Psychiatry and Psychotherapy, 40*, 232–240. https://doi.org/10.1590/2237-6089-2017-0008
Teti, D. M. (2002). Sibling relationships. In J. McHale & W. Grolnick (Eds.), *Interiors: Retrospect and prospect in the psychological study of families* (pp. 193–224). Erlbaum.
Teti, D. M., & Cole, P. M. (2011). Parenting at risk: New perspectives, new approaches. *Journal of Family Psychology, 25*, 625–634. https://psycnet.apa.org/doi/10.1037/a0025287
Teti, D. M., Shimizu, M., Crosby, B., & Kim, B. R. (2016). Sleep arrangements, parent–infant sleep during the first year, and family functioning. *Developmental Psychology, 52*(8), 1169–1181. https://doi.org/10.1037/dev0000148
Thelen, E. (2000). Motor development as foundation and future of developmental psychology. *International Journal of Behavioral Development, 24*, 385–397. https://doi.org/10.1080%2F016502500750037937
Thelen, E. (2001). Dynamic mechanisms of change in early perceptual-motor development. In E. Thelen (Ed.), *Mechanisms of cognitive development: Behavioral and neural perspectives* (pp. 161–184). Erlbaum.
Thomas, A., & Chess, S. (1977). *Temperament and development*. Brunner/Mazel.
Thompson, R. A. (2015). Relationships, regulation, and early development. In M. E. Lamb & R. M. Lerner (Eds.), *Handbook of child psychology and developmental science: Socioemotional processes* (Vol. 3, 7th ed., pp. 201–246). Wiley.
Thompson, R. A., Simpson, J. A., & Berlin, L. J. (2021). *Attachment: The fundamental questions*. Guilford Press.
Thompson, R. A., & Virmani, E. A. (2010). Self and personality. In M. H. Bornstein (Ed.), *Handbook of cultural developmental science* (pp. 195–208). Psychology Press.
Thordardottir, E. (2011). The relationship between bilingual exposure and vocabulary development. *International Journal of Bilingualism, 15*(4), 426–445. https://doi.org/10.1177/1367006911403202
Thurman, S. L., & Corbetta, D. (2017). Spatial exploration and changes in infant–mother dyads around transitions in infant locomotion. *Developmental Psychology, 53*(7), 1207–1221. https://doi.org/10.1037/dev0000328
Tobin, N. H., & Aldrovandi, G. M. (2013). Immunology of pediatric HIV infection. *Immunological Reviews, 254*(1), 143–169. https://doi.org/10.1111/imr.12074
Tooley, U. A., Bassett, D. S., & Mackey, A. P. (2021). Environmental influences on the pace of brain development. *Nature Reviews Neuroscience, 22*(6), 372–384.
Trivers, R. L. (1972). Parental investment and sexual selection. In B. Campbell (Ed.), *Sexual selection and the descent of man, 1871–1971* (pp. 136–179). Aldine. https://doi.org/10.4324/9781315129266–7
Tronick, E. (2007). *The neurobehavioral and social-emotional development in infants and children*. W.W. Norton.

Troseth, G. L., Bloom Pickard, M. E., & DeLoache, J. S. (2007). Young children's use of scale models: Testing an alternative to representational insight. *Developmental Science, 10*(6), 763–769. https://doi.org/10.1111/j.1467–7687.2007.00625.x

Tsang, T., Ogren, M., Peng, Y., Nguyen, B., Johnson, K. L., & Johnson, S. P. (2018). Infant perception of sex differences in biological motion displays. *Journal of Experimental Child Psychology, 173*, 338–350. https://doi.org/10.1016/j.jecp.2018.04.006

Tucker-Drob, E. M., & Briley, D. A. (2014). Continuity of genetic and environmental influences on cognition across the life span: A meta-analysis of longitudinal twin and adoption studies. *Psychological Bulletin, 140*(4), 949–979. https://doi.org/10.1037/a0035893

Turati, C., Macchi Cassia, V., Simion, F., & Leo, I. (2006). Newborns' face recognition: Role of inner and outer facial features. *Child Development, 77*(2), 297–311. https://doi.org/10.1111/j.1467–8624.2006.00871.x

Umemura, T., Jacobvitz, D., Messina, S., & Hazen, N. (2013). Do toddlers prefer their primary caregiver or the parent with whom they feel more secure? The role of toddler emotion. *Infant Behavior and Development, 36*, 102–114. https://doi.org/10.1016/j.infbeh.2012.10.003

UNICEF. (2022). *Global and regional trends*. https://data.unicef.org/topic/hivaids/global-

Væver, M. S., Pedersen, I. E., Smith-Nielsen, J., & Tharner, A. (2020). Maternal postpartum depression is a risk factor for infant emotional variability at 4 months. *Infant Mental Health Journal, 41*(4), 477–494. https://doi.org/10.1002/imhj.21846

Valcan, D. S., Davis, H., & Pino-Pasternak, D. (2018). Parental behaviours predicting early childhood executive functions: A meta-analysis. *Educational Psychology Review, 30*, 607–649. https://doi.org/10.1007/s10648-017-9411-9

Vandell, D. L., Belsky, J., Burchinal, M., Steinberg, L., Vandergrift, N., & NICHD Early Child Care Research Network. (2010). Do effects of early child care extend to age 15 years? Results from the NICHD study of early child care and youth development. *Child Development, 81*, 737–756. https://doi.org/10.1111/j.1467–8624.2010.01431.x

van den Brink, D., & Janzen, G. (2013). Visual spatial cue use for guiding orientation in two-to-three-year-old children. *Frontiers in Psychology, 4*, Article 904. https://doi.org/10.3389/fpsyg.2013.00904

Van IJzendoorn, M. H., & Sagi-Schwartz, A. (2008). Cross-cultural patterns of attachment: Universal and contextual dimensions. In J. Cassidy & P. R. Shaver (Eds.), *Handbook of attachment: Theory, research, and clinical applications* (2nd ed., pp. 880–905). Guilford Press.

Vaurio, L., Crocker, N., & Mattson, S. N. (2011). Fetal alcohol spectrum disorders. In A. S. Davis (Ed.), *Handbook of pediatric neuropsychology* (pp. 877–886). Springer.

Venkatesan, T., Rees, P., Gardiner, J., Battersby, C., Purkayastha, M., Gale, C., & Sutcliffe, A. G. (2023). National trends in preterm infant mortality in the United States by race and socioeconomic status, 1995–2020. *JAMA Pediatrics, 177*(10), 1085–1095. https://doi.org/10.1001/jamapediatrics.2023.3487

Veraksa, N., Colliver, Y., & Sukhikh, V. (2022). Piaget and Vygotsky's play theories: The profile of twenty-first-century evidence. In N. Veraksa & I. Pramling Samuelsson (Eds.), *Piaget and Vygotsky in XXI century. Early childhood research and education: An inter-theoretical focus* (Vol. 4, pp. 165–190). Springer.

Verhage, M. L., Schuengel, C., Madigan, S., Fearon, R. M. P., Oosterman, M., Cassibba, R., Bakermans-Kranenburg, M. J., & van IJzendoorn, M. H. (2016). Narrowing the transmission gap: A synthesis of three decades of research on intergenerational transmission of attachment. *Psychological Bulletin, 142*(4), 337–366. https://doi.org/10.1037/bul0000038

Volling, B. L., & Cabrera, N. J. (2019). Advancing research and measurement on fathering and child development: Introducing the issues and a conceptual framework. *Monographs of the Society for Research in Child Development, 84*, 7–17. https://doi.org/10.1111/mono.12404

Volling, B. L., Gonzalez, R., Oh, W., Song, J.-H., Yu, T., Rosenberg, L., Kuo, P. X., Thomason, E., Beyers-Carlson, E., Safyer, P., & Stevenson, M. M. (2017). Developmental trajectories of children's adjustment across the transition to siblinghood: Pre-birth predictors and sibling outcomes at one year. *Monographs of the Society for Research in Child Development, 82*(3), 1–215.

von Hofsten, C. (1983). Catching skills in infancy. *Journal of Experimental Psychology: Human Perception and Performance, 9*(1), 75–85. https://doi.org/10.1037/0096–1523.9.1.75

Vouloumanos, A., Hauser, M. D., Werker, J. F., & Martin, A. (2010). The tuning of human neonates' preference for speech. *Child Development, 81*(2), 517–527. https://doi.org/10.1111/j.1467–8624.2009.01412.x

Vouloumanos, A., & Werker, J. F. (2007). Listening to language at birth: Evidence for a bias for speech in neonates. *Developmental Science, 10*, 159–171. https://doi.org/10.1111/j.1467–7687.2007.00549.x

Vygotsky, L. S. (1978). *Mind in society*. Cambridge University Press.

Wachs, T. D. (2015). Assessing bioecological influences. In M. H. Bornstein, T. Levanthal, & R. M. Lerner (Eds.), *Handbook of child psychology and developmental science: Ecological settings and processes* (7th ed., vol. 4, pp. 811–846). Wiley.

Walker-Andrews, A. S., Krogh-Jespersen, S., Mayhew, E. M., & Coffield, C. N. (2011). Young infants' generalization of emotional expressions: Effects of familiarity. *Emotion, 11*, 842–851. https://doi.org/10.1037/a0024435

Walle, E. A., & Campos, J. J. (2012). Interpersonal responding to discrete emotions: A functionalist approach to the development of affect specificity. *Emotion Review, 4*(4), 413–422. https://doi.org/10.1177/1754073912445812

Walle, E. A., Main, A., & Morales, S. (2025). Temperament, emotion, and self. In M. H. Bornstein & M. E. Lamb (Eds.), *Developmental science: An advanced textbook* (8th ed., pp. 409–452). Psychology Press.

Wallman, J. (1979). A minimal visual restriction experiment: Preventing chicks from seeing their feet affects later responses to mealworms. *Developmental Psychobiology, 12*(4), 391–397. https://doi.org/10.1002/dev.420120413

Ware, E. A., Uttal, D. H., & DeLoache, J. S. (2010). Everyday scale errors. *Developmental Science, 13*(1), 28–36. https://doi.org/10.1111/j.1467–7687.2009.00853.x

Ware, E. A., Uttal, D. H., Wetter, E. K., & DeLoache, J. S. (2006). Young children make scale errors when playing with dolls. *Developmental Science, 9*(1), 40–45. https://doi.org/10.1111/j.1467–7687.2005.00461.x

Waters, E. (1978). The reliability and stability of individual differences in infant-mother attachment. *Child Development, 49*, 483–494. https://doi.org/10.2307/1128714

Watson, J. B. (1924). *Behaviorism*. W.W. Norton.

Waxman, S., Fu, X., Arunachalam, S., Leddon, E., Geraghty, K., & Song, H. J. (2013). Are nouns learned before verbs? Infants provide insight into a long-standing debate. *Child Development Perspectives, 7*(3), 155–159. https://doi.org/10.1111/cdep.12032

Weinfield, N. S., Sroufe, L. A., Egeland, B., & Carlson, E. (2008). Individual differences in infant-caregiver attachment: Conceptual and empirical aspects of security. In J. Cassidy & P. R. Shaver (Eds.), *Handbook of attachment: Theory, research, and clinical applications* (2nd ed., pp. 78–101). Guilford Press.

Weinraub, M., & Kaufman, R. (2019). Single parenthood. In M. H. Bornstein (Ed.), *Handbook of parenting, Vol. 3: Being and becoming a parent* (3rd ed., pp. 271–310). Routledge.

Wertheimer, M. (1961). Psychomotor coordination of auditory and visual space at birth. *Science, 134*, 1692. https://doi.org/10.1126/science.134.3491.1692.a

Westermann, G., & Mareschal, D. (2012). Mechanisms of developmental change in infant categorization. *Cognitive Development, 27*(4), 367–382. https://doi.org/10.1016/j.cogdev.2012.08.004

Wheeler, A. C. (2018). Development of infants with congenital Zika syndrome: What do we know and what can we expect? *Pediatrics, 141*(2), 154–160. https://doi.org/10.1542/peds.2017–2038D

Whitman, T. L., Borkowski, J. G., Keogh, D. A., & Weed, K. (2001). *Interwoven lives: Adolescent mothers and their children*. Erlbaum.

Whitney, P. G., & Green, J. A. (2011). Changes in infants' affect related to the onset of independent locomotion. *Infant Behavior and Development, 34*, 459–466. https://doi.org/10.1016/j.infbeh.2011.05.001

Williams, L. R. (2020). The impact of infant carrying on adolescent mother-infant interactions during the still-face task. *Infant and Child Development, 29*, e2169. https://doi.org/10.1002/icd.2169

Williams, L. R., & Turner, P. R. (2020). Experiences with "babywearing": Trendy parenting gear or a developmentally attuned parenting tool? *Children and Youth Services Review, 112*, 104918. https://doi.org/10.1016/j.childyouth.2020.104918

Williams, S. T., Mastergeorge, A. M., & Ontai, L. L. (2010). Caregiver involvement in infant peer interactions: Scaffolding in a social context. *Early Childhood Research Quarterly, 25*, 251–266. https://doi.org/10.1016/j.ecresq.2009.11.004

Williams, S. T., Ontai, L. L., & Mastergeorge, A. M. (2007). Reformulating infant and toddler social competence with peers. *Infant Behavior and Development, 30*, 353–365. https://doi.org/10.1016/j.infbeh.2006.10.008

Wilson, E. (1938). *Triple thinkers: Twelve essays on literary subjects*. Oxford University Press.

Winerman, L. (2015). A double life. *Monitor on Psychology, 46*, 30. https://www.apa.org/monitor/2015/01/double-life

Wolfe, C., & Bell, M. A. (2023). The interplay between cognition and emotion during infancy and toddlerhood: Special issue editorial. *Infant Behavior and Development, 72*, 101854. https://doi.org/10.1016/j.infbeh.2023.101845

Wood, D., Bruner, J. S., & Ross, G. (1976). The role of tutoring in problem solving. *Journal of Child Psychology and Psychiatry, 17*, 89–100. https://psycnet.apa.org/doi/10.1111/j.1469–7610.1976.tb00381.x

World Health Organization (WHO). (2018). *Intrapartum care for a positive childbirth experience. WHO guidelines*. https://www.who.int/publications/i/item/9789231550215

World Health Organization (2019, April 24). *To grow up healthy, children need to sit less and play more*. https://www.who.int/news/item/24-04-2019-to-grow-up-healthy-children-need-to-sit-less-and-play-more

Wowdzia, J. B., Hazell, T. J., Berg, E. R. V., Labrecque, L., Brassard, P., & Davenport, M. H. (2023). Maternal and fetal cardiovascular responses to acute high-intensity interval and moderate-intensity continuous training exercise during pregnancy: A randomized crossover trial. *Sports Medicine, 53*(9), 1819–1833. https://doi.org/10.1007/s40279-023-01858-5

Xu, J., Murphy, S., Kochanek, K., & Arias, E. (2022). *Mortality in the United States, 2021*. National Center for Health Statistics (U.S.). https://doi.org/10.15620/cdc:122516

Yonas, A., Granrud, C. E., Chov, M. H., & Alexander, A. J. (2005). Picture perception in infants: Do 9-month-olds attempt to grasp objects depicted in photographs? *Infancy, 8*, 147–166. https://doi.org/10.1207/s15327078in0802_3

Yonas, A., & Hartman, B. (1993). Perceiving the affordance of contact in four- and five-month-old infants. *Child Development, 64*, 298–308. https://doi.org/10.1111/j.1467–8624.1993.tb02911.x

Yu, J. J., & Gamble, W. C. (2008). Pathways of influence: Marital relationships and their association with parenting styles and sibling relationship quality. *Journal of Child and Family Studies, 17*, 757–778. https://doi.org/10.1007/s10826-008-9188-z

Yuan, T. F., Li, J., Ding, F., & Arias-Carrion, O. (2014). Evidence of adult neurogenesis in non-human primates and human. *Cell and Tissue Research, 358*(1), 17–23. https://doi.org/10.1007/s00441-014-1980-z

Zimmer-Gembeck, M. J., Rudolph, J., Kerin, J., & Bohadana-Brown, G. (2022). Parent emotional regulation: A meta-analytic review of its association with parenting and child adjustment. *International Journal of Behavioral Development, 46*(1), 63–82. https://doi.org/10.1177/01650254211051086

Zosuls, K. M., Ruble, D. N., Bornstein, M. H., Tamis-LeMonda, C. S., Shrout, P. E., & Greulich, F. K. (2009). The acquisition of gender labels in infancy: Implications for gender-typed play. *Developmental Psychology, 45*, 688–701. https://psycnet.apa.org/doi/10.1037/a0014053

Zukow-Goldring, P. (2002). Sibling caregiving. In M. H. Bornstein (Ed.), *Handbook of parenting: Being and becoming a parent* (Vol. 3, pp. 253–286). Erlbaum.

Author Index

Subject Index

Note: Page numbers in *italic* indicate a figure and page numbers in **bold** indicate a table on the corresponding page.